CARCINOGENESIS, DIAGNOSIS, AND MOLECULAR TARGETED TREATMENT FOR NASOPHARYNGEAL CARCINOMA

Edited by **Shih-Shun Chen**

Carcinogenesis, Diagnosis, and Molecular Targeted Treatment for Nasopharyngeal Carcinoma
Edited by Shih-Shun Chen

Published by InTech

Janeza Trdine 9, 51000 Rijeka, Croatia

Publishing Process Manager Oliver Kurelic

Technical Editor Teodora Smiljanic

Cover Designer InTech Design Team

Additional hard copies can be obtained from orders@intechopen.com

Carcinogenesis, Diagnosis, and Molecular Targeted Treatment for Nasopharyngeal Carcinoma, Edited by Shih-Shun Chen
p. cm.
ISBN 978-953-307-867-0

For EU product safety concerns:
IN TECH d.o.o., Prolaz Marije Krucifikse Kozulić 3, 51000 Rijeka, Croatia,
info@intechopen.com or visit our website at intechopen.com.

Meet the editor

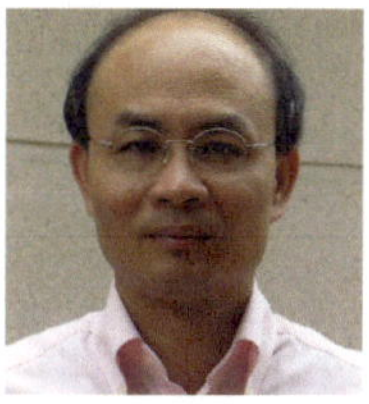

Dr Chen is an associate professor of Medical Laboratory Science and Biotechnology at the Central Taiwan University of Science and Technology, Taiwan. Dr Chen received his PhD from the National Defense Medical Center and in 2004, he was the recipient of the Academia Sinica Distinguished Postdoctoral Scholar Award. Dr Chen specializes in head and neck cancers and has a particular interest in elucidating the molecular mechanisms of action of potential anti-head and neck cancer agents.

Contents

Preface

Nasopharyngeal carcinoma (NPC) is different from other pharyngeal cancers because it has a higher prevalence rate among populations living in South-Eastern Asia. The development of NPC is complex and could be induced by many factors, such as genetic susceptibility, Epstein-Barr virus infection, and environmental exposure to carcinogens. Patients with early-stage cancer have the best chance for long-term survival; therefore, early detection is crucial to the successful treatment of cancer. The sensitivity of magnetic resonance imaging or computer tomography for the detection of cancer is extremely high, but because of the small areas of abnormality, early-stage cancer is frequently not detected on these images. Although NPC is extremely radiosensitive, patients also experience spreading to the lymph node and distant metastasis, which makes the disease difficult to control and results in poor prognosis. Radiation can also damage the hypothalamic-pituitary, the thyroid gland, and the ear, which can result in neuro-endocrine abnormalities and ear-related complications after radiotherapy. Improving NPC detection and diagnosis, developing new cancer therapies, and designing better strategies for NPC are all important practical efforts.

The aim of this book is to provide an overview of the etiologic factors associated with NPC development, to learn more about the effects of radiotherapy and chemotherapy in NPC patients, to provide vital tools for the diagnosis and detection of NPC, and to understand the molecular mechanism of carcinogenesis, which contributes to the development of targeted treatment for NPC.

As the editor, I would like to thank the authors for the high quality of their chapters and for accepting the peer review procedure established for the manual. Finally, I would especially like to thank Oliver Kurelic of the InTech-Open Access Publisher for enabling this project to be realized. I also acknowledge the efforts of the entire staff of the Press who contributed to the editing and production process. I sincerely hope that this book is able to provide valuable advice on professional pursuits.

Shih-Shun Chen
Department of Medical Laboratory Science and Biotechnology,
Central Taiwan University of Science and Technology,
Taiwan

1

Epigenetics of Nasopharyngeal Carcinoma

Zhe Zhang[1], Fu Chen[2], Hai Kuang[3] and Guangwu Huang[1]
[1]*Dept.Otolaryngology-Head & Neck Surgery, First Affiliated Hospital of Guangxi Medical University*
[2]*Dept. Radiation Oncology, Eye Ear Nose & Throat Hospital of Fudan University*
[3]*Dept. Oral & Maxillofacial Surgery, College of Stomatology, Guangxi Medical University*
P.R. China

1. Introduction

Cancer has been previously viewed as a disease exclusively driven by genetic changes, including mutations in tumor suppressor genes and oncogenes, and chromosomal abnormalities. However, recent data have demonstrated that the complexity of human carcinogenesis cannot be accounted for by only genetic machineries, but also involves extensive epigenetic abnormalities. The term "epigenetics" refers to the study of heritable changes in gene regulation that do not involve a change in the DNA sequence or the sequence of the proteins associated with DNA (Egger et al. 2004). Epigenetic machineries plays a fundamental role in several biological processes, such as embryogenesis, imprinting, and X chromosome inactivation, and in disease states such as cancer. Several mechanisms were included in the epigenetic machinery, the most studied of which are DNA methylation; histone modifications; and small, noncoding RNAs (Kargul and Laurent 2009; Jeltsch and Fischle 2011). The molecular mechanisms underlie the epigenetic changes in cancer cells are complicate and only began to be elucidated. The best understood component among which is the transcriptional repression of a growing list of tumor suppressor and candidate tumor suppressor genes (Jones and Laird 1999; Esteller 2007). This suppression is associated with abnormal methylation of DNA at certain CpG islands that often lie in the promoter regions of these genes (Esteller 2006, 2007).

Nasopharyngeal carcinoma (NPC) is a unique head and neck cancer with remarkably distinctive ethnic and geographic distribution among the world. The three major etiologic factors of NPC were well defined as genetic susceptibility, environmental factors and latent infection of the Epstein-Barr Virus (EBV) (Tao and Chan 2007; Lo, To, and Huang 2004). During the passing decade, much attention has been paid to the role of epigenetic alternations occurred in the procedure of tumorigenesis of NPC (Li, Shu, et al. 2011; Tao and Chan 2007).

In this chapter, we will first describe the general mechanisms through which the epigenetic alternations in cancer, then focus on the epigenetic alterations taking place in NPC, with an emphasis on DNA methylation.

2. DNA methylation, histone modifications and chromatin structure

DNA methylation is the only genetically programmed DNA modification in mammals. This postreplication modification is almost exclusively found on the 5′ position of the pyrimidine ring of cytosines in the context of the dinucleotide sequence CpG. 5′-methylcytosine accounts for ~1% of all bases, varying slightly in different tissue types and the majority (75%) of CpG dinucleotides throughout mammalian genomes are methylated (Tost 2010). Sequence regions with a high density of CpG residues are termed as CpG islands. A CpG island is defined as a sequence of 200-plus base pairs with a G+C content of more than 50%, and an observed versus expected ratio for the occurrence of CpGs of more than 0.6 (Jones and Takai 2001). These CpG islands are associated with gene promoters in approximately 50% of genes and are generally maintained in an unmethylated state. DNA methylation can interfere with transcription in several ways. It can inhibit the binding of transcriptional activators with their cognate DNA recognition sequence such as Sp1 and Myc through sterical hindrance. The methylation binding proteins and the DNA methyltransferases (DNMTs) bind to methylated DNA and prevent the binding of potentially activating transcription factors. The methylation binding proteins and DNMTs also recruit additional proteins with repressive function such as histone deacetylases and chromatin remodeling complexes to the methylated DNA to establish a repressive chromatin configuration (Bird 2002).

To date, three major cellular enzymic activities associated with DNA methylation have been characterized (DNMT1, DNMT3A, and DNMT3B) (Malik and Brown 2000). They catalyze the transfer of a methyl group from SAM to the cytosine base. DNMT1 is considered as a maintenance methyltransferase, it is located at the replication fork during the S phase of the cell cycle and catalyze the methylation of the newly synthesized DNA strand using the parent strand as a template. The methyltransferases DNMT3A and DNMT3B are responsible for *De novo* methylation. These enzymes not only targeting specific sequences, they also work cooperatively to methylate the genome (Malik and Brown 2000).

Tumor-specific elevation of DNMTs is a causative step in many cancers. All three DNMTs, were observed modestly overexpressed in many types of tumor cells at the mRNA or protein level (Robertson et al. 1999). Furthermore, modest overexpression of exogenous mouse Dnmt1 in NIH 3T3 cells can promote cellular transformation (Wu et al. 1993). Additionally, genetic inactivation of Dnmt1 in mice decreases the development of gastrointestinal tumors in a mouse model of gastrointestinal cancer (Laird et al. 1995). These evidences indicate a possible role for DNMTs in tumorigenesis. However, the mechanisms that underlie such a role in cancer are still not defined.

Genomic DNA is highly folded and packaged into chromosomes or chromatin by histone and nonhistone proteins in the nuclei of all eukaryotic cells (Jenuwein and Allis 2001). The fundamental repeating unit of chromatin is the nucleosome, in which 146 DNA base pairs are wrapped left handed around a core histone protein, which consists of two of each of the four histone protein subunits: H2A, H2B, H3 and H4. Each core histone has an amino-terminal 'tail' of about 25-40 residues long, where they are frequent targets for various posttranslational modifications (Fischle, Wang, and Allis 2003). The state of chromatin is regulated largely by covalent modifications of the histone tails. The major modifications include the acetylation of specific lysine residues by histone acetyltransferases (HATs), the methylation of lysine and arginine residues by histone methyltransferases (HMTs), and the phosphorylation of specific serine groups by histone kinases (HKs). Other histone modifications include attachment of ubiquitination, and sulmolation. Enzymes responsible for the cleavage of some histone modifications, such as histone deacetylases (HDACs), histone phosphatases (PPs), ubiquitin hydrolases (Ubps) and poly (ADP-ribose)glycohydrolases (PARGs), have already been identified (Biel, Wascholowski, and Giannis 2005).

Posttranslational modifications are closely related to fundamental cellular events like the activation and repression of transcription. In the case of histone H3, in general, acetylation of H3 at lysine 14 (H3-K14), phosphorylation of serine 10 (H3-S10), and methylation of H3-K4 leads to transcriptional activation. In contrast, the repression of certain genes is linked to deacetylation of H3-K14 and methylation of H3-K9. The specific combination of these modifications has been termed the histone code, that determines histone–DNA and histone–histone contacts, which may in turn regulate the on or off state of genes or unfolding/folding state of the chromatin structure (Jenuwein and Allis 2001; Esteller 2007).

Histone modifications and other epigenetic mechanisms such as DNA methylation appear to work together in a coordinated and orderly fashion, to establishing and maintaining gene activity states, thus regulating gene transcription (Fischle, Wang, and Allis 2003; Biel, Wascholowski, and Giannis 2005). In the past decade, more and more attention has been paid on histone modifications, which led to the discovery and characterization of a large number of histone-modifying molecules and protein complexes. Alterations of histone-modifying complexes are believed to disrupt the pattern and levels of histone marks and consequently dysregulate the normal control of chromatin-based cellular processes, ultimately leading to oncogenic transformation and the development of cancer (Esteller 2007).

3. NPC as an epigenetic disease

3.1 Hypermethylation of cellular tumor suppressor genes and the dysregulation of the corresponding cellular pathways

NPC distinguish itself from other malignancies by the number of genes targeted for silencing by promoter methylation. Several classic tumor suppressor genes, such as p53 and Rb, are found to be mutated in more than 50% of all the tumors, but were rarely found to be mutated in NPC (Burgos 2003; Chang et al. 2002; Tao and Chan 2007). On the contrary, hypermethylation of known or candidate tumor suppressor genes involved in various fundamental pathways has been reported in NPC, such as apoptosis, DNA damage repair, tumor invasion and metastasis. The full list of genes which have been found to be aberrantly methylated in NPC was summarized in table 1.

Ras signalling

Activated Ras proteins has been shown to play a key role in the development of human cancers (Bos 1989). Ras proteins serve as a node in the transduction of information from a variety of cell surface receptors to an array of intracellular signaling pathways. Mutated variants of Ras (mutations at residues 12, 13 or 61) are found in 30% of all human cancers

(Bos 1989). Mutations at residues 12, 13 or 61 might lock Ras protein in the active state, which mediate a variety of biological effects associated with enhanced growth and transformation. Ras activity is regulated by cycling between inactive GDP-bound and active GTP-bound forms. When GTP-bound, Ras binds to and activates a plethora of effector molecules. GTPase-activating proteins (GAPs), such as p120GAP and NF1, trigger the hydrolysis of GTP back to the inactive GDP-bound form (Boguski and McCormick 1993). Because Ras GAPs switch off Ras signalling, they have always been considered as potential tumor suppressor genes. Recent study reveal that the Ras GTPase-activating-like protein (RASAL), a Ca2+-regulated Ras GAP that decodes the frequency of Ca2+ oscillations, is silenced through CpG methylation in multiple tumors including NPC (Jin, Wang, Ying, Wong, Cui, et al. 2007). In addition, ectopic expression of catalytically active RASAL leads to growth inhibition of NPC cells by Ras inactivation, thus, epigenetically silencing of RASAL is an alternative mechanism of aberrant Ras activation in NPC (Jin, Wang, Ying, Wong, Cui, et al. 2007).

Although it is widely accepted that Ras functions as an oncoprotein, more and more evidence show that Ras proteins may also induces growth arrest properties of cells, such as senescence, apoptosis, terminal differentiation (Spandidos et al. 2002). The growth inhibitory effects of Ras were induced by a group of proteins with Ras binding domain. These proteins were identified as negative effectors of Ras and designated as Ras association domain family (RASSF). Within this super family, the *RASSF1A* and *RASSF2A* gene are frequently inactivated by promoter hypermethylation (Lo et al. 2001; Zhang et al. 2007), functional studies also support their role as putative tumor suppressors in NPC.

The induction of invasiveness and metastasis by Ras were mediated by downstream effectors which are involved in the regulation of cell adhesion, cell-matrix interaction and cell motility, such as RhoGTPases, RalGEF and components of PI3K pathways (Giehl 2005). Recent studies have further indicated that the Ras/PI3K/AKT pathway is associated in several human cancers. Activation of the Ras/PI3K/AKT pathway can occur by many mechanisms, which include activation of Ras, mutation or amplification of *PI3K*, amplification of *AKT*, and mutation/decreased expression of the tumor-suppressor genes *PTEN* and *HIN-1*. The *HIN-1* gene has various biological functions, including inhibiting cell cycle reentry, suppressing migration and invasion, and inducing apoptosis; these effects are mediated by inhibiting AKT signalling pathway (Krop et al. 2005). *HIN-1* gene is hypermethylated in human NPC. Methylated *HIN-1* promoter was found in 77% of primary NPC tumors and not found in the normal nasopharyngeal biopsies. Moreover, methylated *HIN-1* promoter can be detected in 46% of nasopharyngeal swabs, 19% of throat-rinsing fluids, 18% of plasmas, and 46% of buffy coats of peripheral blood of the NPC patients but was not detectable in all normal controls (Wong, Kwong, et al. 2003).

The Ras family shares at least 30% sequence identity with several other small monomeric G protein families, such as the Rho/Rac/CDC42, Rab/Ypt, Ran, Arf, and Rad families (Adjei 2001). The major 8p22 tumor suppressor Deleted in Liver Cancer 1 (*DLC1*) gene is a homologue of rat p122RhoGAP. It was identified as a major downregulated gene in NPC by expression subtraction. By expression subtraction, Qian Tao's group identified that *DLC1* is an 8p22 TSG as a major downregulated gene in NPC. Their study also demonstrated *DLC1* is hypermethylated not only in NPC, but also in esophageal and cervical carcinomas. Downregulation of *DLC1* contributes to NPC oncogenesis by disrupting

Ras-mediated signalling pathways (Seng et al. 2007). Recently, a novel isoform of the *DLC1* gene was identified, which suppresses tumor growth and frequently silenced in multiple common tumors including NPC. This novel isoform encodes an 1125-aa (amino acid) protein with distinct N-terminus as compared with other known *DLC1* isoforms. Similar to other isoforms, *DLC1-i4* is expressed ubiquitously in normal tissues, and epigenetically inactivated by promoter hypermethylation in NPC. The differential expression of various *DLC1* isoforms suggests interplay in modulating the complex activities of *DLC1* during carcinogenesis (Low et al. 2011).

P53 signalling

Altered p53 pathway is common detected in NPC, even though NPC rarely presents abnormality in the p53 gene itself, p53 function may be inactivated by either overexpression of ΔN-p63 or loss of p14/ARF. ΔN-p63 is a p53 homolog. It can block p53's function as transcription factor. P14 functions as a stabilizer of p53 as it can interact with, and sequester, MDM1, a protein responsible for the degradation of p53 (Ozenne et al. 2010). *p14* is methylated in 20% on NPC, the epigenetic inactivation of *p14/ARF* may facilitate p53 degradation in NPC cells (Kwong et al. 2002). Loss of p53 function may affect cell cycle arrest at the G1 or G2/M phase and p53-mediated apoptosis in response to DNA damage (Kwong et al. 2002; Crook et al. 2000).

Recently, Qian Tao et al. found that *UCHL1* was frequently silenced by promoter CpG methylation in nasopharyngeal carcinoma; and acts as a functional tumor suppressor gene for NPC through stabilizing p53 through deubiquitinating p53 and p14ARF and ubiquitinating MDM2, which is mediated by its hydrolase and ligase activities, further resulting in the induction of tumor cell apoptosis (Li et al. 2010).

Wnt signalling

The Wnt signalling pathway is important for normal development and is frequently aberrantly activated in a variety of cancers. Although the role of the Wnt pathway in NPC has not been fully explored, there is abundant evidence that aberrant Wnt signalling plays a role in NPC development. In a recent study by gene expression profiling, the aberrant expression of the Wnt signalling pathway components, such as wingless-type MMTV integration site family, member 5A, Frizzled homolog 7, casein kinase II beta, β-catenin, CREB-binding protein, and dishevelled-associated activator of morphogenesis 2 was identified and further validated on NPC tissue microarrays (Zeng et al. 2007). Furthermore, most NPC tumors exhibit Wnt pathway protein dysregulation: 93% have increased Wnt protein expression and 75% have decreased expression of Wnt inhibitory factor (WIF), an endogenous Wnt antagonist (Shi et al. 2006; Zeng et al. 2007). These results indicate that aberrant Wnt signalling is a critical component of NPC.

The Wnt inhibitory factor 1 (*WIF1*) gene acts as a Wnt antagonist factor by direct binding to Wnt ligands. In NPC, methylation was frequently observed in 85% of NPC primary tumors, with *WIF1* expressed and unmethylated in normal cell lines and normal tissues. Ectopic expression of WIF1 in NPC cells resulted in significant inhibition of tumor cell colony formation, and significant downregulation of β-catenin protein level in NPC cells. Indicates that epigenetic inactivation of *WIF1* contributes to the aberrant activation of Wnt pathway and is involved in the pathogenesis of NPC (Chan et al. 2007).

Cell cycle and DNA repair

Aberrant apoptosis, as in all malignancies, is also required for NPC development. Inhibition of apoptosis seems to be critical to NPC tumorigenesis. Death-associated protein kinase (*DAPK*) is a Ca/calmodulin-regulated serine/threonine kinase and a positive mediator of apoptosis. Loss of *DAPK* expression was shown to be associated with promoter region methylation in NPC. Methylation of the promoter was found in 76% of NPC, as well as plasma of patients with NPC (Chang et al. 2003). A demethylating agent, 5-aza-2'-deoxycytidine, might slow the growth of NPC cells in vitro and in vivo by reactivating the *DAPK* gene silenced by de novo methylation (Kong et al. 2006).

Like all cancers, development of NPC requires the derangement of the normal cell cycle. Several classical CDK inhibitors in G1 -S checkpoint, such as p16/INK4A, p15/INK4A, and p14/ARF, were demonstrated to be hypermethylated in NPC and act as tumor suppressors during NPC development (Li, Shu, et al. 2011).

Dysregulation of the DNA repair system by DNA methylation is also an essential event in NPC development (Lo, To, and Huang 2004; Tao and Chan 2007). MGMT is a DNA repair protein that removes mutagenic and cytotoxic adducts from O6-guanine in DNA. Frequent methylation of *MGMT* associated with gene silencing occurs in human cancers. However, only a small portion (28%) of primary NPC were *MGMT* hypermethylated (Wong, Tang, et al. 2003). A rather high frequency (40%) of hypermethylation of the DNA mismatch repair gene *hMLH1* was observed in NPC primary tumors (Wong, Tang, et al. 2003). But methylation of *hMLH1* cannot be detected in the plasma of NPC patients (Wong et al. 2004).

Chromosomal instability (CIN) is a cytogenetic hallmark of human cancers (Cheung et al. 2005; Lengauer, Kinzler, and Vogelstein 1998). Increasing evidence suggests that impairment of mitotic checkpoint is causally associated with CIN. Several chromosomal aberrations have been identified in NPC. Some sites correspond to proteins key to NPC development, including p16, RASSF1A, and CKIs, while a number of sites do not correspond to any known tumor suppressors or oncogenes (Li, Shu, et al. 2011). CHFR is one of the mitotic checkpoint regulators and it delays chromosome condensation in response to mitotic stress. *CHFR* mRNA was significantly decreased or undetectable in NPC cell lines as well as human NPC xenografts, hypermethylation of *CHFR* promoter was strongly correlated with decreased CHFR expression in NPC cell lines and xenografts (Cheung et al. 2005). And hypermethylation of *CHFR* promoter region was detected in 61.1% (22 out of 36) of primary NPC tumors while it was absent in non-malignant tissues (Cheung et al. 2005).

Cell adhesion

Multiple cell adhesion molecules involve in intercellular and cell-extracellular matrix interactions of cancer. Cancer progression is a multi-step process in which some adhesion molecules play a pivotal role in the development of recurrent, invasion, and metastasis. Alterations in the adhesion properties of cancer cells play an essential role in the development and progression of cancer. Loss of intercellular adhesion allows malignant cells to escape from their site of origin, degrade the extracellular matrix, acquire a more motile and invasion phenotype, and finally, invade and metastasize. In NPC, epigenetic mechanism was involved in the abnormal cell adhesion, a diverse of molecules such as cadherins, connexins, and other components of cell adhesion are dysregulated (Du et al. 2011; Sun et al. 2007; Ying et al. 2006; Huang et al. 2001; Lou, Chen, Lin, et al. 1999; Xiang et al. 2002).

Cadherins have strong implications in tumorigenesis through cadherin-mediated cell–cell adhesion, which maintains tissue integrity and homeostasis. Disruption of this organized adhesion by genetic and epigenetic mechanisms during carcinogenesis might result in changes in signal transduction, loss of contact inhibition, and altered cell migration and stromal interactions. Some of the cadherins, such as E-cadherin and H-cadherin, were characterized as TGSs, which inhibit tumor invasion and metastasis (Berx and van Roy 2009; Jeanes, Gottardi, and Yap 2008). Disruption of cadherin expression and inappropriate switching among cadherin family members by genetic or epigenetic mechanisms are key events in the acquisition of the invasive phenotype for many tumors. The E-cadherin gene is silenced by promoter hypermethylation in human NPC because of aberrant expression of DNMT induced by the Epstein-Barr virus-encoded oncoprotein latent membrane 1 (Tsai et al. 2002). Moreover, loss of E-cadherin expression is significantly associated with histological grade, intracranial invasion and lymph node and distant metastasis (Lou, Chen, Sheen, et al. 1999). Three other members of the cadherin family: *CDH13*, *CDH4* and *PCDH10*, are involved in NPC owing to promoter methylation (Sun et al. 2007; Ying et al. 2006; Du et al. 2011). This evidence indicates a deep involvement of epigenetic regulation of the cadherin family in the carcinogenesis of NPC.

Intercellular communication through gap junction (GJIC) have a significant role in maintaining tissue homeostasis and has long been proposed as a mechanism to regulate growth control, development and differentiation. Reduced GJIC activity has long been implicated in carcinogenesis. Loss of GJIC leads to aberrant proliferation and an enhanced neoplastic phenotype. Reduced expression of the connexin (Cx) genes dysregulation of GJIC activity were observed in a series of human cancers. Thus, some Cx genes have been suggested as tumor suppressor genes (Pointis et al. 2007). Down-regulation of connexin 43 (*Cx43*) expression and dysfunctional GJIC were demonstrated in NPC tissues and cells, suggesting that dysfunctional GJIC plays a key role in nasopharyngeal carcinogenesis (Shen et al. 2002; Xiang et al. 2002). Further study revealed that inactivation of *Cx43* gene was mediated by epigenetic mechanism of promoter hypermethylation in NPC. Treatment of DNA methyltransferase inhibitor 5-aza-2′-deoxycytidine could induce restoration of GJIC and an inhibition of tumor phenotype of CNE-1 cells (Yi et al. 2007).

MMPs are type IV collagenases whose overexpression has been implicated in a number of cancers. MMPs can not only degrade basement membranes and extracellular matrices to allow for tumor invasion, they are also involved in activation of growth factors to promote cell growth and angiogenesis, and also protect tumor cells from apoptotic signals (Gialeli, Theocharis, and Karamanos 2011). In NPC, MMP1, MMP3 and MMP9 were shown to be up-regulated by LMP1 (Stevenson, Charalambous, and Wilson 2005; Kondo et al. 2005; Lee et al. 2007). While MMP19 appears to be down-regulated in 69.7% of primary NPC specimens (Chan et al. 2010). Allelic deletion and promoter hypermethylation contribute to MMP19 down-regulation. The catalytic activity of MMP19 plays an important role in anti-tumor and anti-angiogenesis activities (Chan et al. 2010).

OPCML (opioid binding protein/cell adhesion molecule-like gene), also known as *OBCAM* (opioid binding cell adhesion molecule), belonging to the IgLON family of glycosylphosphatidylinositol (GPI)-anchored cell adhesion molecules involved in cell adhesion and cell-cell recognition. Located at 11q25, *OPCML* was the first IgLON member linked to tumorigenesis. In NPC, the *OPCML-v1* were observed to be epigenetically inactivated, what's more, the methylation was detected in a remarkable frequency: 98% of NPC tumor tissues. The high incidence of epigenetic inactivation of *OPCML* in NPC indicates that *OPCML* methylation could be an epigenetic biomarker for the molecular diagnosis of NPC (Cui et al. 2008).

Cancer-related process	Gene	Full name	Chromosomal location	Function	Refs
Cell cycle	*CDKN2B/ P15/MTS2/T P15/ INK4B*	Cyclin-dependent kinase inhibitor 2B	9p21	Cyclin-dependent kinase inhibitor for CDK4 and CDK6, a cell growth regulator of cell cycle G1 progression	(Wong, Tang, et al. 2003; Chang et al. 2003; Wong et al. 2004; Li, Shu, et al. 2011)
	CDKN2A/ P16/INK4A/ MTS1/ CDK4I/ CDKN2	Cyclin-dependent kinase inhibitor 2A	9p21	Cell cycle regulation	(Wong et al. 2004; Chang et al. 2003; Wong, Tang, et al. 2003; Lo et al. 1996; Li, Shu, et al. 2011)
	CHFR/ RNF116/ RNF196	Checkpoint with forkhead and ring finger domains	12q24.33	Mitotic checkpoint regulator early in G2-M transition	(Cheung et al. 2005; Li, Shu, et al. 2011)
	BRD7	Bromodomain containing 7	16q12	Transcriptional regulation, inhibits G1-S transition	(Liu et al. 2008)
	FHIT/ FRA3B/ 3P3Aase	Fragile histidine triad gene	3P14.2	Cell-cycle regulation, G1-S phase checkpoint, DNA-damage response, nucleotide and nucleic acid metabolism	(Loyo et al. 2011)
	GADD45G	Growth arrest and DNA-damage-inducible, gamma	9q22	Inhibits G1-S and G2-M transition, apoptosis	(Ying et al. 2005)
	DLEC1	Deleted in lung and esophageal cancer1	3p22-21.3	G1 cell cycle arrest	(Ayadi et al. 2008)
	ZMYND10/ BLU	Zinc finger, MYND-type containing 10	3P21.3	Cell cycle	(Liu et al. 2003)
	MIPOL1	Mirror-image polydactyly1	14q13.1	Negative regulator of G1 progression	(Cheung et al. 2009)
	PRDM2/ PRDM2	PR domain containing 2, with ZNF domain	1p36.21	G2-M cell cycle arrest	(Chang et al. 2003)

Cancer-related process	Gene	Full name	Chromo-somal location	Function	Refs
	LTF	Lactoferrin	3p21.3	Cell cycle regulation	(Yi et al. 2006; Zhang et al. 2011)
	CCNA1	Cyclin A1	13q12.3-q13	An important regulator of the cell cycle required for S phase and passage through G_2	(Yanatatsaneejit et al. 2008)
	PTPRG	Receptor-type tyrosine-protein phosphatase gamma	3p14-21	Cell cycle regulator via inhibition of pRB phosphorylation through down-regulation of cyclin D1	(Cheung et al. 2008)
	TP73	Tumor protein p73	1p36.3	Cell cycle, DNA damage response, apoptosis, transcription factor	(Wong, Tang, et al. 2003)
Apoptosis	*DAPK*	Death-associated protein kinase	9p34.1	Positive mediator of gamma-interferon induced apoptosis	(Wong et al. 2004; Chang et al. 2003; Kwong et al. 2002; Li, Shu, et al. 2011)
	CASP8/CAP 4/MACH/M CH5/ FLICE	Caspase 8, apoptosis-related cysteine peptidase	2q33-q34	Apoptosis	(Li, Shu, et al. 2011; Wong, Tang, et al. 2003)
	GSTP1/ DFN7/ GST3	Glutathione S-transferase pi 1	11q13	Apoptosis, metobolism, energy pathways	(Kwong et al. 2002; Li, Shu, et al. 2011)
	CMTM3	CKLF like MARVEL transmembrane domain-containing member 3	16q21	Induces apoptosis with caspase-3 activation	(Wang et al. 2009)
	CMTM5	CKLF like MARVEL transmembrane domain-containing member 5	14q11.2	Induces apoptosis with activation of caspase 3, 8 and 9, synergistic effects with TNF-α.	(Shao et al. 2007)
	ZNF382	Zinc finger protein 382	19q13.12	Key regulator of cell proliferation, differentiation, and apoptosis, repress NF-kB and AP-1 signaling	(Cheng et al. 2010)
	TNFRSF11B /OPG	Tumor necrosis factor receptor superfamily, member 11b	8q24	Induced apoptosis, inhibits tumor growth specifically in bones	(Lu et al. 2009)
	PLA2G16/H RASLS3	Phospholipase A2, group XVI	11q12.3	Proapoptotic function through the inhibition of PP2A	(Yanatatsaneejit et al. 2008)

Cancer-related process	Gene	Full name	Chromo-somal location	Function	Refs
Invasion and metastasis	*CDH1*	Cadherin 1, type 1, E-cadherin (epithelial)	16q22.1	Calcium-dependent adhesion and cell migration	(Wong, Tang, et al. 2003; Wong et al. 2004)
	CDH13	Cadherin 13, H-cadherin (heart)	16q23.3	Calcium-dependent adhesion and cell migration	(Sun et al. 2007)
	PCDH10 /OL-PCDH /KIAA1400	Protocadherin 10	4q28.3	Calcium-dependent adhesion and cell migration	(Ying et al. 2006)
	CDH4	Cadherin 4, type 1, R-cadherin (retinal)	20q13.3	Calcium-dependent adhesion and cell migration	(Du et al. 2011)
	OPCML	Opioid binding protein/cell adhesion molecule	11q25	Cell adhesion, cell-cell recognition	(Cui et al. 2008)
	TFPI-2	Tissue factor pathway inhibitor-2	7q22	Serine protease inhibitor	(Wang et al. 2010)
	MMP19	Matrix metalloproteinase-19	12q14	Extra cellular matrix	(Chan et al. 2010)
	THBS1	Thrombospondin 1	15q15	An adhesive glycoprotein that mediates cell-to-cell and cell-to-matrix interactions	(Wong, Tang, et al. 2003)
	Cx43	Connexin 43	20q11	Gap junction and intercellular communication	(Yi et al. 2007)
	TSLC1 /CADM1	Tumor suppressor in lung cancer 1	11q23	Cell adhesion molecules, mediate cell-cell interaction	(Hui et al. 2003; Lung et al. 2004)
	ADAMTS18	ADAM metallopeptidase with thrombospondin type 1 motif, 18	16q23.1	Cell adhesion modulator, inhibits growth factor-independent cell proliferation	(Jin, Wang, Ying, Wong, Li, et al. 2007; Wei et al. 2010)
	THY1/CD90	Thy-1 cell surface antigen	11q23.3	Regulates cytoskeletal organization, focal adhesion and migration by modulating the activity of p190 RhoGAP and Rho GTPase	(Lung et al. 2005)
DNA repair	*MGMT*	O-6-methyoguanine-DNA methyltransferase	10q26	Repair alkylated guanine	(Kwong et al. 2002)
	MLH1 /hMLH1 /HNPCC /FCC2	MutL homolog 1, colon cancer, nonpolyposis type 2 (E. coli)	3p21.3	DNA mismatch repair protein, cell cycle G2-M arrest	(Wong, Tang, et al. 2003; Wong et al. 2004)

Cancer-related process	Gene	Full name	Chromosomal location	Function	Refs
Signal transduction	*ARF/P14*	Alternate open reading frame	9p21	Stabilizes p53, interacts with MDM2	(Li, Shu, et al. 2011; Wong, Tang, et al. 2003)
	RASSF1A	Ras association (RalGDS/AF-6) domain family member 1A	3p21.3	Regulate Ras signaling pathway	(Chow et al. 2004; Zhou et al. 2005)
	RASFF2A	Ras association (RalGDS/AF-6) domain family member 2A	20p12.1	Regulate Ras signaling pathway	(Zhang et al. 2007)
	WIF-1	Wnt inhibitory factor-1	12q14	Antagonist of Wnt signaling	(Lin et al. 2006; Chan et al. 2007)
	DLC-1	Deleted in liver cancer-1	8p21.3-22	GTPase-activating protein specific for RhoA and Cdc42	(Peng et al. 2006)
	DAB2	Disabled homolog 2, mitogen-responsive phosphoprotein (Drosophila)	5p13	Adaptor molecule involved in multiple receptor-mediated signaling pathways	(Tong et al. 2010)
	RASAL1	RAS protein activator like 1 (GAP1 like)	12q23-q24	Ras GTPase-activating protein, negatively regulates RAS signaling	(Jin, Wang, Ying, Wong, Cui, et al. 2007)
	UCHL1	Ubiquitin carboxyl-terminal esterase L1	4p14	Stabilize p53 and activate the p14^{ARF}-p53 signaling pathway	(Li et al. 2010)
	SFN/14-3-3 σ	Stratifin	1p36.11	Downstream target of p53, negative regulator of G2-M phase checkpoint	(Yi et al. 2009)
Angiogenesis	*EDNRB*	Endothelin receptor type B	13q22	Negative regulator of ET/ETAR pathway	(Lo et al. 2002; Zhou et al. 2007)
	ADAMTS9	A disintegrin-like and metallopeptidase with thrombospondin type 1 motif 9	3p14.1	Anti-angiogenesis	(Lung, Lo, Xie, et al. 2008)
	FBLN2	Fibulin 2	3p25.1	Angiogenesis suppression via concomitant downregulation of vascular endothelial growth factor and matrix metalloproteinase 2	(Law et al. 2011)

Cancer-related process	Gene	Full name	Chromo-somal location	Function	Refs
Vitamin response	*RARβ2*	Retinoic acid receptor beta 2	3q24	Binds retinoic acid to mediates cellular signaling during embryonic morphogenesis, cell growth and differentiation	(Kwong, Lo, Chow, To, et al. 2005; Kwong et al. 2002; Seo, Kim, and Jang 2008)
	RARRES1 /TIG1	Retinoic acid receptor responder (tazarotene induced) 1	3q25	Retinoic acid target gene	(Yanatatsaneejit et al. 2008; Kwong, Lo, Chow, Chan, et al. 2005; Kwok et al. 2009)
	CRBP I /RBP1	Cellular retinol binding protein 1	3q23	Draws retinol from blood stream into cells, solubilizes retinol and retinal, protects cells from membranolytic retinoid action	(Kwong, Lo, Chow, To, et al. 2005)
	CRBPIV	Cellular retinol binding protein 4	1p36.22	Similar to CRBP1	(Kwong, Lo, Chow, To, et al. 2005)
Tissue develo-pment and differe-ntiation	*Myocd*	Myocardin	17p11.2	Transcription factor, involved in smooth muscle cell differentiation	(Chen et al. 2011)
	HIN1 /SCGB3A1	High-in-normal-1	5q35	Involved in epithelial cell differentiation, cell-cycle reentry regulator, suppresses tumor cell migration and invasion, induces apoptosis	(Wong, Kwong, et al. 2003)
Others	*NOR1*	Oxidored-nitro domain-contrining protein 1	1p34.3	Interaction partner of the mitochondrial ATP synthase subunit OSCP/ATP5O protein, a stress-responsive gene	(Li, Li, et al. 2011)
	LARS2	Leucyl-tRNA synthetase 2, mitochondrial	3p21.3	Essential roles in group I intron RNA splicing and protein synthesis within the mitochondria, indirectly required for mitochondrial genome maintenance	(Zhou et al. 2009)
	CRYAB	Crystallin,alpha B	11q23.1	An important nuclear role in maintaining genomic integrity	(Lung, Lo, Wong, et al. 2008)

Table 1. List of methylated tumor suppressor genes involved in nasopharyngeal carcinoma (NPC)

3.2 Epstein-Barr virus and DNA methylation

EBV is a prototype of gamma herpes virus which was discovered more than 40 years ago from Burkitt's lymphoma, a childhood tumor that is common in sub-Saharan Africa. Further studies reveal that EBV was widespread in all human populations, which infects more than 90% of the world's adult population. Human are the only natural host for EBV. Once infected with EBV, the individual remains a lifelong asymptomatic carrier of the virus (Young and Rickinson 2004).

EBV was implicated in a variety of human malignancies, such as post-transplant lymphoma, AIDS-associated lymphomas, Burkitt lymohoma, Hodgkin's disease, T-cell lymphoma, NPC, parotid gland carcinoma and gastric carcinoma (Young and Rickinson 2004; Pattle and Farrell 2006). The association between EBV infection and NPC was well documented by the fact that EBV genome presents in virtually all the NPC cells (Lo and Huang 2002; Lo, To, and Huang 2004). Tumorigenesis of NPC is proposed to be a multistep process. EBV may play an important role in the etiology of the NPC, involving activation of oncogenes and/or the inactivation of tumor suppressor genes. Early genetic changes may predispose the epithelial cells to EBV infection or persistent maintenance of latent cycle. Expression of latent genes in the EBV-infected cells may enhance its transformation capacities, and subsequently, clonal expansion may result in the rapid progression to invasive carcinoma.

There are two alternative states of EBV infection: lytic and latent (Young and Rickinson 2004; Fernandez et al. 2009). In EBV-infected cells, virus replication with production of infectious virus is a rare event. Typically, EBV establishes a latent infection. This is characterized by the expression of a limited set of viral products, including six EBV-encoded nuclear antigens (EBNA1, 2, 3A, 3B, 3C, -LP), three latent membrane proteins (LMP1, 2A, 2B) and two EBV-encoded nuclear RNAs (EBER1, EBER2). Expression of different panels of latent gene transcripts is controlled by usage of three distinct EBV nuclear antigen (EBNA) promoters (Wp, Cp, and Qp). In established lymphoblastoid cell lines (LCLs), the EBNA transcripts are initiated at the C promoter, Cp, located to the BamHI C fragment of the viral genome. In EBV genome, W promoter (Wp) is the first promoter to be activated immediately after EBV infection of human B cells, but it undergoes progressively methylation and switches off in LCLs. In parallel, an unmethylated promoter, Cp, is switched on. In other EBV-carrying cell types, Cp is switched off. These include memory B cells, Burkitt's lymphomas (BLs), EBV-associated carcinomas (NPC, gastric carcinoma) and Hodgkin's lymphomas; these cells typically use the Q promoter (Qp) for expression of EBNA1 transcripts, but not the transcripts coding for the other five EBNAs, and may differ from each other regarding the expression of LMPs, BARTs (BARF0 and BARF1) and EBV-encoded microRNAs (Li and Minarovits 2003). LMP1 is the major EBV oncoprotein in NPC (Tao and Chan 2007; Lo, To, and Huang 2004). By activating several important cellular signalling pathways like NF-κB, JNK, JAK/STAT and PI-3K pathway, LMP1 could upregulate anti-apoptotic gene products, such as BCL2, A20, AP-1, CD40, CD54 and also cytokines IL-6 and IL-8; thereby exhibit its oncogenic characteristics (Eliopoulos and Young 2001). LMP1-expressing NPCs show different growth pattern and prognosis from those without LMP1 expression (Hu et al. 1995). Although EBV genome presents in virtually all the NPC cells, expression of LMP1 is variable in NPC: LMP1 is expressed in only approximately 65% of NPC biopsies (Fahraeus et al. 1988; Young et al. 1988). This variability can be related to the methylation status of the regulatory sequences (LRS, LMP1 regulatory sequence) located 5′ from LMP1p, as LMP1 is expressed in NPCs with unmethylated LRS but is absent from NPCs with highly methylated LRS. A good correlation exists between LRS methylation and silencing of LMP1p in EBV-carrying lymphoid cell lines and tumors as well (Li and Minarovits 2003)).

On the other hand, EBV regulates the expression of critical cellular genes using cellular DNA methylation machinery. LMP1 has been shown to interacting with methyltransferase and further induce the cellular gene E-cadherin (*CDH1*) promoter methylation. Increased methylation may occur through the activity of DNA methyltransferases 1, 3a, and 3b that in turn are induced through JNK/AP1 signalling by LMP1. Transfection of LMP1 into cancer cells suppressed E-cadherin expression, thereby facilitating a more invasive growth of NPC cells (Tsai et al. 2006). It will be interesting to discover novel target genes regulated by epigenetic mechanism of EBV.

3.3 MicroRNAs in the development of NPC

MicroRNAs (miRNAs) are short non-coding RNA molecules of about 20-23 nucleotides in length, involved in post-transcriptional gene regulation. In animals, miRNAs control the expression of target genes by inhibiting translation or degradating target mRNAs through binding to their 3'UTR. MicroRNAs are involved in regulating a broad range of biological processes, such as development, differentiation, proliferation, apoptosis, and signal transduction pathways often deregulated in cancers. Some miRNAs can function as tumor suppressors or oncogenes (McManus 2003; Ventura and Jacks 2009).

Several biological pathways that are well characterised in cancer are significantly targeted by the downregulated miRNAs. These pathways include TGF-Wnt pathways, G1-S cell cycle progression, VEGF signalling pathways, apoptosis and survival pathways, and IP3 signalling pathways (Chen et al. 2009). Several known oncogenic miRNAs, such as miR-141 (Zhang et al. 2010) miR-17-92 cluster and miR-155 (Chen et al. 2009)were found to significantly up-regulated in NPC tumors. While some tumor suppressive miRNAs, including miR-34 family, miR-143, and miR-145, miR-218 (Alajez et al. 2011), mir-29c, miR-200a, miR-26a and let-7 (Wong et al. 2011) are significantly down-regulated in NPC. Among them, let-7 inhibits cell proliferation through down-regulation of c-Myc expression while miR-26a inhibits cell growth and tumorigenesis through repression of another oncogene: *EZH2* (Lu et al. 2011).

EBV is reported to be present in almost all NPCs and can transform cells, which subsequently induces cell proliferation and tumor growth. In addition to EBV-encoded protein-coding genes such as EBNA1 and LMP1, NPC cells and tissues also express high levels of non-coding EBV RNAs, including EBER1, EBER2 and multiple microRNAs (miRNAs). EBV was the first human virus found to encode microRNAs (Barth, Meister, and Grasser 2011). By small RNA cloning and sequencing, Zhu JY et al. characterized the miRNA expression profile of NPC tissues. Their study revealed an NPC-specific miRNA signature. EBV expresses all miRNAs from the BART cluster in NPC tissues, while no miRNA originating from the BHRF1 region of the EBV genome was found. Their study suggested that BART-derived miRNAs may have an important function in maintaining the virus in NPC tissues, whereas BHRF1 origin miRNAs might not be required for NPC pathogenesis. In the same study, they also identified two novel and highly abundant EBV miRNA genes, namely, miR-BART21 and miR-BART22 (Zhu et al. 2009). A parallel study demonstrated that LMP2A is the putative target of miR-BART22 in NPC. LMP2A is a potent immunogenic viral antigen that is recognized by the cytotoxic T cells, down-modulation of LMP2A expression by miR-BART22 may permit escape of EBV-infected cells from host immune surveillance (Lung et al. 2009). Similar regulations were also addressed on LMP1: EBV-encoded BART miRNAs target the 3' UTR of the LMP1 gene and negatively regulate LMP1 protein expression. These miRNAs also modulate LMP1-induced NF-κB signalling and alleviate the cisplatin sensitivity of LMP1-expressing NPC cells (Lo et al. 2007).

4. Epigenetic alternations in relation to clinical parameters of NPC, and their roles as biomarkers

Frequent aberrantly methylated TSGs in tumors have been used as molecular markers for the detection of malignant cells from various clinical materials. It provides possibilities of both cancer early detection and dynamic monitoring of cancer patients after treatment (Schulz 2005).

DNA methylation biomarkers hold a number of advantages over other biomarker types, such as proteins, gene expression and DNA mutations (Balch et al. 2009; Laird 2003). Methylated DNA sequences are more chemically and biologically stable, and more easier to be amplified, thus greatly enhancing detection sensitivity. DNA methylation are often cancer specific, and restriction to limited regions of DNA in the CpG islands. Compared to genetic alternations such as gene mutation or amplification, aberrant methylation on TSG promoters is rather prevalent and tumor-specific among NPCs. As mentioned above, NPC tumor progression is well characterized by a number of combinatorial epigenetic aberrations distinct to other malignancy, including DNA methylation of more than 30 genes. Consequently, these methylated DNA sequences represent potential biomarkers for diagnosis, staging, prognosis and monitoring of response to therapy or tumor recurrence (Balch et al. 2009; Laird 2003).

4.1 DNA methylation, results from tumor tissues

It has been shown that some genes are high frequently methylated in tumor tissue DNA obtained from NPC primary tumors, but not in normal tissues (Pan et al. 2005; Sun et al. 2007; Zhang et al. 2007; Li, Shu, et al. 2011). These genes are ideal candidate to serve as biomarkers for detection of NPC. Some of these TSGs are not only methylated in NPC, but also commonly methylated in other cancers. So methylation assessment of single genes lacks sufficient specificity for NPC diagnosis. It is believed that panels of multiple methylation biomarkers may achieve higher accuracy required for discriminate NPC from other cancers (Kwong et al. 2002; Hutajulu et al. 2011). This notion was supported by a study of Esteller et al, which showed that a panel of three to four markers could define an abnormality in 70–90% of each cancer type through detecting their aberrant methylation (Esteller et al. 2001). Some studies have been conducted using different combination of gene panels, though there is overlap among them. Combination of methylation markers not only improved the discrimination between NPC and non-NPC diseases, but also the sensitivity of cancer detection. The detection rate can reach 98% when combined analysis of five methylation markers (*RASSF1A, p16, WIF1, CHFR* and *RIZ1*) in a recent study (Hutajulu et al. 2011).

4.2 Methylation markers in circulating DNA

Cancer specific DNA methylation can be detected in tumor-derived free DNA in the bloodstream, e.g. in serum or plasma. High frequency of methylated *DAPK* gene were found not only in NPC tumors, but also could be detected in plasma and buffy coat of NPC patients (Wong et al. 2002). Methylated DNA was detectable in plasma of NPC patients before treatment including 46% for *CDH1*,42% for *CDH1*, 42% for *p16*, 20% for *DAPK* ,20% for *p15 and 5%* for *RASSF1A*. Aberrantly hypermethylated promoter DNA of at least one of the five genes was detectable in 71% of plasma of NPC patients before treatment. Hypermethylated promoter DNA of at least one of the three genes (*CDH1, DAPK1,* and p16) was detectable in post-treatment plasma of 38% recurrent NPC patients and none of the patients in remission. Suggesting that cell-free circulating methylated DNA might be a useful serological marker in assisting in screening of primary and potentially salvageable local or regional recurrent NPC (Wong et al. 2004).

4.3 Methylation markers in other body fluids and nasopharyngeal swabs

In addition to tissue analysis, methylated DNA has been detected in the mouth and throat rinsing fluid, saliva and nasopharyngeal swabs of NPC patients. Methylated DNA found in cancer patient serum correlated reasonably well with methylation levels in tumor tissue, and it is also believed that the source of serum DNA is necrotic tumor cells. Hypermethylated *RIZ1* gene was detected in 60% of NPC primary tumors, but not in any of the normal controls. Of 30 matched body fluid samples, methylated *RIZ1* DNA was found in 37% of NP swabs, 30% of rinsing fluid, 23% of plasma, and 10% of buffy coat samples. The results in NPC tumor and NP swab samples from the same patients show good concordance. Our early study also reported that the high sensitivity (81%) and specificity (0% false positives) of detecting aberrant methylation of *CDH13* (encoded a cell adhesion molecule H-cadherin) from nasopharyngeal swabs suggested it could be utilized as a tool for early diagnosis.

5. DNA methylation modification as therapeutic targets in NPC

DNA methylation plays important roles in NPC carcinogenesis, including the silencing of cellular TSGs and some EBV encoded genes. The EBV encoded oncoprotein, LMP1, has been shown to interacting with methyltransferase (DNMT) and further induce the cellular gene E-cadherin promoter methylation (Tsai et al. 2006). And DNA methylation also suppresse EBV encoded genes, including the LMP1, immediate-early lytic antigens Zta and Rta, and some EBV immunodominant antigens (EBNA2,3A, 3B, 3C) (Paulson and Speck 1999; Tierney et al. 2000; Salamon et al. 2001). Thus, DNA methylation also plays an important role in the maintenance of specific EBV latency programmers and regulating EBV lifecycle and latency in NPC cells.

DNA methylation is a reversible phenomenon. Reactivating methylated and silenced cellular tumor suppressor genes and immunodominant tumor/viral antigens by demethylating agents might restore normal cell growth control, or induce cell immunity against cancer cells. Demethylating agents would also reactivate the expression of EBV early and lytic genes in latently infected NPC cells, which will lead to further tumor cell death.

Epigenetic therapeutic agents include DNA methyltransferase inhibitors and histone deacetylase (HDAC) inhibitors. 5-Azacytidine and 5-aza-2′-deoxycytidine are the most widely studied DNMT inhibitors. Clinical trials using such agents have been carried out on a series of cancer patients. In several phase I/II/III studies, decitabine (5-aza-2′-deoxycytidine) has also shown promising data in patients with MDS and AML (Kantarjian et al. 2007; Issa et al. 2004). In patients with NPC and EBV-positive AIDS-associated Burkitt lymphoma, azacitidine effectively induces demethylation of all the latent and early lytic EBV promoters and some viral antigens, indicated the potential of epigenetic therapy for NPC (Chan et al. 2004).

6. References

Adjei, A. A. 2001. Blocking oncogenic Ras signaling for cancer therapy. *J Natl Cancer Inst* 93 (14):1062-74.

Ayadi, W., H. Karray-Hakim, A. Khabir, L. Feki, S. Charfi, T. Boudawara, A. Ghorbel, J. Daoud, M. Frikha, P. Busson, and A. Hammami. 2008. Aberrant methylation of p16, DLEC1, BLU and E-cadherin gene promoters in nasopharyngeal carcinoma biopsies from Tunisian patients. *Anticancer Res* 28 (4B):2161-7.

Balch, C., F. Fang, D. E. Matei, T. H. Huang, and K. P. Nephew. 2009. Minireview: epigenetic changes in ovarian cancer. *Endocrinology* 150 (9):4003-11.

Barth, S., G. Meister, and F. A. Grasser. 2011. EBV-encoded miRNAs. *Biochim Biophys Acta.*

Berx, G., and F. van Roy. 2009. Involvement of members of the cadherin superfamily in cancer. *Cold Spring Harb Perspect Biol* 1 (6):a003129.

Biel, M., V. Wascholowski, and A. Giannis. 2005. Epigenetics--an epicenter of gene regulation: histones and histone-modifying enzymes. *Angew Chem Int Ed Engl* 44 (21):3186-216.

Bird, A. 2002. DNA methylation patterns and epigenetic memory. *Genes Dev* 16 (1):6-21.

Boguski, M. S., and F. McCormick. 1993. Proteins regulating Ras and its relatives. *Nature* 366 (6456):643-54.

Bos, J. L. 1989. ras oncogenes in human cancer: a review. *Cancer Res* 49 (17):4682-9.

Burgos, J. S. 2003. Absence of p53 alterations in nasopharyngeal carcinoma Spanish patients with Epstein-Barr virus infection. *Virus Genes* 27 (3):263-8.

Chan, K. C., J. M. Ko, H. L. Lung, R. Sedlacek, Z. F. Zhang, D. Z. Luo, Z. B. Feng, S. Chen, H. Chen, K. W. Chan, S. W. Tsao, D. T. Chua, E. R. Zabarovsky, E. J. Stanbridge, and M. L. Lung. 2010. Catalytic activity of matrix metalloproteinase-19 is essential for tumor suppressor and anti-angiogenic activities in nasopharyngeal carcinoma. *Int J Cancer.*

Chan, S. L., Y. Cui, A. van Hasselt, H. Li, G. Srivastava, H. Jin, K. M. Ng, Y. Wang, K. Y. Lee, G. S. Tsao, S. Zhong, K. D. Robertson, S. Y. Rha, A. T. Chan, and Q. Tao. 2007. The tumor suppressor Wnt inhibitory factor 1 is frequently methylated in nasopharyngeal and esophageal carcinomas. *Lab Invest* 87 (7):644-50.

Chang, H. W., A. Chan, D. L. Kwong, W. I. Wei, J. S. Sham, and A. P. Yuen. 2003. Detection of hypermethylated RIZ1 gene in primary tumor, mouth, and throat rinsing fluid, nasopharyngeal swab, and peripheral blood of nasopharyngeal carcinoma patient. *Clin Cancer Res* 9 (3):1033-8.

———. 2003. Evaluation of hypermethylated tumor suppressor genes as tumor markers in mouth and throat rinsing fluid, nasopharyngeal swab and peripheral blood of nasopharygeal carcinoma patient. *Int J Cancer* 105 (6):851-5.

Chang, K. P., S. P. Hao, S. Y. Lin, K. C. Tsao, T. T. Kuo, M. H. Tsai, C. K. Tseng, and N. M. Tsang. 2002. A lack of association between p53 mutations and recurrent nasopharyngeal carcinomas refractory to radiotherapy. *Laryngoscope* 112 (11):2015-9.

Chen, F., Y. Mo, H. Ding, X. Xiao, S. Y. Wang, G. Huang, Z. Zhang, and S. Z. Wang. 2011. Frequent epigenetic inactivation of Myocardin in human nasopharyngeal carcinoma. *Head Neck* 33 (1):54-9.

Chen, H. C., G. H. Chen, Y. H. Chen, W. L. Liao, C. Y. Liu, K. P. Chang, Y. S. Chang, and S. J. Chen. 2009. MicroRNA deregulation and pathway alterations in nasopharyngeal carcinoma. *Br J Cancer* 100 (6):1002-11.

Cheng, Y., H. Geng, S. H. Cheng, P. Liang, Y. Bai, J. Li, G. Srivastava, M. H. Ng, T. Fukagawa, X. Wu, A. T. Chan, and Q. Tao. 2010. KRAB zinc finger protein ZNF382 is a proapoptotic tumor suppressor that represses multiple oncogenes and is commonly silenced in multiple carcinomas. *Cancer Res* 70 (16):6516-26.

Cheung, A. K., H. L. Lung, S. C. Hung, E. W. Law, Y. Cheng, W. L. Yau, D. K. Bangarusamy, L. D. Miller, E. T. Liu, J. Y. Shao, C. W. Kou, D. Chua, E. R. Zabarovsky, S. W. Tsao, E. J. Stanbridge, and M. L. Lung. 2008. Functional analysis of a cell cycle-associated, tumor-suppressive gene, protein tyrosine phosphatase receptor type G, in nasopharyngeal carcinoma. *Cancer Res* 68 (19):8137-45.

Cheung, A. K., H. L. Lung, J. M. Ko, Y. Cheng, E. J. Stanbridge, E. R. Zabarovsky, J. M. Nicholls, D. Chua, S. W. Tsao, X. Y. Guan, and M. L. Lung. 2009. Chromosome 14 transfer and functional studies identify a candidate tumor suppressor gene, mirror image polydactyly 1, in nasopharyngeal carcinoma. *Proc Natl Acad Sci U S A* 106 (34):14478-83.

Cheung, H. W., Y. P. Ching, J. M. Nicholls, M. T. Ling, Y. C. Wong, N. Hui, A. Cheung, S. W. Tsao, Q. Wang, P. W. Yeun, K. W. Lo, D. Y. Jin, and X. Wang. 2005. Epigenetic inactivation of CHFR in nasopharyngeal carcinoma through promoter methylation. *Mol Carcinog* 43 (4):237-45.

Chow, L. S., K. W. Lo, J. Kwong, K. F. To, K. S. Tsang, C. W. Lam, R. Dammann, and D. P. Huang. 2004. RASSF1A is a target tumor suppressor from 3p21.3 in nasopharyngeal carcinoma. *Int J Cancer* 109 (6):839-47.

Crook, T., J. M. Nicholls, L. Brooks, J. O'Nions, and M. J. Allday. 2000. High level expression of deltaN-p63: a mechanism for the inactivation of p53 in undifferentiated nasopharyngeal carcinoma (NPC)? *Oncogene* 19 (30):3439-44.

Cui, Y., Y. Ying, A. van Hasselt, K. M. Ng, J. Yu, Q. Zhang, J. Jin, D. Liu, J. S. Rhim, S. Y. Rha, M. Loyo, A. T. Chan, G. Srivastava, G. S. Tsao, G. C. Sellar, J. J. Sung, D. Sidransky, and Q. Tao. 2008. OPCML is a broad tumor suppressor for multiple carcinomas and lymphomas with frequently epigenetic inactivation. *PLoS One* 3 (8):e2990.

Du, C., T. Huang, D. Sun, Y. Mo, H. Feng, X. Zhou, X. Xiao, N. Yu, B. Hou, G. Huang, I. Ernberg, and Z. Zhang. 2011. CDH4 as a novel putative tumor suppressor gene epigenetically silenced by promoter hypermethylation in nasopharyngeal carcinoma. *Cancer Lett.*

———. 2011. CDH4 as a novel putative tumor suppressor gene epigenetically silenced by promoter hypermethylation in nasopharyngeal carcinoma. *Cancer Lett* 309 (1):54-61.

Egger, G., G. Liang, A. Aparicio, and P. A. Jones. 2004. Epigenetics in human disease and prospects for epigenetic therapy. *Nature* 429 (6990):457-63.

Eliopoulos, A. G., and L. S. Young. 2001. LMP1 structure and signal transduction. *Semin Cancer Biol* 11 (6):435-44.

Esteller, M. 2006. Epigenetics provides a new generation of oncogenes and tumour-suppressor genes. *Br J Cancer* 94 (2):179-83.

———. 2007. Cancer epigenomics: DNA methylomes and histone-modification maps. *Nat Rev Genet* 8 (4):286-98.

Esteller, M., P. G. Corn, S. B. Baylin, and J. G. Herman. 2001. A gene hypermethylation profile of human cancer. *Cancer Res* 61 (8):3225-9.

Fernandez, A. F., C. Rosales, P. Lopez-Nieva, O. Grana, E. Ballestar, S. Ropero, J. Espada, S. A. Melo, A. Lujambio, M. F. Fraga, I. Pino, B. Javierre, F. J. Carmona, F. Acquadro, R. D. Steenbergen, P. J. Snijders, C. J. Meijer, P. Pineau, A. Dejean, B. Lloveras, G. Capella, J. Quer, M. Buti, J. I. Esteban, H. Allende, F. Rodriguez-Frias, X. Castellsague, J. Minarovits, J. Ponce, D. Capello, G. Gaidano, J. C. Cigudosa, G. Gomez-Lopez, D. G. Pisano, A. Valencia, M. A. Piris, F. X. Bosch, E. Cahir-McFarland, E. Kieff, and M. Esteller. 2009. The dynamic DNA methylomes of double-stranded DNA viruses associated with human cancer. *Genome Res* 19 (3):438-51.

Fischle, W., Y. Wang, and C. D. Allis. 2003. Histone and chromatin cross-talk. *Curr Opin Cell Biol* 15 (2):172-83.

Gialeli, C., A. D. Theocharis, and N. K. Karamanos. 2011. Roles of matrix metalloproteinases in cancer progression and their pharmacological targeting. *FEBS J* 278 (1):16-27.

Giehl, K. 2005. Oncogenic Ras in tumour progression and metastasis. *Biol Chem* 386 (3):193-205.

Hu, L. F., F. Chen, Q. F. Zhen, Y. W. Zhang, Y. Luo, X. Zheng, G. Winberg, I. Ernberg, and G. Klein. 1995. Differences in the growth pattern and clinical course of EBV-LMP1 expressing and non-expressing nasopharyngeal carcinomas. *Eur J Cancer* 31A (5):658-60.

Huang, G. W., W. N. Mo, G. Q. Kuang, H. T. Nong, M. Y. Wei, M. Sunagawa, and T. Kosugi. 2001. Expression of p16, nm23-H1, E-cadherin, and CD44 gene products and their significance in nasopharyngeal carcinoma. *Laryngoscope* 111 (8):1465-71.

Hui, A. B., K. W. Lo, J. Kwong, E. C. Lam, S. Y. Chan, L. S. Chow, A. S. Chan, P. M. Teo, and D. P. Huang. 2003. Epigenetic inactivation of TSLC1 gene in nasopharyngeal carcinoma. *Mol Carcinog* 38 (4):170-8.

Hutajulu, S. H., S. R. Indrasari, L. P. Indrawati, A. Harijadi, S. Duin, S. M. Haryana, R. D. Steenbergen, A. E. Greijer, and J. M. Middeldorp. 2011. Epigenetic markers for early detection of nasopharyngeal carcinoma in a high risk population. *Mol Cancer* 10:48.

Jeanes, A., C. J. Gottardi, and A. S. Yap. 2008. Cadherins and cancer: how does cadherin dysfunction promote tumor progression? *Oncogene* 27 (55):6920-9.

Jeltsch, A., and W. Fischle. 2011. Molecular epigenetics: connecting human biology and disease with little marks. *Chembiochem* 12 (2):183-4.

Jenuwein, T., and C. D. Allis. 2001. Translating the histone code. *Science* 293 (5532):1074-80.

Jin, H., X. Wang, J. Ying, A. H. Wong, Y. Cui, G. Srivastava, Z. Y. Shen, E. M. Li, Q. Zhang, J. Jin, S. Kupzig, A. T. Chan, P. J. Cullen, and Q. Tao. 2007. Epigenetic silencing of a Ca (2+)-regulated Ras GTPase-activating protein RASAL defines a new mechanism of Ras activation in human cancers. *Proc Natl Acad Sci U S A* 104 (30):12353-8.

Jin, H., X. Wang, J. Ying, A. H. Wong, H. Li, K. Y. Lee, G. Srivastava, A. T. Chan, W. Yeo, B. B. Ma, T. C. Putti, M. L. Lung, Z. Y. Shen, L. Y. Xu, C. Langford, and Q. Tao. 2007. Epigenetic identification of ADAMTS18 as a novel 16q23.1 tumor suppressor frequently silenced in esophageal, nasopharyngeal and multiple other carcinomas. *Oncogene* 26 (53):7490-8.

Jones, P. A., and P. W. Laird. 1999. Cancer epigenetics comes of age. *Nat Genet* 21 (2):163-7.

Jones, P. A., and D. Takai. 2001. The role of DNA methylation in mammalian epigenetics. *Science* 293 (5532):1068-70.

Kargul, J., and G. J. Laurent. 2009. Epigenetics and human disease. *Int J Biochem Cell Biol* 41 (1):1.

Kondo, S., N. Wakisaka, M. J. Schell, T. Horikawa, T. S. Sheen, H. Sato, M. Furukawa, J. S. Pagano, and T. Yoshizaki. 2005. Epstein-Barr virus latent membrane protein 1 induces the matrix metalloproteinase-1 promoter via an Ets binding site formed by a single nucleotide polymorphism: enhanced susceptibility to nasopharyngeal carcinoma. *Int J Cancer* 115 (3):368-76.

Kong, W. J., S. Zhang, C. K. Guo, Y. J. Wang, X. Chen, S. L. Zhang, D. Zhang, Z. Liu, and W. Kong. 2006. Effect of methylation-associated silencing of the death-associated protein kinase gene on nasopharyngeal carcinoma. *Anticancer Drugs* 17 (3):251-9.

Krop, I., M. T. Parker, N. Bloushtain-Qimron, D. Porter, R. Gelman, H. Sasaki, M. Maurer, M. B. Terry, R. Parsons, and K. Polyak. 2005. HIN-1, an inhibitor of cell growth, invasion, and AKT activation. *Cancer Res* 65 (21):9659-69.

Kwok, W. K., J. C. Pang, K. W. Lo, and H. K. Ng. 2009. Role of the RARRES1 gene in nasopharyngeal carcinoma. *Cancer Genet Cytogenet* 194 (1):58-64.

Kwong, J., K. W. Lo, L. S. Chow, F. L. Chan, K. F. To, and D. P. Huang. 2005. Silencing of the retinoid response gene TIG1 by promoter hypermethylation in nasopharyngeal carcinoma. *Int J Cancer* 113 (3):386-92.

Kwong, J., K. W. Lo, L. S. Chow, K. F. To, K. W. Choy, F. L. Chan, S. C. Mok, and D. P. Huang. 2005. Epigenetic silencing of cellular retinol-binding proteins in nasopharyngeal carcinoma. *Neoplasia* 7 (1):67-74.

Kwong, J., K. W. Lo, K. F. To, P. M. Teo, P. J. Johnson, and D. P. Huang. 2002. Promoter hypermethylation of multiple genes in nasopharyngeal carcinoma. *Clin Cancer Res* 8 (1):131-7.

Laird, P. W. 2003. The power and the promise of DNA methylation markers. *Nat Rev Cancer* 3 (4):253-66.

Laird, P. W., L. Jackson-Grusby, A. Fazeli, S. L. Dickinson, W. E. Jung, E. Li, R. A. Weinberg, and R. Jaenisch. 1995. Suppression of intestinal neoplasia by DNA hypomethylation. *Cell* 81 (2):197-205.

Law, E. W., A. K. Cheung, V. I. Kashuba, T. V. Pavlova, E. R. Zabarovsky, H. L. Lung, Y. Cheng, D. Chua, D. Lai-Wan Kwong, S. W. Tsao, T. Sasaki, E. J. Stanbridge, and M. L. Lung. 2011. Anti-angiogenic and tumor-suppressive roles of candidate tumor-suppressor gene, Fibulin-2, in nasopharyngeal carcinoma. *Oncogene.*

Lee, D. C., D. T. Chua, W. I. Wei, J. S. Sham, and A. S. Lau. 2007. Induction of matrix metalloproteinases by Epstein-Barr virus latent membrane protein 1 isolated from nasopharyngeal carcinoma. *Biomed Pharmacother* 61 (9):520-6.

Lengauer, C., K. W. Kinzler, and B. Vogelstein. 1998. Genetic instabilities in human cancers. *Nature* 396 (6712):643-9.

Li, H., and J. Minarovits. 2003. Host cell-dependent expression of latent Epstein-Barr virus genomes: regulation by DNA methylation. *Adv Cancer Res* 89:133-56.

Li, L. L., X. S. Shu, Z. H. Wang, Y. Cao, and Q. Tao. 2011. Epigenetic disruption of cell signaling in nasopharyngeal carcinoma. *Chin J Cancer* 30 (4):231-9.

Li, L., Q. Tao, H. Jin, A. van Hasselt, F. F. Poon, X. Wang, M. S. Zeng, W. H. Jia, Y. X. Zeng, A. T. Chan, and Y. Cao. 2010. The tumor suppressor UCHL1 forms a complex with p53/MDM2/ARF to promote p53 signaling and is frequently silenced in nasopharyngeal carcinoma. *Clin Cancer Res* 16 (11):2949-58.

Li, W., X. Li, W. Wang, Y. Tan, M. Yi, J. Yang, J. B. McCarthy, Z. Zhang, B. Su, Q. Liao, M. Wu, W. Xiong, J. Ma, B. Xiang, and G. Li. 2011. NOR1 is an HSF1- and NRF1-regulated putative tumor suppressor inactivated by promoter hypermethylation in nasopharyngeal carcinoma. *Carcinogenesis.*

Lin, Y. C., L. You, Z. Xu, B. He, I. Mikami, E. Thung, J. Chou, K. Kuchenbecker, J. Kim, D. Raz, C. T. Yang, J. K. Chen, and D. M. Jablons. 2006. Wnt signaling activation and WIF-1 silencing in nasopharyngeal cancer cell lines. *Biochem Biophys Res Commun* 341 (2):635-40.

Liu, H., L. Zhang, Z. Niu, M. Zhou, C. Peng, X. Li, T. Deng, L. Shi, Y. Tan, and G. Li. 2008. Promoter methylation inhibits BRD7 expression in human nasopharyngeal carcinoma cells. *BMC Cancer* 8:253.

Liu, X. Q., H. K. Chen, X. S. Zhang, Z. G. Pan, A. Li, Q. S. Feng, Q. X. Long, X. Z. Wang, and Y. X. Zeng. 2003. Alterations of BLU, a candidate tumor suppressor gene on chromosome 3p21.3, in human nasopharyngeal carcinoma. *Int J Cancer* 106 (1):60-5.

Lo, K. W., S. T. Cheung, S. F. Leung, A. van Hasselt, Y. S. Tsang, K. F. Mak, Y. F. Chung, J. K. Woo, J. C. Lee, and D. P. Huang. 1996. Hypermethylation of the p16 gene in nasopharyngeal carcinoma. *Cancer Res* 56 (12):2721-5.

Lo, K. W., and D. P. Huang. 2002. Genetic and epigenetic changes in nasopharyngeal carcinoma. *Semin Cancer Biol* 12 (6):451-62.

Lo, K. W., J. Kwong, A. B. Hui, S. Y. Chan, K. F. To, A. S. Chan, L. S. Chow, P. M. Teo, P. J. Johnson, and D. P. Huang. 2001. High frequency of promoter hypermethylation of RASSF1A in nasopharyngeal carcinoma. *Cancer Res* 61 (10):3877-81.

Lo, K. W., K. F. To, and D. P. Huang. 2004. Focus on nasopharyngeal carcinoma. *Cancer Cell* 5 (5):423-8.

Lo, K. W., Y. S. Tsang, J. Kwong, K. F. To, P. M. Teo, and D. P. Huang. 2002. Promoter hypermethylation of the EDNRB gene in nasopharyngeal carcinoma. *Int J Cancer* 98 (5):651-5.

Lou, P., W. Chen, T. Sheen, J. Ko, M. Hsu, and J. Wu. 1999. Expression of E-cadherin/catenin complex in nasopharyngeal carcinoma: correlation with clinicopathological parameters. *Oncol Rep* 6 (5):1065-71.

Lou, P. J., W. P. Chen, C. T. Lin, R. M. DePhilip, and J. C. Wu. 1999. E-, P-, and N-cadherin are co-expressed in the nasopharyngeal carcinoma cell line TW-039. *J Cell Biochem* 76 (1):161-72.

Low, J. S., Q. Tao, K. M. Ng, H. K. Goh, X. S. Shu, W. L. Woo, R. F. Ambinder, G. Srivastava, M. Shamay, A. T. Chan, N. C. Popescu, and W. S. Hsieh. 2011. A novel isoform of the 8p22 tumor suppressor gene DLC1 suppresses tumor growth and is frequently silenced in multiple common tumors. *Oncogene* 30 (16):1923-35.

Loyo, M., M. Brait, M. S. Kim, K. L. Ostrow, C. C. Jie, A. Y. Chuang, J. A. Califano, N. J. Liegeois, S. Begum, W. H. Westra, M. O. Hoque, Q. Tao, and D. Sidransky. 2011. A survey of methylated candidate tumor suppressor genes in nasopharyngeal carcinoma. *Int J Cancer* 128 (6):1393-403.

Lu, T. Y., C. F. Kao, C. T. Lin, D. Y. Huang, C. Y. Chiu, Y. S. Huang, and H. C. Wu. 2009. DNA methylation and histone modification regulate silencing of OPG during tumor progression. *J Cell Biochem* 108 (1):315-25.

Lung, H. L., D. K. Bangarusamy, D. Xie, A. K. Cheung, Y. Cheng, M. K. Kumaran, L. Miller, E. T. Liu, X. Y. Guan, J. S. Sham, Y. Fang, L. Li, N. Wang, A. I. Protopopov, E. R. Zabarovsky, S. W. Tsao, E. J. Stanbridge, and M. L. Lung. 2005. THY1 is a candidate tumour suppressor gene with decreased expression in metastatic nasopharyngeal carcinoma. *Oncogene* 24 (43):6525-32.

Lung, H. L., Y. Cheng, M. K. Kumaran, E. T. Liu, Y. Murakami, C. Y. Chan, W. L. Yau, J. M. Ko, E. J. Stanbridge, and M. L. Lung. 2004. Fine mapping of the 11q22-23 tumor suppressive region and involvement of TSLC1 in nasopharyngeal carcinoma. *Int J Cancer* 112 (4):628-35.

Lung, H. L., C. C. Lo, C. C. Wong, A. K. Cheung, K. F. Cheong, N. Wong, F. M. Kwong, K. C. Chan, E. W. Law, S. W. Tsao, D. Chua, J. S. Sham, Y. Cheng, E. J. Stanbridge, G. P. Robertson, and M. L. Lung. 2008. Identification of tumor suppressive activity by irradiation microcell-mediated chromosome transfer and involvement of alpha B-crystallin in nasopharyngeal carcinoma. *Int J Cancer* 122 (6):1288-96.

Lung, H. L., P. H. Lo, D. Xie, S. S. Apte, A. K. Cheung, Y. Cheng, E. W. Law, D. Chua, Y. X. Zeng, S. W. Tsao, E. J. Stanbridge, and M. L. Lung. 2008. Characterization of a novel epigenetically-silenced, growth-suppressive gene, ADAMTS9, and its association with lymph node metastases in nasopharyngeal carcinoma. *Int J Cancer* 123 (2):401-8.

Malik, K., and K. W. Brown. 2000. Epigenetic gene deregulation in cancer. *Br J Cancer* 83 (12):1583-8.

McManus, M. T. 2003. MicroRNAs and cancer. *Semin Cancer Biol* 13 (4):253-8.

Ozenne, P., B. Eymin, E. Brambilla, and S. Gazzeri. 2010. The ARF tumor suppressor: structure, functions and status in cancer. *Int J Cancer* 127 (10):2239-47.

Pan, Z. G., V. I. Kashuba, X. Q. Liu, J. Y. Shao, R. H. Zhang, J. H. Jiang, C. Guo, E. Zabarovsky, I. Ernberg, and Y. X. Zeng. 2005. High frequency somatic mutations in RASSF1A in nasopharyngeal carcinoma. *Cancer Biol Ther* 4 (10):1116-22.

Pattle, S. B., and P. J. Farrell. 2006. The role of Epstein-Barr virus in cancer. *Expert Opin Biol Ther* 6 (11):1193-205.

Peng, D., C. P. Ren, H. M. Yi, L. Zhou, X. Y. Yang, H. Li, and K. T. Yao. 2006. Genetic and epigenetic alterations of DLC-1, a candidate tumor suppressor gene, in nasopharyngeal carcinoma. *Acta Biochim Biophys Sin (Shanghai)* 38 (5):349-55.

Pointis, G., C. Fiorini, J. Gilleron, D. Carette, and D. Segretain. 2007. Connexins as precocious markers and molecular targets for chemical and pharmacological agents in carcinogenesis. *Curr Med Chem* 14 (21):2288-303.

Robertson, K. D., E. Uzvolgyi, G. Liang, C. Talmadge, J. Sumegi, F. A. Gonzales, and P. A. Jones. 1999. The human DNA methyltransferases (DNMTs) 1, 3a and 3b: coordinate mRNA expression in normal tissues and overexpression in tumors. *Nucleic Acids Res* 27 (11):2291-8.

Schulz, W. 2005. Qualified promise: DNA methylation assays for the detection and classification of human cancers. *J Biomed Biotechnol* 2005 (3):227-9.

Seng, T. J., J. S. Low, H. Li, Y. Cui, H. K. Goh, M. L. Wong, G. Srivastava, D. Sidransky, J. Califano, R. D. Steenbergen, S. Y. Rha, J. Tan, W. S. Hsieh, R. F. Ambinder, X. Lin, A. T. Chan, and Q. Tao. 2007. The major 8p22 tumor suppressor DLC1 is frequently silenced by methylation in both endemic and sporadic nasopharyngeal, esophageal, and cervical carcinomas, and inhibits tumor cell colony formation. *Oncogene* 26 (6):934-44.

Seo, S. Y., E. O. Kim, and K. L. Jang. 2008. Epstein-Barr virus latent membrane protein 1 suppresses the growth-inhibitory effect of retinoic acid by inhibiting retinoic acid receptor-beta2 expression via DNA methylation. *Cancer Lett* 270 (1):66-76.

Shao, L., Y. Cui, H. Li, Y. Liu, H. Zhao, Y. Wang, Y. Zhang, K. M. Ng, W. Han, D. Ma, and Q. Tao. 2007. CMTM5 exhibits tumor suppressor activities and is frequently silenced by methylation in carcinoma cell lines. *Clin Cancer Res* 13 (19):5756-62.

Shen, Z., J. Lin, M. Li, and Q. Zeng. 2002. [Study on the expression of connexin 43 in human nasopharyngeal carcinoma]. *Lin Chuang Er Bi Yan Hou Ke Za Zhi* 16 (8):402-3, 406.

Shi, W., C. Bastianutto, A. Li, B. Perez-Ordonez, R. Ng, K. Y. Chow, W. Zhang, I. Jurisica, K. W. Lo, A. Bayley, J. Kim, B. O'Sullivan, L. Siu, E. Chen, and F. F. Liu. 2006. Multiple dysregulated pathways in nasopharyngeal carcinoma revealed by gene expression profiling. *Int J Cancer* 119 (10):2467-75.

Spandidos, D. A., G. Sourvinos, C. Tsatsanis, and A. Zafiropoulos. 2002. Normal ras genes: their onco-suppressor and pro-apoptotic functions (review). *Int J Oncol* 21 (2):237-41.

Stevenson, D., C. Charalambous, and J. B. Wilson. 2005. Epstein-Barr virus latent membrane protein 1 (CAO) up-regulates VEGF and TGF alpha concomitant with hyperlasia, with subsequent up-regulation of p16 and MMP9. *Cancer Res* 65 (19):8826-35.

Sun, D., Z. Zhang, N. Van do, G. Huang, I. Ernberg, and L. Hu. 2007. Aberrant methylation of CDH13 gene in nasopharyngeal carcinoma could serve as a potential diagnostic biomarker. *Oral Oncol* 43 (1):82-7.

Tao, Q., and A. T. Chan. 2007. Nasopharyngeal carcinoma: molecular pathogenesis and therapeutic developments. *Expert Rev Mol Med* 9 (12):1-24.
Tong, J. H., D. C. Ng, S. L. Chau, K. K. So, P. P. Leung, T. L. Lee, R. W. Lung, M. W. Chan, A. W. Chan, K. W. Lo, and K. F. To. 2010. Putative tumour-suppressor gene DAB2 is frequently down regulated by promoter hypermethylation in nasopharyngeal carcinoma. *BMC Cancer* 10:253.
Tost, J. 2010. DNA methylation: an introduction to the biology and the disease-associated changes of a promising biomarker. *Mol Biotechnol* 44 (1):71-81.
Tsai, C. L., H. P. Li, Y. J. Lu, C. Hsueh, Y. Liang, C. L. Chen, S. W. Tsao, K. P. Tse, J. S. Yu, and Y. S. Chang. 2006. Activation of DNA methyltransferase 1 by EBV LMP1 Involves c-Jun NH (2)-terminal kinase signaling. *Cancer Res* 66 (24):11668-76.
Tsai, C. N., C. L. Tsai, K. P. Tse, H. Y. Chang, and Y. S. Chang. 2002. The Epstein-Barr virus oncogene product, latent membrane protein 1, induces the downregulation of E-cadherin gene expression via activation of DNA methyltransferases. *Proc Natl Acad Sci U S A* 99 (15):10084-9.
Ventura, A., and T. Jacks. 2009. MicroRNAs and cancer: short RNAs go a long way. *Cell* 136 (4):586-91.
Wang, S., X. Xiao, X. Zhou, T. Huang, C. Du, N. Yu, Y. Mo, L. Lin, J. Zhang, N. Ma, M. Murata, G. Huang, and Z. Zhang. 2010. TFPI-2 is a putative tumor suppressor gene frequently inactivated by promoter hypermethylation in nasopharyngeal carcinoma. *BMC Cancer* 10:617.
Wang, Y., J. Li, Y. Cui, T. Li, K. M. Ng, H. Geng, H. Li, X. S. Shu, W. Liu, B. Luo, Q. Zhang, T. S. Mok, W. Zheng, X. Qiu, G. Srivastava, J. Yu, J. J. Sung, A. T. Chan, D. Ma, Q. Tao, and W. Han. 2009. CMTM3, located at the critical tumor suppressor locus 16q22.1, is silenced by CpG methylation in carcinomas and inhibits tumor cell growth through inducing apoptosis. *Cancer Res* 69 (12):5194-201.
Wei, X., T. D. Prickett, C. G. Viloria, A. Molinolo, J. C. Lin, I. Cardenas-Navia, P. Cruz, S. A. Rosenberg, M. A. Davies, J. E. Gershenwald, C. Lopez-Otin, and Y. Samuels. 2010. Mutational and functional analysis reveals ADAMTS18 metalloproteinase as a novel driver in melanoma. *Mol Cancer Res* 8 (11):1513-25.
Wong, T. S., H. W. Chang, K. C. Tang, W. I. Wei, D. L. Kwong, J. S. Sham, A. P. Yuen, and Y. L. Kwong. 2002. High frequency of promoter hypermethylation of the death-associated protein-kinase gene in nasopharyngeal carcinoma and its detection in the peripheral blood of patients. *Clin Cancer Res* 8 (2):433-7.
Wong, T. S., D. L. Kwong, J. S. Sham, S. W. Tsao, W. I. Wei, Y. L. Kwong, and A. P. Yuen. 2003. Promoter hypermethylation of high-in-normal 1 gene in primary nasopharyngeal carcinoma. *Clin Cancer Res* 9 (8):3042-6.
Wong, T. S., D. L. Kwong, J. S. Sham, W. I. Wei, Y. L. Kwong, and A. P. Yuen. 2004. Quantitative plasma hypermethylated DNA markers of undifferentiated nasopharyngeal carcinoma. *Clin Cancer Res* 10 (7):2401-6.
Wong, T. S., K. C. Tang, D. L. Kwong, J. S. Sham, W. I. Wei, Y. L. Kwong, and A. P. Yuen. 2003. Differential gene methylation in undifferentiated nasopharyngeal carcinoma. *Int J Oncol* 22 (4):869-74.

Wu, J., J. P. Issa, J. Herman, D. E. Bassett, Jr., B. D. Nelkin, and S. B. Baylin. 1993. Expression of an exogenous eukaryotic DNA methyltransferase gene induces transformation of NIH 3T3 cells. *Proc Natl Acad Sci U S A* 90 (19):8891-5.

Xiang, Q., S. Q. Fan, J. Li, C. Tan, J. J. Xiang, Q. H. Zhang, R. Wang, and G. Y. Li. 2002. [Expression of connexin43 and connexin45 in nasopharyngeal carcinoma]. *Ai Zheng* 21 (6):593-6.

Yanatatsaneejit, P., T. Chalermchai, V. Kerekhanjanarong, K. Shotelersuk, P. Supiyaphun, A. Mutirangura, and V. Sriuranpong. 2008. Promoter hypermethylation of CCNA1, RARRES1, and HRASLS3 in nasopharyngeal carcinoma. *Oral Oncol* 44 (4):400-6.

Yi, B., S. X. Tan, C. E. Tang, W. G. Huang, A. L. Cheng, C. Li, P. F. Zhang, M. Y. Li, J. L. Li, H. Yi, F. Peng, Z. C. Chen, and Z. Q. Xiao. 2009. Inactivation of 14-3-3 sigma by promoter methylation correlates with metastasis in nasopharyngeal carcinoma. *J Cell Biochem* 106 (5):858-66.

Yi, H. M., H. Li, D. Peng, H. J. Zhang, L. Wang, M. Zhao, K. T. Yao, and C. P. Ren. 2006. Genetic and epigenetic alterations of LTF at 3p21.3 in nasopharyngeal carcinoma. *Oncol Res* 16 (6):261-72.

Yi, Z. C., H. Wang, G. Y. Zhang, and B. Xia. 2007. Downregulation of connexin 43 in nasopharyngeal carcinoma cells is related to promoter methylation. *Oral Oncol* 43 (9):898-904.

Ying, J., H. Li, T. J. Seng, C. Langford, G. Srivastava, S. W. Tsao, T. Putti, P. Murray, A. T. Chan, and Q. Tao. 2006. Functional epigenetics identifies a protocadherin PCDH10 as a candidate tumor suppressor for nasopharyngeal, esophageal and multiple other carcinomas with frequent methylation. *Oncogene* 25 (7):1070-80.

Ying, J., G. Srivastava, W. S. Hsieh, Z. Gao, P. Murray, S. K. Liao, R. Ambinder, and Q. Tao. 2005. The stress-responsive gene GADD45G is a functional tumor suppressor, with its response to environmental stresses frequently disrupted epigenetically in multiple tumors. *Clin Cancer Res* 11 (18):6442-9.

Young, L. S., and A. B. Rickinson. 2004. Epstein-Barr virus: 40 years on. *Nat Rev Cancer* 4 (10):757-68.

Zeng, Z. Y., Y. H. Zhou, W. L. Zhang, W. Xiong, S. Q. Fan, X. L. Li, X. M. Luo, M. H. Wu, Y. X. Yang, C. Huang, L. Cao, K. Tang, J. Qian, S. R. Shen, and G. Y. Li. 2007. Gene expression profiling of nasopharyngeal carcinoma reveals the abnormally regulated Wnt signaling pathway. *Hum Pathol* 38 (1):120-33.

Zhang, H., X. Feng, W. Liu, X. Jiang, W. Shan, C. Huang, H. Yi, B. Zhu, W. Zhou, L. Wang, C. Liu, L. Zhang, W. Jia, W. Huang, G. Li, J. Shi, S. Wanggou, K. Yao, and C. Ren. 2011. Underlying mechanisms for LTF inactivation and its functional analysis in nasopharyngeal carcinoma cell lines. *J Cell Biochem* 112 (7):1832-43.

Zhang, Z., D. Sun, N. Van do, A. Tang, L. Hu, and G. Huang. 2007. Inactivation of RASSF2A by promoter methylation correlates with lymph node metastasis in nasopharyngeal carcinoma. *Int J Cancer* 120 (1):32-8.

Zhou, L., X. Feng, W. Shan, W. Zhou, W. Liu, L. Wang, B. Zhu, H. Yi, K. Yao, and C. Ren. 2007. Epigenetic and genetic alterations of the EDNRB gene in nasopharyngeal carcinoma. *Oncology* 72 (5-6):357-63.

Zhou, L., W. Jiang, C. Ren, Z. Yin, X. Feng, W. Liu, Q. Tao, and K. Yao. 2005. Frequent hypermethylation of RASSF1A and TSLC1, and high viral load of Epstein-Barr

Virus DNA in nasopharyngeal carcinoma and matched tumor-adjacent tissues. *Neoplasia* 7 (9):809-15.

Zhou, W., X. Feng, H. Li, L. Wang, B. Zhu, W. Liu, M. Zhao, K. Yao, and C. Ren. 2009. Inactivation of LARS2, located at the commonly deleted region 3p21.3, by both epigenetic and genetic mechanisms in nasopharyngeal carcinoma. *Acta Biochim Biophys Sin (Shanghai)* 41 (1):54-62.

Zhu, J. Y., T. Pfuhl, N. Motsch, S. Barth, J. Nicholls, F. Grasser, and G. Meister. 2009. Identification of novel Epstein-Barr virus microRNA genes from nasopharyngeal carcinomas. *J Virol* 83 (7):3333-41.

2

Pathologic Significance of EBV Encoded RNA in NPC

Zhi Li, Lifang Yang and Lun-Quan Sun
Center for Molecular Medicine, Xiangya Hospital, Central South University, Changsha, China

1. Introduction

The EBV-encoded RNAs (EBERs) are the most abundant EBV transcripts (about 10^7 copies per cell) during latent infection by EBV in a variety of cells. Owing to its expression abundance and universal existence in all of the 3 forms of latent infection, EBERs have been under intensive studies since they were discovered by Lernar (Lerner et al., 1981) for the first time. Looking back over the past 30 years, great efforts have been made to unveil the accurate role of EBERs in the latency and transformation process, the definite secondary structure and the signaling pathways they participate in. Despite significant achievements were achieved in these fields, most pioneer work was conducted in lymphoma cells. Bearing this in mind, we explore the similarities between lymphoma and carcinoma to fill the gaps in our knowledge of EBERs' roles in nasopharyngeal carcinoma (NPC). However, it remains to be clarified whether the same scenario accurately applies to the pathological significance of EBERs in NPC.

Epstein-Barr virus (EBV) is consistently detected in NPC from regions of both high and low incidence. In EBV infected cells, there exist some polyribosomal virus-specific RNAs which are the most abundant RNAs (Rymo, 1979). Initial transcription mapping studies by Kieff and colleagues indicated that polyribosomal virus-specific RNA was encoded primarily by the internal repeat region of EBV DNA and, to a lesser extent, by certain other regions of the genome (Orellana & Kieff, 1977; Powell et al., 1979). Making use of cloned restriction endonuclease fragments of EBV, Arrand discovered that the major cytoplasmic RNA in these cells was specified by part of the EcoRI J fragment, which was consistent with Rymo's observation (Arrand & Rymo, 1982). Meanwhile, there were reports that revealed SLE antibodies anti-La, but not the other sera tested, identified two new small RNAs, which corresponded to the most actively transcribed portion of EBV DNA in Rymo's investigation and they were termed EBERs for the first time. In the following 1980's, emphasis were put on the structure, transcription regulation and the function of EBER-La complex. After these preliminary explorations, intensive research was focused on the role of EBERs in the oncogenesis of lymphoma, the involvement of EBERs in the process of lymphoblastoid cell line (LCL) transformation and the potential anti-apoptosis response triggered by EBERs. With these inspiring achievements, some scholars were intrigued by the autocrine growth of several tumor cells and successfully discovered the link between cytokine induction and EBERs in B and T lymphocyte, gastric carcinoma and nasopharyngeal carcinoma in the following decade. More recently, our knowledge has been deepened by unveiling the TLR3 and RIG-I signaling pathways induced by EBERs, which are responsible for the autocrine growth of lymphomas and some EBV associated pathogenesis (Iwakiri et al., 2005; Samanta et al., 2008). However, the accurate role of EBERs in the pathogenesis of NPC is still obscure. There have been some contradictory reports with respect to the contribution of EBERs to the oncogenesis of NPC and the relationship between EBERs and anti-apoptosis response. What makes these dilemmas more complicated is the existence of EBERs in various stages of NPC. Interestingly, expression of the EBERs seems to be down-regulated during differentiation. Thus examples of NPC that have differing degrees of differentiation lack EBER expression in differentiated areas (Pathmanathan et al., 1995). The EBERs are also not detected in the permissive EBV infection, hairy leukoplakia, and are downregulated during viral replication (Gilligan et al., 1990). Collecting the previous data together, despite that the EBERs have been studied over 3 decades and some observations indicate they may play important roles in the transformation of lymphoma (Yajima et al., 2005) and NPC (Yoshizaki et al., 2007), the exact function of EBERs in NPC are still controversial.

2. Structure, transcription and clinical significance of EBERs

EBERs, the most abundant cytoplasmic RNA species identified in five lymphoid cell lines and a Burkitt lymphoma biopsy, are encoded by the right-hand 1,000 base pairs of the EcoRI J fragment of EBV DNA (Rosa et al., 1981). EBER1 is 166 (167) nucleotides long and EBER2 is 172 ± 1 nucleotides long with the heterogeneity resides at the 3' termini (Fig. 1). Striking similarities are apparent both between the EBERs and the two adenovirus-associated RNAs, VAI and VAII, and between the regions of the two viral genomes that specify these small RNAs (Arrand et al., 1989). The EBER genes are separated by 161 base pairs and are transcribed from the same DNA strand. Both EBER genes carry intragenic transcription control regions A and B boxes which can be transcribed by RNA polymerase III (pol III). However, both EBER1 and 2 contain upstream elements and TATA-like sequences typical of pol II promoters including Sp1 and ATF binding sites (Howe & Shu, 1989). Within 1 kilo base EBER region, 10 single base changes which group the strains into two families (1 and 2) have been identified. The EBER1 sequences are completely conserved, two base changes are within EBER2-coding sequence and eight are outside the coding regions (Arrand et al., 1989). EBV has been shown to induce the cellular transcription factors TFIIIB and TFIIIC (leading to induction of general pol III-mediated transcription) and the typical pol II transcription factor ATF-2, that enhance expression of EBER1 and EBER2 (Felton-Edkins et al., 2006), which may account for the low expression of transfected EBERs plasmids in EBV-negative cells (Komano et al., 1999). To elucidate transcription regulation of EBERs more exactly, Thomas J Owen discovered that transient expression of EBNA1 in Ad/AH cells stably expressing the EBERs led to induction of both EBER1 and EBER2 through transcription factors used by EBER genes, including TFIIIC, ATF-2 and c-Myc (Owen et al., 2010). To shed more light on the transcription of EBERs, Hans Helmut Niller analyzed protein binding at the EBER locus of EBV by genomic footprinting electrophoretic mobility shift, reporter gene assay, and chromatin immunoprecipitation in a panel of six B-cell lines. With these methods, 130 base pairs upstream of the EBER1 gene, contains two E-boxes providing a consensus sequence for binding of the transcription factor and oncoprotein c-Myc to the EBV genome. Translocated and deregulated c-myc directly activates and maintains the antiapoptotic functions of the EBER locus in a single EBV-infected B cell which is undergoing the germinal center (GC) reaction. This single translocated and surviving cell is the founder cell of an endemic BL, which accounts for the oncogenic role of EBV in lymphoma (Niller et al., 2003). What's more, Ferenc Banati found that in vitro methylation blocked binding of the cellular proteins c-Myc and ATF to the 50-region of the EBER-1 gene, which indicated a complicated transcription regulation of EBERs (Banati et al., 2008). With the special transcription elements of EBERs, Choy had devised shRNA plasmid to silence gene expression, which achieves better effect in some cases (Choy et al., 2008).

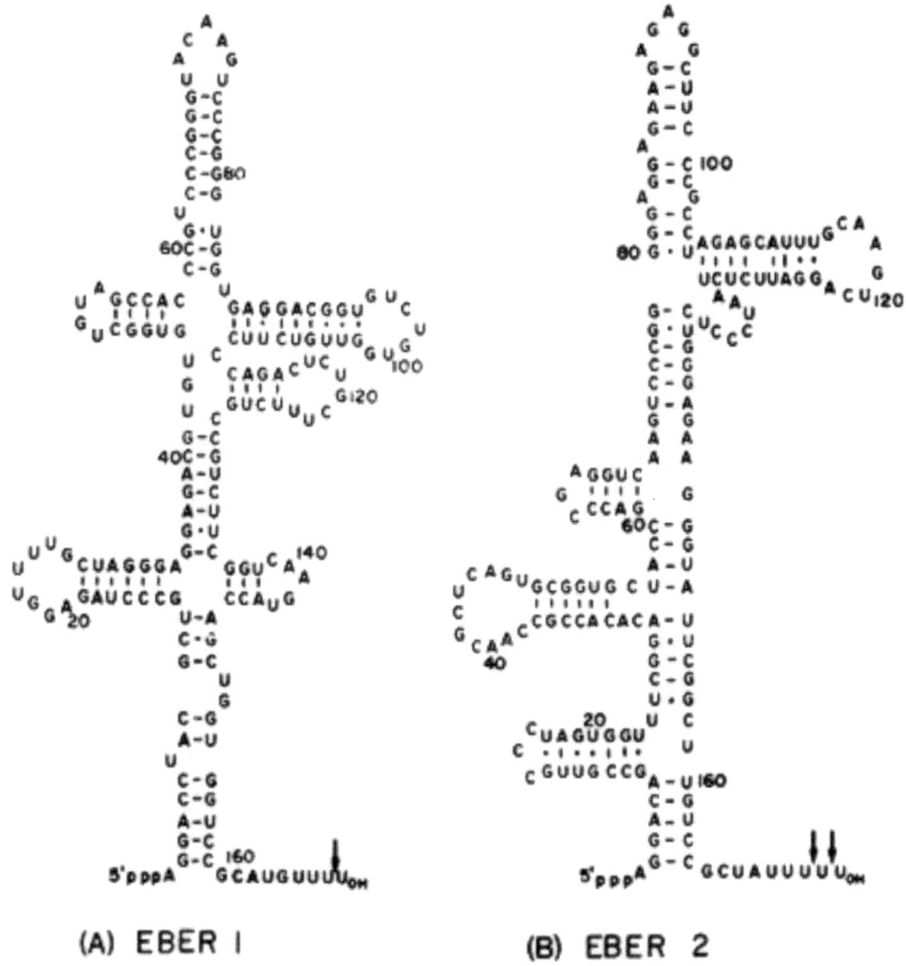

Fig. 1. Potential secondary structures of EBERs. The arrows indicate alternate 3' termini. (A) EBER 1; (B) EBER 2. Adapted from Rosa *et al.* (1981)

EBER in situ hybridization is considered the gold standard for detecting and localizing latent EBV in tissue samples (Ambinder & Mann, 1994). After all, EBER transcripts are consistently expressed in virtually all the EBV positive tumors, and they are likewise expressed in lymphoid tissues taken from patients with infectious mononucleosis, and in the rare infected cell representing normal flora in healthy virus carriers. The only EBV-related lesion that lacks EBERs is oral hairy leukoplakia, a purely lytic infection of oral epithelial cells. (Gilligan et al., 1990). Recently, researchers have discovered that EBERs could be used as a sensitive marker to monitor NPC cells at various metastatic sites by techniques of in situ hybridization. In cases of metastatic cancer of unknown origin, it is thus reasonable to consider NPC if EBV is present in the tumor cells (Chao et al., 1996). Kimura has established a novel flow cytometric in situ hybridization assay to detect EBV+ suspension cells using a peptide nucleic acid probe specific for EBERs. With this method, they can not only decide the EBV load but also locate EBV-infected cells, which will be beneficial for diagnosis of Epstein-Barr virus (EBV)–associated diseases and exploration of the pathogenesis of EBV infection (Kimura et al., 2009).

3. Localization and potential function of EBERs involved RNP complexes

EBERs are believed to be confined in the nucleus by ISH according to several early publications (Barletta et al., 1993; Chang et al., 1992; Howe & Steitz, 1986). In contrast, Schwemmle *et al.* traced EBERs localization in interphase and mitotic phase and they discovered both RNAs were found in the cytoplasm as well as in the nuclei of interphase cells. The cytoplasm distribution of the EBERs was similar to that of the double-stranded RNA-dependent protein kinase, to which these RNAs could bind, and the location was coincident with the rough endoplasmic reticulum. Thus a cytoplasmic location for EBER-1 and EBER-2 in interphase cells is consistent with the evidence for a role for these small RNAs in translational control (Schwemmle et al., 1992). Despite this sole publication in accord with the potential function of EBERs involved RNP complexes, a recent report (Fok et al., 2006) indicated that EBERs are confined to the nucleus. They carried out heterokaryon assays and oocyte assays, the outcomes of which indicated EBERs did not shutter out of the nucleus under any circumstances and speculated that the report of cytoplasmic localization of EBERs (Schwemmle et al., 1992) was probably due to the complement between the probe and regions including conserved polymerase III promoter elements A and B. EBER1 was shown to have a half-life of 25-30 hours, and was more stable than RNAs that did undergo shuttling, indicating that rapid cytoplasmic degradation was not responsible for the inability to detect shuttling.

While the accurate localization of EBERs is still controversial, the scenario of the function of EBERs involved RNP complexes is perhaps more complicated. EBERs, which resemble another virus encoded RNA VA RNAs (adenovirus virus-associated RNAs) , were firstly found to be complexed with La. Although there is no striking nucleotide sequence homology between EBERs and VAs, similarities exist in their size, degree of secondary structure, and genomic organization (Bhat & Thimmappaya, 1983). The many shared features of the two RNA molecules enumerated above and the fact that they bind a common antigenic host protein supports the supposition that these RNPs play similar roles in virus-infected cells. A specific role in the splicing of adenovirus messenger RNAs has been proposed for the VA RNAs (Murray & Holliday, 1979). The demonstration of a direct physical association between the VA RNAs and certain adenovirus late messenger RNAs supports this proposal (Mathews, 1980). Thus, EBERs could well perform comparable functions in splicing of EBV messenger RNAs. Furthermore, VA RNAs play an important role in adenovirus replication by rescuing cells from inhibition of protein translation mediated by the cellular kinase PKR, which is induced by interferon and activated by double-stranded RNAs produced during replication of many viruses (Ghadge et al., 1994;

Hovanessian, 1989). Considering the resemblance, Bhat and Thimmappaya successfully proved that EBERs can functionally substitute for the VA RNAs in the lytic growth of Ad5 (Bhat & Thimmappaya, 1983, 1985). What's more, EBERs could directly bind PKR and inhibit its activity, then block phosphorylation of eIF2a, thus resulting in the blockage of inhibition of protein synthesis by eIF2a (Clarke et al., 1991; Sharp et al., 1993). When added to reticulocyte lysates at high concentrations, EBER-1 could prevent inhibition of translation by double-stranded RNA (Clarke et al., 1990). However, EBER-1 enhanced overall protein synthesis in the absence of PKR expression (Laing et al., 2002; Laing et al., 1995). In support of EBERs function regardless of PKR, EBER-deleted recombinant EBV transformed primary B lymphocytes into LCLs, which were indistinguishable from LCLs transformed by wildtype EBV in their proliferation, in latency-associated EBV gene expression, and in their permissiveness for EBV replication cycle gene expression (Swaminathan et al., 1991). Especially, another publication indicated EBERs could support replication of the defective adenovirus in vivo but PKR phosphorylation status wasn't influenced (Wang et al., 2005). This difference is likely a result of distinct subcellular compartmentalization of these two molecules, with the EBERs being exclusively nuclear, while PKR is predominately found in the cytoplasm.

Furthermore, it was speculated EBERs could partly restores resistance to both spontaneous and interferon-induced apoptosis (Komano et al., 1999) and PKR probably act as the mediator of the EBER protective effect against apoptosis despite controversial observation provided by Ruf et al. (Ruf et al., 2000). According to Komano et al., Transfection of the EBER genes into EBV-negative Akata clones restored the capacity for growth in soft agar, tumorigenicity in SCID mice, resistance to apoptotic inducers, and upregulated expression of bcl-2 oncoprotein that were originally retained in parental EBV-positive Akata cells and lost in EBV-negative subclones. To support this hypothesis, researchers have made it clear that when EBV-negative Akata cells transfected with EBERs were analysed, PKR autophosphorylation *in vitro* was inhibited (Nanbo et al., 2002). However, Ruf reported that EBERs did posses a modest ability to protect the cell against interferon-induced apoptosis, but this process was independent of PKR-eIF-2α activation (Ruf et al., 2005). Thus Swaminathan suggested that EBERs might inhibit apoptosis while it was unlikely that inhibition of PKR was the primary mechanism for this effect (Swaminathan, 2010).

EBER-1 also interacts with the ribosomal protein L22, a componenet of the 60S eukaryotic ribosomal subunit unique to eukaryotes (Dobbelstein & Shenk, 1995; Toczyski et al., 1994; Toczyski & Steitz, 1991, 1993). In EBV-infected BL cells, roughly 50% of the cellular pool of L22 is found in association with EBER-1 ribonucleoprotein (RNP) particles, and a substantial fraction of L22 is physically relocalized from nucleoli to the nucleoplasm. Using the recombinant viruses and novel EBER expression vectors, the nuclear redistribution of rpL22 protein by EBER1 in 293 cells was confirmed (Gregorovic et al., 2011). Binding to 28S rRNA likely serves to target L22 to nucleoli, while binding to EBER-1 RNA likely results in sequestration or retention of L22 in the nucleoplasm. In truth, BL cells expressing mutated EBER-1 RNAs incapable of binding to and relocalizing L22 have significantly reduced capacity to enhance cell growth potential relative to BL cells expressing wild-type EBERs (Houmani et al., 2009), which indicated that the EBER1-L22 complex may be beneficial for lymphoma growth.

Intriguingly, to date there has been no investigation with respect to the function of EBERs involved RNP complexes in NPC and whether the same machinery in lymphomas readily applies to NPC remains to be seen.

4. EBERs associated oncogenesis and cell transformation

Comparison of EBV-positive and -negative cell clones revealed that the presence of EBV in Akata cells was required for the cells to be more malignant and apoptosis resistant, which underlined the oncogenic role of EBV in the genesis of BL (Komano et al., 1998; Ruf et al., 1999). Subsequent studies revealed that EBERs were responsible for these phenotypes (Komano et al., 1999; Ruf et al., 2005). Transfection of the EBER genes into EBV-negative Akata clones restored the capacity for growth in soft agar, tumorigenicity in SCID mice, resistance to apoptotic inducers, and upregulated expression of bcl-2 that was originally retained in parental EBV-positive Akata cells but lost in EBV-negative subclones. More recently, a new investigation indicated that in vivo expression of a polymerase III driven non-coding viral EBER-1 construct led to the transgenic mouse more inclined to develop tumor. In Repellin's reports, they provided the first evidence by producing ten transgenic mouse lines expressing EBER1 in the lymphoid compartment, and discovered the transgenic mice developed lymphoid hyperplasia, which in some cases proceeded to B cell malignancy (Repellin et al., 2010).

Because EBERs are expressed in large amounts in latently infected cells and virtually all EBV-associated tumors, it had long been speculated that they may play a vital role in the process of transformation. To support this hypothesis, EBER-negative recombinants generated by Yajima in 2005 provided a quantitative advantage in transformation ability. Transformation assays performed with high titres of recombinant EBV generated from the EBER knockout and knock-in strains revealed that the EBER knock-in recombinant possessed approximately 20-fold more transforming ability than the EBER-negative recombinant. Furthermore, growth of the EBER-negative LCLs was impaired compared with that of the revertants under low serum conditions. In contrast, Swaminathan *et al* demonstrated that EBERs were not essential for the immotalization of B lymphocytes or for the replication of the virus. In their experiments, strains of EBV with deletions of the small RNA (EBER) genes were made by homologous recombination using the EBV P3HR-1 strain, which has undergone deletion of the essential transforming gene that encoded the EBV nuclear antigen, EBNA-2, and a DNA fragment that was wild type at the EBNA-2 locus but from which the EBER genes had been deleted. EBER-deleted recombinants transformed primary B lymphocytes into LCLs, which were indistinguishable from LCLs transformed by wildtype EBV. However, they were not able to produce a large quantity of pure EBER-deleted EBV, which may lead to the false negative outcome. To address this issue more specifically, Wu *et al.* (Wu et al., 2007) demonstrated that the transforming ability of recombinant EBVs expressing EBER2 was as high as that of EBVs expressing both EBER1 and EBER2. In contrast, the transforming ability of recombinant EBVs carrying EBER1 was impaired and was similar to that of EBV lacking both EBER1 and EBER2. Gregorovic *et al.* (Gregorovic et al., 2011)recently reported there was little effect of either EBER deletion on the transformation efficiency. This contrasts with the results of a previous study (Wu et al., 2007) where deletion of EBER2 caused a 50-fold reduction of transformation efficiency. It should be noted that a different EBV strain background was used in the two experiments.

With respect to the role of EBER in the carcinogenesis of NPC, it was reported that EBERs expression may confer an apoptotic-resistant phenotype in immortalized nasopharyngeal epithelial cells. The EBER-expressing NP69 cells attained a higher growth rate compared to cells transfected with control plasmid (pcDNA3). However, the EBER-expressing NP69 cells did not form colonies in soft agar and were non-tumorigenic in nude mice (Wong et al., 2005). Iwakiri, however, reported that EBV infection induces IGF-1 expression in NPC cell lines, and that the secreted IGF-1 acts as an autocrine growth factor. These findings seem to be operative in vivo, as NPC biopsies consistently express IGF-1 (Iwakiri et al., 2005). Recently, in contrast, there are somewhat contradictive observations from Tomokazu. In their experimets, MDCK cells transfected with EBERs-high-expression vector showed an enhanced growth ability in soft agar compared with the MDCK transfected with EBERs-low-expression vector-transfected or untransfected MDCK cells. However, they did not show the acquisition of any anti-apoptotic potential against either IFN-α or serum deprivation. Introduction of EBERs-low-expression vector into MDCK cells did not show anchor independent growth characteristics (Yoshizaki et al., 2007). The reasons for these contrary outcomes are not clear and whether EBERs could transform cells or even be tumorigenic are still obscure. It may be attributable to the origin of the cell line. For instance, NPC-KT, the parental cell line of EBV-neg-KT, was derived from NPC, whereas MDCK is derived from normal epitheliumand (Yoshizaki et al., 2007).

It has long been believed that both EBER1 and EBER2 play similar roles in the pathologic process. Microarray expression profiling, however, identified genes whose expression correlates with the presence of EBER1 or EBER2 (Gregorovic et al., 2011). To researchers' surprise, although most emphasis has previously been given to EBER1 because it is more abundant than EBER2, the differences in cellular gene expression were greater with EBER2 deletion. The number of genes and degree to which the regulated genes were unique to EBER1 or EBER2 was further analyzed, showing that the greater number of differences in cell gene expression was observed in EBER2 deletion. To look more specifically at some of the cellular genes whose expression correlated with EBER2 expression, the expression values from individual cell lines were derived. In each case, the expression level in parental and revertant was similar, but the expression in the EBER2 deletion was consistently different. Some additional data from an earlier comparison of del-EBER2 and parental LCLs were consistent. LCL gene expression was modified according to the presence of EBER2. The examples include genes involved in receptor function and signaling (CNKRS3, CXCL12, CXCR3, DACT1, GDF15, GPR125, IGF1, and IL12RB2A), cellular adhesion (IGSF4), a transcription factor (TBX15), an RNA binding protein (MEX3A), and a proposed tumor suppressor gene (SASH1). This comprehensive description of EBER2 related genes indicates many facets of biological process related to EBER2. Especially there seems to be a link between EBER2 and lymphoma invasion and metastasis. Hopefully this microarray analysis may lead to new insight into the EBERs' research in EBV related carcinomas.

5. EBERs participate in cytokine secretion pathway through TLR3 and RIG-I

Expression of a variety of cytokines and growth factors is enhanced in several types of EBERs-expressing cells. It was demonstrated that IL-10 induced by EBERs acts as an autocrine growth factor for BL (Kitagawa et al., 2000). It was found that EBV-positive Akata and Mutu cell clones expressed higher levels of interleukin (IL)-10 than their EBV-negative subclones at the transcription level. Transfection of an individual EBV latent gene into EBV-negative Akata cells revealed that EBERs were responsible for IL-10 induction. Recombinanat IL-10 enabled EBV-negative Akata cells to grow in low (0.1%) serum conditions. Likewise, Iwakiri *et al.* reported infection of EBV-negative gastric carcinoma cell lines with EBV led to expression of a limited number of EBV genes including EBERs and was correlated with increased IGF-1 production, as was transfection of EBERs genes (Iwakiri et al., 2003). Using the recombinant virus, Yang *et al.* (Yang et al., 2004) found that a human T-cell line, MT-2, was susceptible to EBV infection, and succeeded in isolating EBV-infected cell clones with type II EBV latency, which was identical with those seen in EBV-infected T cells in vivo. EBV-positive MT-2 cells expressed higher levels of interleukin (IL)-9 than EBV-negative MT-2 cells at the transcriptional level. It was also demonstrated that EBV-encoded small RNA was responsible for IL-9 expression. Addition of recombinant IL-9 accelerated the growth of MT-2 cells, whereas growth of the EBV-converted MT-2 cells was blocked by treatment with an anti-IL-9 antibody. These results suggest that IL-9 induced by EBV-encoded small RNA acts as an autocrine growth factor for EBV-infected T cells.

Since EBERs are expected to form dsRNA structure, it's believed they activate RIG (Yoneyama et al., 2004), a specific pattern-recognition receptors (PRR) that specifically recognize pathogen-associated molecular patterns (PAMPs) within microbes and induce interferon induction. Recently this hypothesis was experimentally tested by Samanta *et al* (Samanta et al., 2006). According to their observation, transfection of RIG-I plasmid induced IFNs and IFN-stimulated genes (ISGs) in EBV-positive Burkitt's lymphoma (BL) cells, but not in their EBV-negative counterparts or EBER-knockout EBV-infected BL cells. Transfection of EBER plasmid or in vitro synthesized EBERs induced expression of type I IFNs and ISGs in RIG-I-expressing, EBV-negative BL cells, but not in RIG-I-minus counterparts. (Samanta et al., 2006). EBERs are recognized by RIG-I through the RNA helicase domain, and following recognition, RIG-I associates with the adaptor IPS-1 via CARD. IPS-1 is localized to mitochondria and initiates signaling leading to activation of IRF3 and NF-κB to induce type-I IFNs and inflammatory cytokines. Furthermore, they indicated that EBERs induce an anti-inflammatory cytokine IL-10 through RIG-I-mediated IRF-3 but not NF-κB signaling (FIG. 2) (Samanta et al., 2008).

Toll-like receptors (TLRs) constitute distinct families of PRRs that sense nucleic acids derived from viruses and trigger antiviral innate immune responses through activation of signaling cascades via Toll/IL-1 receptor (TIR) domain-containing adaptors (Akira & Takeda, 2004). Iwakiri et al. (Iwakiri et al., 2009) reported that EBERs were released extracellulary and recognized by TLR3, leading to induction of type-I IFN and inflammatory cytokines. A substantial amount of EBER, which was sufficient to induce TLR3 signaling involving IRF3 and NF-B activation, was released from EBV-infected cells. Thus, EBERs can contribute to the pathogenesis of EBV infection through interaction with RIG-I and TLR3.

TLRs and RIG-I as PRRs could trigger the innate immune response, as first line of defense against pathogens and tissue injury. This response i.e. inflammation, is a complex response to infection, trauma, and other conditions of homeostatic imbalance (Nathan, 2002). An acute inflammatory response is usually beneficial, especially in response to microbial

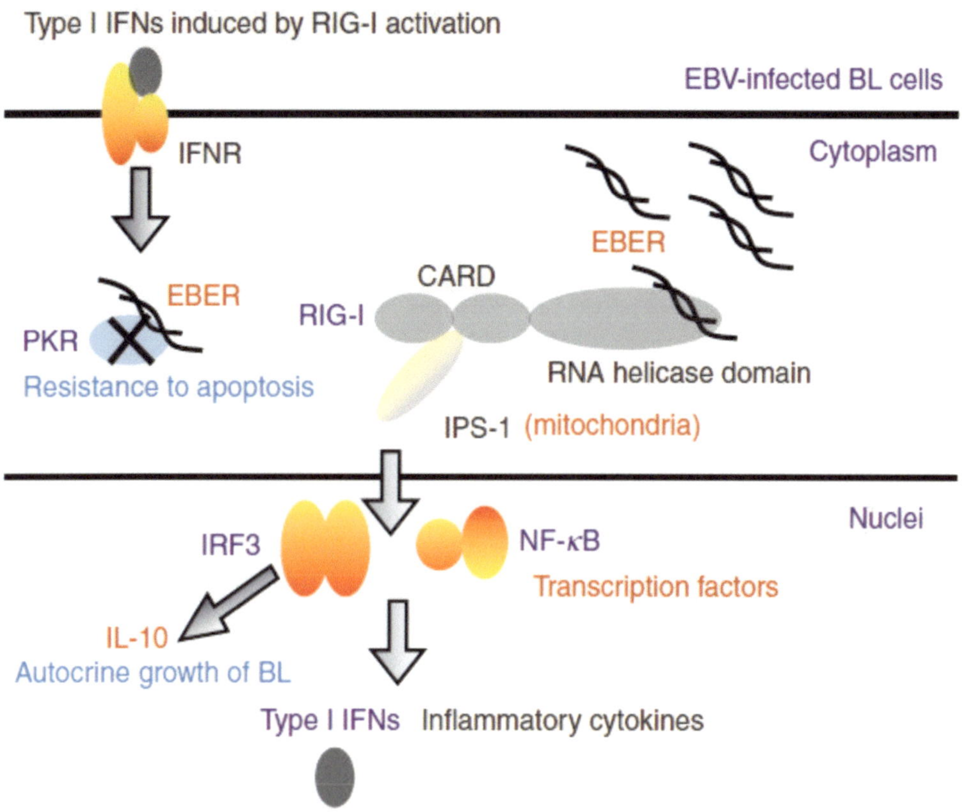

Fig. 2. Modulation of RIG-I signaling by EBERs contributes to EBV-mediated oncogenesis in BL cells. What's more, EBERs bind PKR and inhibit its phosphorylation, which disturb PKR mediated apoptosis. Adapted from Iwakiri & Takada, 2010.

infections and tissue damage. A well-regulated inflammatory response can also be anti-tumorigenic and have a role in tumorsuppression (Mantovani et al., 2008). Chronic inflammation, however, is detrimental and, among other deleterious effects, will frequently predispose cells for an oncogenic transformation. Various mechanisms account for the oncogenic role of chronic inflammation. These include induction of genomic instability, increasing angiogenesis, altering the genomic epigenetic state and increasing cell proliferation. Over-production of reactive oxygen and nitrogen species (RONS), aberrant inflammatory cytokine and chemokine expression, increased (COX-2) and NFκB expression are just some of the molecular factors that contribute to inflammation-induced carcinogenesis (Schetter et al., 2010). Considering the emerging link between EBERs and TLR and RIG-I in lymphoma and the involvement of PRR in the subsequent inflammation associated cancer, it was intriguing to investigate this potential interaction in other carcinoma. For instance, we demonstrated that EBERs' expression could instantly trigger acute accumulation of inflammation cytokines and this response was impaired in EBERs knock-down NPC cell lines (unpublished data). Furthermore, EBERs induced this inflammation response through TLR3 and RIG-I signaling, as was the scenario in lymphoma. To dissect the exact role of the EBER induced signaling pathway, we have established a positive feedback loop between NF-κB and the EBV encoded oncogenic protein LMP1, which constitute the cascade downstream of EBERs activated NF-κB (Fig. 3).

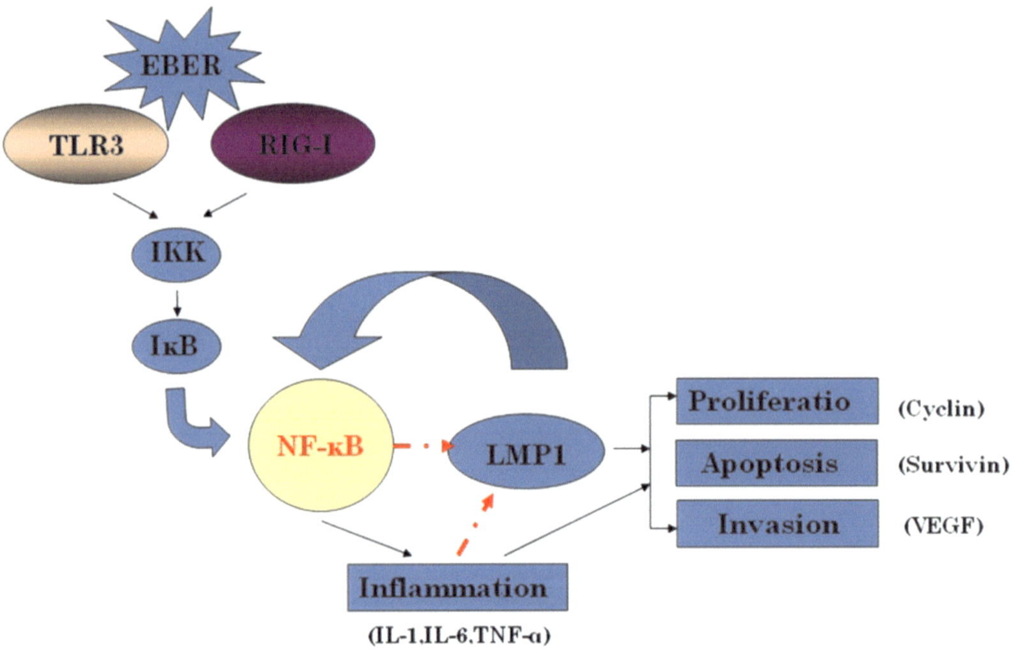

Fig. 3. EBERs induced inflammation response in NPC is intensified by the feedback loop composed of NF-κB and LMP1. Dotted line represents tentative transcription activation. Refer to main text for details.

In light of this model, When nasopharyngeal epithelial cells were infected by EBV, EBERs could initiate NF-κB induced pro-inflammatory cytokines production through PRRs TLR3 and RIG-I. Thus cellular physiological status is shifted in several avenues such as proliferation and apoptosis due to the pro-inflammatory cytokines. Meanwhile, NF-κB could induce oncogenic protein LMP1 transcription, which in turn trigger the NF-κB pathway thus intensify the pro-inflammatory cytokines production. Cooperation between this pro-inflammatory cytokine production and LMP-1 probably potentiate risk of developing NPC.

6. References

Akira, S. & Takeda, K. (2004). Toll-like receptor signalling. *Nat Rev Immunol*, Vol. 4, No. 7, pp. 499-511

Ambinder, R. F. & Mann, R. B. (1994). Epstein-Barr-encoded RNA in situ hybridization: diagnostic applications. *Hum Pathol*, Vol. 25, No. 6, pp. 602-605

Arrand, J. R. & Rymo, L. (1982). Characterization of the major Epstein-Barr virus-specific RNA in Burkitt lymphoma-derived cells. *J Virol*, Vol. 41, No. 2, pp. 376-389

Arrand, J. R., Young, L. S. & Tugwood, J. D. (1989). Two families of sequences in the small RNA-encoding region of Epstein-Barr virus (EBV) correlate with EBV types A and B. *J Virol*, Vol. 63, No. 2, pp. 983-986

Banati, F., Koroknai, A., Salamon, D., Takacs, M., Minarovits-Kormuta, S., Wolf, H., Niller, H. H. & Minarovits, J. (2008). CpG-methylation silences the activity of the RNA polymerase III transcribed EBER-1 promoter of Epstein-Barr virus. *FEBS Lett*, Vol. 582, No. 5, pp. 705-709

Barletta, J. M., Kingma, D. W., Ling, Y., Charache, P., Mann, R. B. & Ambinder, R. F. (1993). Rapid in situ hybridization for the diagnosis of latent Epstein-Barr virus infection. *Mol Cell Probes*, Vol. 7, No. 2, pp. 105-109

Bhat, R. A. & Thimmappaya, B. (1983). Two small RNAs encoded by Epstein-Barr virus can functionally substitute for the virus-associated RNAs in the lytic growth of adenovirus 5. *Proc Natl Acad Sci U S A*, Vol. 80, No. 15, pp. 4789-4793

Bhat, R. A. & Thimmappaya, B. (1985). Construction and analysis of additional adenovirus substitution mutants confirm the complementation of VAI RNA function by two small RNAs encoded by Epstein-Barr virus. *J Virol*, Vol. 56, No. 3, pp. 750-756

Chang, K. L., Chen, Y. Y., Shibata, D. & Weiss, L. M. (1992). Description of an in situ hybridization methodology for detection of Epstein-Barr virus RNA in paraffin-embedded tissues, with a survey of normal and neoplastic tissues. *Diagn Mol Pathol*, Vol. 1, No. 4, pp. 246-255

Chao, T. Y., Chow, K. C., Chang, J. Y., Wang, C. C., Tsao, T. Y., Harn, H. J. & Chi, K. H. (1996). Expression of Epstein-Barr virus-encoded RNAs as a marker for metastatic undifferentiated nasopharyngeal carcinoma. *Cancer*, Vol. 78, No. 1, pp. 24-29

Choy, E. Y., Kok, K. H., Tsao, S. W. & Jin, D. Y. (2008). Utility of Epstein-Barr virus-encoded small RNA promoters for driving the expression of fusion transcripts harboring short hairpin RNAs. *Gene Ther*, Vol. 15, No. 3, pp. 191-202

Clarke, P. A., Schwemmle, M., Schickinger, J., Hilse, K. & Clemens, M. J. (1991). Binding of Epstein-Barr virus small RNA EBER-1 to the double-stranded RNA-activated protein kinase DAI. *Nucleic Acids Res*, Vol. 19, No. 2, pp. 243-248

Clarke, P. A., Sharp, N. A. & Clemens, M. J. (1990). Translational control by the Epstein-Barr virus small RNA EBER-1. Reversal of the double-stranded RNA-induced inhibition of protein synthesis in reticulocyte lysates. *Eur J Biochem*, Vol. 193, No. 3, pp. 635-641

Dobbelstein, M. & Shenk, T. (1995). In vitro selection of RNA ligands for the ribosomal L22 protein associated with Epstein-Barr virus-expressed RNA by using randomized and cDNA-derived RNA libraries. *J Virol*, Vol. 69, No. 12, pp. 8027-8034

Felton-Edkins, Z. A., Kondrashov, A., Karali, D., Fairley, J. A., Dawson, C. W., Arrand, J. R., Young, L. S. & White, R. J. (2006). Epstein-Barr virus induces cellular transcription factors to allow active expression of EBER genes by RNA polymerase III. *J Biol Chem*, Vol. 281, No. 45, pp. 33871-33880

Fok, V., Friend, K. & Steitz, J. A. (2006). Epstein-Barr virus noncoding RNAs are confined to the nucleus, whereas their partner, the human La protein, undergoes nucleocytoplasmic shuttling. *J Cell Biol*, Vol. 173, No. 3, pp. 319-325

Ghadge, G. D., Malhotra, P., Furtado, M. R., Dhar, R. & Thimmapaya, B. (1994). In vitro analysis of virus-associated RNA I (VAI RNA): inhibition of the double-stranded RNA-activated protein kinase PKR by VAI RNA mutants correlates with the in vivo phenotype and the structural integrity of the central domain. *J Virol*, Vol. 68, No. 7, pp. 4137-4151

Gilligan, K., Rajadurai, P., Resnick, L. & Raab-Traub, N. (1990). Epstein-Barr virus small nuclear RNAs are not expressed in permissively infected cells in AIDS-associated leukoplakia. *Proc Natl Acad Sci U S A*, Vol. 87, No. 22, pp. 8790-8794

Gregorovic, G., Bosshard, R., Karstegl, C. E., White, R. E., Pattle, S., Chiang, A. K., Dittrich-Breiholz, O., Kracht, M., Russ, R. & Farrell, P. J. (2011). Cellular gene expression that correlates with EBER expression in Epstein-Barr Virus-infected lymphoblastoid cell lines. *J Virol*, Vol. 85, No. 7, pp. 3535-3545

Houmani, J. L., Davis, C. I. & Ruf, I. K. (2009). Growth-promoting properties of Epstein-Barr virus EBER-1 RNA correlate with ribosomal protein L22 binding. *J Virol*, Vol. 83, No. 19, pp. 9844-9853

Hovanessian, A. G. (1989). The double stranded RNA-activated protein kinase induced by interferon: dsRNA-PK. *J Interferon Res*, Vol. 9, No. 6, pp. 641-647

Howe, J. G. & Shu, M. D. (1989). Epstein-Barr virus small RNA (EBER) genes: unique transcription units that combine RNA polymerase II and III promoter elements. *Cell*, Vol. 57, No. 5, pp. 825-834

Howe, J. G. & Steitz, J. A. (1986). Localization of Epstein-Barr virus-encoded small RNAs by in situ hybridization. *Proc Natl Acad Sci U S A*, Vol. 83, No. 23, pp. 9006-9010

Iwakiri, D., Eizuru, Y., Tokunaga, M. & Takada, K. (2003). Autocrine growth of Epstein-Barr virus-positive gastric carcinoma cells mediated by an Epstein-Barr virus-encoded small RNA. *Cancer Res*, Vol. 63, No. 21, pp. 7062-7067

Iwakiri, D., Sheen, T. S., Chen, J. Y., Huang, D. P. & Takada, K. (2005). Epstein-Barr virus-encoded small RNA induces insulin-like growth factor 1 and supports growth of nasopharyngeal carcinoma-derived cell lines. *Oncogene*, Vol. 24, No. 10, pp. 1767-1773

Iwakiri, D. & Takada, K. (2010). Role of EBERs in the pathogenesis of EBV infection. *Adv Cancer Res*, Vol. 107, No. pp. 119-136

Iwakiri, D., Zhou, L., Samanta, M., Matsumoto, M., Ebihara, T., Seya, T., Imai, S., Fujieda, M., Kawa, K. & Takada, K. (2009). Epstein-Barr virus (EBV)-encoded small RNA is released from EBV-infected cells and activates signaling from Toll-like receptor 3. *J Exp Med*, Vol. 206, No. 10, pp. 2091-2099

Kimura, H., Miyake, K., Yamauchi, Y., Nishiyama, K., Iwata, S., Iwatsuki, K., Gotoh, K., Kojima, S., Ito, Y. & Nishiyama, Y. (2009). Identification of Epstein-Barr virus (EBV)-infected lymphocyte subtypes by flow cytometric in situ hybridization in EBV-associated lymphoproliferative diseases. *J Infect Dis*, Vol. 200, No. 7, pp. 1078-1087

Kitagawa, N., Goto, M., Kurozumi, K., Maruo, S., Fukayama, M., Naoe, T., Yasukawa, M., Hino, K., Suzuki, T., Todo, S. & Takada, K. (2000). Epstein-Barr virus-encoded poly(A)(-) RNA supports Burkitt's lymphoma growth through interleukin-10 induction. *Embo J*, Vol. 19, No. 24, pp. 6742-6750

Komano, J., Maruo, S., Kurozumi, K., Oda, T. & Takada, K. (1999). Oncogenic role of Epstein-Barr virus-encoded RNAs in Burkitt's lymphoma cell line Akata. *J Virol*, Vol. 73, No. 12, pp. 9827-9831

Komano, J., Sugiura, M. & Takada, K. (1998). Epstein-Barr virus contributes to the malignant phenotype and to apoptosis resistance in Burkitt's lymphoma cell line Akata. *J Virol*, Vol. 72, No. 11, pp. 9150-9156

Laing, K. G., Elia, A., Jeffrey, I., Matys, V., Tilleray, V. J., Souberbielle, B. & Clemens, M. J. (2002). In vivo effects of the Epstein-Barr virus small RNA EBER-1 on protein synthesis and cell growth regulation. *Virology*, Vol. 297, No. 2, pp. 253-269

Laing, K. G., Matys, V. & Clemens, M. J. (1995). Effects of expression of the Epstein-Barr virus small RNA EBER-1 in heterologous cells on protein synthesis and cell growth. *Biochem Soc Trans*, Vol. 23, No. 2, pp. 311S

Lerner, M. R., Andrews, N. C., Miller, G. & Steitz, J. A. (1981). Two small RNAs encoded by Epstein-Barr virus and complexed with protein are precipitated by antibodies from patients with systemic lupus erythematosus. *Proc Natl Acad Sci U S A*, Vol. 78, No. 2, pp. 805-809

Mantovani, A., Romero, P., Palucka, A. K. & Marincola, F. M. (2008). Tumour immunity: effector response to tumour and role of the microenvironment. *Lancet*, Vol. 371, No. 9614, pp. 771-783

Mathews, M. B. (1980). Binding of adenovirus VA RNA to mRNA: a possible role in splicing? *Nature*, Vol. 285, No. 5766, pp. 575-577

Murray, V. & Holliday, R. (1979). Mechanism for RNA splicing of gene transcripts. *FEBS Lett*, Vol. 106, No. 1, pp. 5-7

Nanbo, A., Inoue, K., Adachi-Takasawa, K. & Takada, K. (2002). Epstein-Barr virus RNA confers resistance to interferon-alpha-induced apoptosis in Burkitt's lymphoma. *Embo J*, Vol. 21, No. 5, pp. 954-965

Nathan, C. (2002). Points of control in inflammation. *Nature*, Vol. 420, No. 6917, pp. 846-852

Niller, H. H., Salamon, D., Ilg, K., Koroknai, A., Banati, F., Bauml, G., Rucker, O., Schwarzmann, F., Wolf, H. & Minarovits, J. (2003). The in vivo binding site for oncoprotein c-Myc in the promoter for Epstein-Barr virus (EBV) encoding RNA (EBER) 1 suggests a specific role for EBV in lymphomagenesis. *Med Sci Monit*, Vol. 9, No. 1, pp. 1-9

Orellana, T. & Kieff, E. (1977). Epstein-barr virus-specific RNA. II. Analysis of polyadenylated viral RNA in restringent, abortive, and prooductive infections. *J Virol*, Vol. 22, No. 2, pp. 321-330

Owen, T. J., O'Neil, J. D., Dawson, C. W., Hu, C., Chen, X., Yao, Y., Wood, V. H., Mitchell, L. E., White, R. J., Young, L. S. & Arrand, J. R. (2010). Epstein-Barr virus-encoded EBNA1 enhances RNA polymerase III-dependent EBER expression through induction of EBER-associated cellular transcription factors. *Mol Cancer*, Vol. 9, No. pp. 241

Pathmanathan, R., Prasad, U., Chandrika, G., Sadler, R., Flynn, K. & Raab-Traub, N. (1995). Undifferentiated, nonkeratinizing, and squamous cell carcinoma of the nasopharynx. Variants of Epstein-Barr virus-infected neoplasia. *Am J Pathol*, Vol. 146, No. 6, pp. 1355-1367

Powell, A. L., King, W. & Kieff, E. (1979). Epstein-Barr virus-specific RNA. III. Mapping of DNA encoding viral RNA in restringent infection. *J Virol*, Vol. 29, No. 1, pp. 261-274

Repellin, C. E., Tsimbouri, P. M., Philbey, A. W. & Wilson, J. B. (2010). Lymphoid hyperplasia and lymphoma in transgenic mice expressing the small non-coding RNA, EBER1 of Epstein-Barr virus. *PLoS One*, Vol. 5, No. 2, pp. e9092

Rosa, M. D., Gottlieb, E., Lerner, M. R. & Steitz, J. A. (1981). Striking similarities are exhibited by two small Epstein-Barr virus-encoded ribonucleic acids and the adenovirus-associated ribonucleic acids VAI and VAII. *Mol Cell Biol*, Vol. 1, No. 9, pp. 785-796

Ruf, I. K., Lackey, K. A., Warudkar, S. & Sample, J. T. (2005). Protection from interferon-induced apoptosis by Epstein-Barr virus small RNAs is not mediated by inhibition of PKR. *J Virol*, Vol. 79, No. 23, pp. 14562-14569

Ruf, I. K., Rhyne, P. W., Yang, C., Cleveland, J. L. & Sample, J. T. (2000). Epstein-Barr virus small RNAs potentiate tumorigenicity of Burkitt lymphoma cells independently of an effect on apoptosis. *J Virol*, Vol. 74, No. 21, pp. 10223-10228

Ruf, I. K., Rhyne, P. W., Yang, H., Borza, C. M., Hutt-Fletcher, L. M., Cleveland, J. L. & Sample, J. T. (1999). Epstein-barr virus regulates c-MYC, apoptosis, and tumorigenicity in Burkitt lymphoma. *Mol Cell Biol*, Vol. 19, No. 3, pp. 1651-1660

Rymo, L. (1979). Identification of transcribed regions of Epstein-Barr virus DNA in Burkitt lymphoma-derived cells. *J Virol*, Vol. 32, No. 1, pp. 8-18

Samanta, M., Iwakiri, D., Kanda, T., Imaizumi, T. & Takada, K. (2006). EB virus-encoded RNAs are recognized by RIG-I and activate signaling to induce type I IFN. *Embo J*, Vol. 25, No. 18, pp. 4207-4214

Samanta, M., Iwakiri, D. & Takada, K. (2008). Epstein-Barr virus-encoded small RNA induces IL-10 through RIG-I-mediated IRF-3 signaling. *Oncogene*, Vol. 27, No. 30, pp. 4150-4160

Schetter, A. J., Heegaard, N. H. & Harris, C. C. (2010). Inflammation and cancer: interweaving microRNA, free radical, cytokine and p53 pathways. *Carcinogenesis*, Vol. 31, No. 1, pp. 37-49

Schwemmle, M., Clemens, M. J., Hilse, K., Pfeifer, K., Troster, H., Muller, W. E. & Bachmann, M. (1992). Localization of Epstein-Barr virus-encoded RNAs EBER-1 and EBER-2 in interphase and mitotic Burkitt lymphoma cells. *Proc Natl Acad Sci U S A*, Vol. 89, No. 21, pp. 10292-10296

Sharp, T. V., Schwemmle, M., Jeffrey, I., Laing, K., Mellor, H., Proud, C. G., Hilse, K. & Clemens, M. J. (1993). Comparative analysis of the regulation of the interferon-inducible protein kinase PKR by Epstein-Barr virus RNAs EBER-1 and EBER-2 and adenovirus VAI RNA. *Nucleic Acids Res*, Vol. 21, No. 19, pp. 4483-4490

Swaminathan, S., Tomkinson, B. & Kieff, E. (1991). Recombinant Epstein-Barr virus with small RNA (EBER) genes deleted transforms lymphocytes and replicates in vitro. *Proc Natl Acad Sci U S A*, Vol. 88, No. 4, pp. 1546-1550

Swaminathan, S. (2010). The role of non-coding RNAs in EBV-induced cell growth and transformation, in: *Epstein-Barr Virus: Latency and Transformation*, Erle S. Robertson. 155-166. Caister Academic Press, ISBN 978-1-904455-62-2, Norfolk , UK.

Toczyski, D. P., Matera, A. G., Ward, D. C. & Steitz, J. A. (1994). The Epstein-Barr virus (EBV) small RNA EBER1 binds and relocalizes ribosomal protein L22 in EBV-infected human B lymphocytes. *Proc Natl Acad Sci U S A*, Vol. 91, No. 8, pp. 3463-3467

Toczyski, D. P. & Steitz, J. A. (1991). EAP, a highly conserved cellular protein associated with Epstein-Barr virus small RNAs (EBERs). *Embo J*, Vol. 10, No. 2, pp. 459-466

Toczyski, D. P. & Steitz, J. A. (1993). The cellular RNA-binding protein EAP recognizes a conserved stem-loop in the Epstein-Barr virus small RNA EBER 1. *Mol Cell Biol*, Vol. 13, No. 1, pp. 703-710

Wang, Y., Xue, S. A., Hallden, G., Francis, J., Yuan, M., Griffin, B. E. & Lemoine, N. R. (2005). Virus-associated RNA I-deleted adenovirus, a potential oncolytic agent targeting EBV-associated tumors. *Cancer Res*, Vol. 65, No. 4, pp. 1523-1531

Wong, H. L., Wang, X., Chang, R. C., Jin, D. Y., Feng, H., Wang, Q., Lo, K. W., Huang, D. P., Yuen, P. W., Takada, K., Wong, Y. C. & Tsao, S. W. (2005). Stable expression of EBERs in immortalized nasopharyngeal epithelial cells confers resistance to apoptotic stress. *Mol Carcinog*, Vol. 44, No. 2, pp. 92-101

Wu, Y., Maruo, S., Yajima, M., Kanda, T. & Takada, K. (2007). Epstein-Barr virus (EBV)-encoded RNA 2 (EBER2) but not EBER1 plays a critical role in EBV-induced B-cell growth transformation. *J Virol*, Vol. 81, No. 20, pp. 11236-11245

Yajima, M., Kanda, T. & Takada, K. (2005). Critical role of Epstein-Barr Virus (EBV)-encoded RNA in efficient EBV-induced B-lymphocyte growth transformation. *J Virol*, Vol. 79, No. 7, pp. 4298-4307

Yang, L., Aozasa, K., Oshimi, K. & Takada, K. (2004). Epstein-Barr virus (EBV)-encoded RNA promotes growth of EBV-infected T cells through interleukin-9 induction. *Cancer Res*, Vol. 64, No. 15, pp. 5332-5337

Yoneyama, M., Kikuchi, M., Natsukawa, T., Shinobu, N., Imaizumi, T., Miyagishi, M., Taira, K., Akira, S. & Fujita, T. (2004). The RNA helicase RIG-I has an essential function in double-stranded RNA-induced innate antiviral responses. *Nat Immunol*, Vol. 5, No. 7, pp. 730-737

Yoshizaki, T., Endo, K., Ren, Q., Wakisaka, N., Murono, S., Kondo, S., Sato, H. & Furukawa, M. (2007). Oncogenic role of Epstein-Barr virus-encoded small RNAs (EBERs) in nasopharyngeal carcinoma. *Auris Nasus Larynx*, Vol. 34, No. 1, pp. 73-78

3

Role of the Epstein-Barr Virus ZEBRA Protein and HPV in the Carcinogenesis of Nasopharyngeal Carcinoma

Moumad Khalid[1,4], Laantri Nadia[1], Attaleb Mohammed[2], Dardari R'kia[1], Benider Abdellatif[3], Benchakroun Nadia[3], Ennaji Mustapha[4] and Khyatti Meriem[1]

[1]*Laboratory of Oncovirology, Institut Pasteur du Maroc, Casablanca,*
[2]*Biology and Medical Research Unit, Centre National de l'Energie, des Sciences et Techniques Nucléaires (CNESTEN), Rabat,*
[3]*Service de Radiothérapie, Centre d'Oncologie IBN Rochd, Casablanca,*
[4]*Laboratoire de Biologie Moléculaire, Institut Pasteur du Maroc, Casablanca*
Morocco

1. Introduction

Approximately 15% of all cancers worldwide appear to be associated with viral infections, and several human DNA viruses are now accepted as causative factors of specific malignancies. Human papillomaviruses (HPVs) cause cervical and anogenital cancers (zur Hausen 1999) and is now associated with oral cancers (Gillison & Shah 2001), but, the natural history of oncogenic HPV infections in the oral cavity is poorly understood. Epstein-Barr virus (EBV) causes infectious mononucleosis and is closely associated with Burkitt's lymphoma, nasopharyngeal carcinoma (NPC), and Hodgkin's disease (Raab-Traub 1996).

NPC is a malignant tumour that originates within the post nasal space (Pathmanathan et al. 1995). The etiologic factors of endemic NPC include environmental risk factors, genetic susceptibility and viral infection (Yu 1991). Evidence of EBV DNA in almost all NPC cells that were studied supports the association of NPC with EBV, while, HPV has been detected in a variety of head and neck tumours including NPC. Current data suggest that approximately 15-20% of head and neck squamous cell carcinomas (HNSCC) are linked to HPV infection. To date, different degrees of associations between HPV and NPC have been described, yet no conclusive data have been obtained. Given the particular characteristics of NPC in the Moroccan population in terms of incidence, age distribution and the predominance of specific EBV strains, and HPV genotype we describe in this chapter the role of the Epstein-Barr virus ZEBRA protein and HPV in the carcinogenesis of NPC.

1.1 Nasopharyngeal carcinoma

NPC is a malignancy of the head and neck region that arises in the epithelium surface of the posterior nasopharynx, and shows a peculiar geographic and ethnic distribution. The highest incidence rates of NPC are found among the southern Chinese population and in isolated northern populations such as Eskimos and Greenlanders (30 to 80 cases per 100,000 per year) (Parkin & Muir 1992). Intermediate incidence (8 to 12 cases per 100,000 per year) was reported in the Mediterranean basin, especially among the Arabic populations of North Africa (7-10% of all cancers among men), where NPC is also the commonest tumour of the ear, nose and throat region (Benider et al. 1995). The aetiology of NPC seems to be multifactorial with evidence that genetic susceptibility, environmental factors and viral infection with EBV reactivation and HPV infection are involved together or separately, simultaneously or consecutively (Hildesheim & Levine 1993).

The increased risk of NPC in North African population was associated with the consumption of rancid butter and rancid sheep fat. In fact, higher level of N-nitrosamines in rancid fat has not been demonstrated, which suggests some other disease causing chemicals in this population. A possible compound is butyric acid, which is also named n-Butanoic Acid. The glyceride form of butyric acid makes up 3 to 4% of butter, and is released into free butyric acid by hydrolysis when it becomes rancid (Feng et al. 2007). Butyric acid is known to be able to activate EBV in the B-lymphoid cells into lyric cycle (Takimoto et al. 1984), and therefore, could be related to NPC. In addition, Marijuana smoking was associated significantly to high NPC risk independently of cigarette smoking which suggests dissimilar carcinogenic mechanisms between cannabis and tobacco.

Genetic traits play a significant role in the development of NPC. Specific human leukocyte antigen (HLA) haplotypes have been reported to be associated with high risk for NPC, namely HLA-B13 in Tunisians, HLA-A3, B5 and B15 in Algerians and HLA-B18 allele in Moroccans population. In contrast, HLA-Aw33, -B14 and A9 were associated to low risk of NPC in Tunisians, Algerians and Moroccans, respectively.

Retrospectives and prospectives epidemiologic studies have indicated that assocaition between EBV, an ubiquitous human herpesvirus, and the development of different malignancies, such as Burkitt's lymphoma, 40%-50% of Hodgkin's disease, B-cell lymphoma in immunocompromised individuals, and NPC (Rickinson 2002). Undifferentiated NPC is one of the most striking examples of human malignancies that have been found strongly associated with the EBV, and interest in HPV as a cofactor in NPC occurrences has emerged over the last few years (Punwaney et al. 1999).

2. EBV life cycle in brief

During primary infection, EBV initially undergoes a brief replication in the epithelial cells of the oropharynx and salivary glands (Young & Rickinson 2004). The virus subsequently infects trafficking B-cells where the virus establishes a lifelong persistence and proceeds periodic spontaneous reactivation, resulting in lytic replication, infectious virus production and transmission (Cohen 2000). Upon reactivation, EBV can productively infect oropharyngeal epithelium, leading to infectious virus production and transmission (Jenkins, Binne & Farrell 2000). In latent infection, EBV genomic DNA exists as an episome, replicating only once during S phase and partitioning accurately into daughter cells during the mitotic phase. In lytic state, the EBV genomic DNA is linear. The initiation of lytic replication process greatly depends on the expression of two EBV immediate-early (IE) genes, BZLF1 and BRLF1, whose protein products (Zta and Rta) function as transcriptional transactivators and induce the lytic cascade of viral gene expression (Flemington & Speck 1990). Interestingly, a variety of important proteins encoded by EBV show the homology of sequences and functions to diverse human cellular proteins. Furthermore, the EBV proteins can modulate the expressions of a large number of cellular proteins.

2.1 ZEBRA on the scene

In cancer cells, EBV is also present in a latent state. During latency, EBV is effectively hidden from the immune system but if viral replication is initiated and lytic replication ensues, the cells express EBV genes that are more readily recognized by the immune system. The lytic DNA replication of EBV requires many viral proteins, including ZEBRA, polymerase, polymerase processivity factor, single-stranded DNA binding protein, primase, helicase and primase-associated factor. Among them ZEBRA (also called BZLF1, EB1 and Zta) is a lytic switch transactivator for expression of many early lytic genes and plays a critical role in both viral gene transcription and viral replication (Fixman, Hayward & Hayward 1995). Of all the viral transactivators, ZEBRA is unique in initiation of the ordered cascade of EBV gene expression, resulting in the expression of an estimated over 100 viral replication associated genes including those encoding early antigens, viral capsid antigens and membrane antigens (Baer et al. 1984). Many target genes of ZEBRA, such as BZLF1, BRLF1 and BMLF1 encoding the transactivators, BHRF1 and BHLF1 encoding the viral homologues of Bcl-2 (Marshall et al. 1999), and BMRF1 encoding EBV DNA polymerase accessory protein (Zhang et al. 1997), have been identified in the EBV genome. Through binding to cis-acting AP-1 or ZEBRA responsive elements (ZREs) in lytic cycle promoters ZEBRA activates the transcription of the target genes (Lieberman et al. 1990). Recently, some cellular genes modulated by ZEBRA have also been revealed. The products of these cellular genes are fundamentally linked to the viral life cycle, virus-host interactions, hosT-cell environment, cell cycle progression and immunomodulation.

2.2 ZEBRA structure

ZEBRA or Zta is a member of the family of bZIP transcription factors (Sinclair 2003); it contains adjacent DNA contact (approximately amino acids 175 to 195) and multimerization domains (approximately amino acids 196 to 245) (figure 1) (Sinclair 2006) and can interact directly with specific DNA sequence elements, i.e., ZREs as a multimer . By analogy with other members of the bZIP family, the multimerization interface of ZEBRA has been predicted to fold through a coiled-coil structure (Sinclair & Farrell 1992). Biophysical evidence that this prediction holds true was recently provided (Hicks et al. 2001).

The DNA binding region and dimerization region partly conform to the well-characterized bZIP (basic/leucine zipper) domain that is found in a family of cellular transcription factors such as fos/jun, C/EBPa and GCN4. Interestingly, ZEBRA recognizes a wider range of DNA binding sites than other bZIP members. bZIP proteins are homo- or heterodimers that contain highly basic DNA binding regions adjacent to regions of a-helix that fold together as coiled coils (Sinclair 2006); the interaction with DNA is dependent on dimer formation (Busch & Sassone-Corsi 1990).

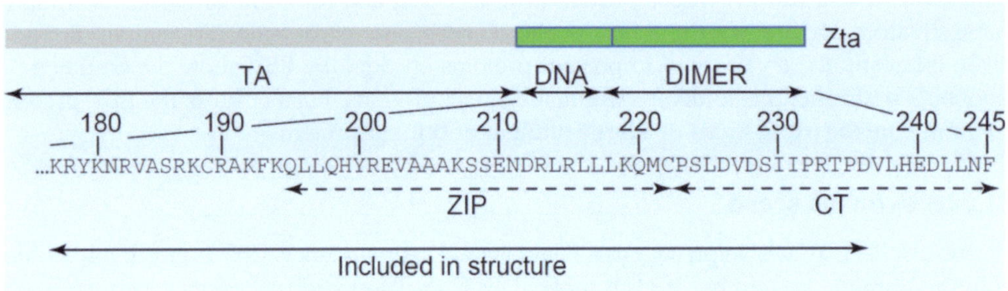

Fig. 1. Schematic representation of the functional regions of ZEBRA and its structure. The transactivation (TA) domain is shown in grey and the DNA contact region and the dimerization region are shown in green and blue. The amino acid sequence of the DNA binding and dimerization domain is expanded below. The location of the region with homology to leucine zippers (ZIP) and the additional region required for dimerization function (CT) are indicated below the sequence

2.3 Role of ZEBRA during viral replication

During the lytic phase of the EBV life cycle, the activation of viral DNA synthesis is related to ZEBRA efficient recognition of a large (~1 kb) complex intergenic region that serves as the origin of replication. This region, known as oriLyt, consists of essential and auxiliary segments (Hammerschmidt & Sugden 1988).The two essential components of oriLyt, the upstream and downstream elements, together constitute the minimal origin of DNA replication (Rennekamp, Wang & Lieberman 2010). The auxiliary component serves as an enhancer element that augments DNA replication (Cox, Leahy & Hardwick 1990). ZEBRA recognizes the origin of lytic DNA replication (oriLyt) by interacting with seven ZEBRA-binding sites (Schepers, Pich & Hammerschmidt 1993). Mutation of all seven binding motifs in the background of a recombinant virus drastically reduces production of infectious virus particles (Feederle & Delecluse 2004).These ZEBRA binding elements are located in two noncontiguous regions of oriLyt. Four elements are present in the upstream core region of oriLyt and overlap with the promoter of the BHLF1 open reading frame and three additional ZEBRA binding elements located mainly in the enhancer region are dispensable for viral replication (Schepers, Pich & Hammerschmidt 1996).

The current model for the role of ZEBRA in lytic DNA replication suggests that the protein serves as a physical link between oriLyt and core components of the replication machinery. The six core replication factors encoded by EBV are the DNA polymerase (BALF5); the polymerase processivity factor (BMRF1); the helicase (BBLF4); the primase (BSLF1); the primase associated factor (BBLF2/3), and the single-stranded DNA binding protein (BALF2) (El-Guindy, Heston & Miller 2010). The function of tethering replication proteins to oriLyt is not limited to ZEBRA; the transactivation domains of Sp1 and ZBP89 interact with BMRF1 and BALF5 and target them to the downstream region of oriLyt (Baumann et al. 1999). Similarly, ZBRK1, a cellular DNA binding zinc finger protein, serves as a contact point for BBLF2/3 on oriLyt (Liao et al. 2005).

2.4 Cellular genes induction

The EBV lytic transactivator ZEBRA not only initiates expression cascade of viral lytic genes but also induces some cellular genes involved in immune regulation (Cayrol & Flemington 1995; Chen, C., Li & Guo 2009). ZEBRA can turn on gene expression through binding to and activation of the target promoters. Notably, a previous study shows that ZEBRA induces transcription of human interleukin 10 (IL-10) in B cells (Mahot et al. 2003).

Table 2 lists a number of genes whose expression is perturbed by ZEBRA. In each case, the regulation occurs in the absence of other viral genes. Regulation at the RNA level implies that ZEBRA may act as transcription factors on the cellular promoters by direct binding or via their associations with other transcription factors. However, the mechanisms of regulation of the cellular genes have not been assessed further as yet. Several of these genes have also been shown to be regulated at the protein level, suggesting relevance. Of special note is the identification of a series of cell cycle regulatory genes such as p21CIP1, p53, CDC25A and E2F1.

RNA changes	Proteins changes
TGFβ inh3 (Cayrol & Flemington 1995)	C/EBPα (Wu et al. 2003)
TGFβ (Cayrol & Flemington 1995)	p21 (Cayrol & Flemington 1996)
α1 collagen (Cayrol & Flemington 1995)	p53 (Wu et al. 2003)
TKT tyrosine kinase (Lu, J. et al. 2000)	p27 (Cayrol & Flemington 1996)
MMP1 (Lu, J. et al. 2000)	E2F1 (MauserHolley-Guthrie, et al. 2002)
IFN-γ receptor (Morrison et al. 2001)	Stem-loop binding protein (MauserHolley-Guthrie, et al. 2002)
E2F1 (MauserHolley-Guthrie, et al. 2002)	CDC25 (MauserHolley-Guthrie, et al. 2002)
Stem-loop binding protein (MauserHolley-Guthrie, et al. 2002)	Cyclin E (MauserHolley-Guthrie, et al. 2002)
CDC25A (MauserHolley-Guthrie, et al. 2002)	
Cyclin E (MauserHolley-Guthrie, et al. 2002)	
C/EBPα (Wu et al. 2003)	
p21 (Wu et al. 2003)	

Table 1. Cell genes regulated by ZEBRA

In NPC, ZEBRA was found to be a potent inducer of IL-8, increasing IL-8 at both protein and RNA levels and activating the IL-8 promoter suggesting that the EBV lytic infection may contribute to the inflammation-like microenvironment of NPC by the upregulation of chemokines (Hsu et al. 2008).

During EBV reactivation in NPC cells, the lytic protein ZEBRA not only induces GM-CSF expression but also upregulates COX-2 that increases production of PGE2 (Dolcetti et al. 2010; Kared et al. 2008). The secreted GM-CSF and PGE2 may cooperatively promote IL-10 production from monocytes (Lee et al. 2011). Thus, through the Zta-induced immunomodulators, EBV lytic infection in NPC cells may drive nearby monocytes into IL-10 producing cells, facilitating local immunosuppression.

By initiating or enhancing leukocyte infiltration, the lytic-cycle-induced chemokines may contribute to an inflammation-like microenvironment, where the interaction between immune infiltrates and tumour cells is crucial for NPC development (Sbih-Lammali et al. 1999). The contribution possibly occurs not only in the developed NPC tumours but also at the precancer stage where an inflammation like microenvironment predisposes precancerous cells to tumour formation (Lu, H., Ouyang & Huang 2006), which may account for how EBV reactivation serves as a risk factor before the onset of NPC (Chien et al. 2001).

2.5 Prognostic value of ZEBRA

Antibodies against ZEBRA are produced during primary EBV infection, and thus, the detection of ZEBRA-specific antibodies may allow an early diagnosis of EBV infections. In 1991, Joab and al were able to detect IgG anti-ZEBRA antibodies (IgG/ZEBRA) in 87% of NPC patients. These antibodies were absent in control sera (Joab et al. 1991). In a more recent study, IgG-ZEBRA antibodies have been shown to represent a sensitive marker for the diagnosis of NPC in children than IgA-VCA and IgA-EA antibodies, which have been recognized as specific markers for this tumour. This study also indicates that Zp125, identified as the most immunogenic epitope of the activation domain of ZEBRA protein, showed a high degree of immunoreactivity with sera from children, young adult and older adult patients with NPC (Dardari et al. 2008). The analysis of antibody patterns in patients with NPC indicates that IgG-ZEBRA had better prognostic value than IgA-EA and IgA-VCA. Stable low IgG-ZEBRA antibody titer, or a striking decline in IgG-ZEBRA antibodies, was observed in children during treatment (Gutierrez et al. 2001; Schaade, Kleines & Hausler 2001). Of note, children showing low IgG-ZEBRA titers were also negative for IgAVCA and IgA-EA; the latter have been identified as being produced following frequent reactivation of latent EBV, repeated EBV infection, or both (Gutierrez et al. 2001; Yip et al. 1994).

Epigenetic dysregulation plays significant role in oncogenesis. Methylation changes in both global and targeted genes have been attributed to EBV+ lymphomas and carcinomas (Niller, Wolf & Minarovits 2009). These studies suggest the contribution of EBV genome in the epigenetic dysregulation of genes involved in tumorigenesis. Systemic analyses of epigenetic alterations under the expression of specific viral gene that may help to specify the contribution of EBV genome. Although results from the Ying-Fan Chen (Chen, Y. F. et al. 2011) suggest that the expression of major viral lytic protein Zta has no effect on changing DNA methylation in the host genome, the comprehensive methods established by him provide a useful platform to investigate genomic methylation changes upon various conditions. These results from these studies will lead to a better understanding of the EBV pathogenesis and may facilitate the development of new therapies.

3. Human Papilloma Virus

The papilloma viruses and its viral nature were first seen in human warts in 1907, and the first papilloma virus was isolated from a rabbit that was identified by Richard Shoppe in the year 1983. Even it was an early start for the detection of human papilloma viruses; this topic remained closed till 1970's. Studies related with papilloma viruses were allowed to move forth only when cervical cancer's proximity with HPV was proved and with its increasing significance in the field of molecular virology (Levinson, 2008).

HPVs are small non enveloped virus containing double stranded DNA as their genetic material and are about 55 nm in size. HPV are strictly epitheliotropic viruses infecting skin or mucosal surfaces, and displaying a very high selectivity for the specific epithelium infected [7,8], and are one of the most common viruses which are transmitted sexually and are found in both men and women. Its ratio is much higher in western countries as compared to other regions of the world. The genome is a circular molecule of double-stranded DNA 8000 base pairs or so. Ten open reading frames (POL) are grouped in a region L (early) coding non-structural protein and an L (late) region encoding the capsid proteins. The non-coding region (NCR of 850 bp for HPV 16) is located between the POL L1 and E6/E7. It contains the promoters of early genes, regulatory sequences (original site) and transcription (cis sequence).

According to their ability to transform epithelial cells, HPV genotypes are divided into low-risk and high-risk types. Low-risk types are associated with benign lesions such as warts, while infections with high-risk types progress to malignant lesions (Munoz et al. 2003). More than 100 different HPV genotypes have been described, but only 30 genotypes identified in the female genital tract are associated with epithelial neoplasms ranging from benign common warts to malignant carcinoma of the uterine cervix (McGlennen 2000). It is widely reported that in addition to HPV 16 and 18, which are frequently found in association with cervical cancer (CC), HPVs 31, 33, 35, 39, 45, 51, 52, 56, 58, 59, 68, 73 and 82, while other three as probable high-risk types (types 26, 53, and 66) are also considered as carcinogenic (Munoz et al. 2003).

3.1 HPV and head and neck cancer

Approximately 15% of malignant diseases are caused by infectious agents. HPV can be frequently found in oral carcinomas, especially tonsillar cancer. A group of HPV-infected tumours shows clear signs for a virally induced transformation process: high-risk HPVs can be detected in all tumour cells, the viral oncogenes E6 and E7 are constantly expressed and lead to upregulation of cellular p16(INK4a), a cyclin-dependent kinase inhibitor. The patients frequently lack typical risk factors associated with head and neck cancers such as drinking and smoking. An association of herpes viruses with head and neck cancer has been for long time suspected and there is good evidence there, but only for a relationship of EBV nasopharyngeal carcinoma. HPV aetiology is now accepted for up to 20% of head and neck cancer. However, the relationship between carcinogenesis and HPV infection is not as clear as with cervical cancer. HPV is not detectable in many head and neck cancers, and it is frequently detected in normal oral mucosa, which is why HPV infections were in head and neck cancer is often regarded only as an accompanying infection. Initial investigations into a causal role for HPV in the aetiology of head and neck lesions relied upon electron microscopy (EM) or immunohistochemical staining. Human papillomavirus virions could be identified by EM from specimens of papillomas (Frithiof & Wersall 1967), fibromas (Gross et al. 1982), verruca, condyloma acuminatav (Shaffer, Reimann & Gysland 1980; Syrjanen, K. J. & Surjanen 1981), focal epithelial hyperplasia, and oral nodular leukoplakias (Jenson et al. 1982). Immunohistochemical staining has revealed the presence of HPV capsid antigens in HPV-infected cells (Loning et al. 1984). Capsid antigen, however, has rarely been detected in high-grade neoplasias or invasive cancer, probably because such tissue contains limited numbers of highly differentiated squamous cell epithelial cells. Consequently, the majority of head and neck lesions that contained HPV structural antigens were either benign or precancerous. Inconsistencies in antigen detection also resulted from sampling error, variable expression or lack of HPV capsid antigens, destruction of antigens during cellular processing or long term storage, or lack of sensitivity to a particular assay (Koutsky, Galloway & Holmes 1988; Syrjanen, S. M. 1990). From published studies, the overall antigen positivity in noncancerous head and neck lesions was about 34.4% (Adler-Storthz et al. 1986; Syrjanen, K., Syrjanen & Pyrhonen 1982). Whereas light microscopy, EM, and immunohistochemistry have resulted in inconsistent or irreproducible findings, the use of DNA hybridization has revolutionized the detection of HPV DNA types in benign and malignant lesions.

New data from case-control studies suggest that HPV is an independent risk factor for oral and oropharyngeal squamous-cell carcinomas (Rosenquist et al. 2005; Schwartz et al. 1998). Moreover, a systematic review showed an overall prevalence of HPV infection of 25.9% in specimens obtained from 5046 patients with head and neck squamous-cell carcinoma that had been analyzed in 60 separate studies (Kreimer et al. 2005). Using PCR detection from 26 countries which included 5046 cases of squamous cell cancers; 2642 oral cancers, 969 oropharyngeal cancers and 1435 laryngeal cancers. HPV prevalence was 35.6% in oropharyngeal cancers, 23.5% in oral cancers and 24.0% in laryngeal cancers. Overall prevalence of HPV in HNSCC was estimated at 26%. HPV 16 was by far the commonest subtype in all types of HPV+ cancers; 86.7% of oropharyngeal, 68.2% of oral and 69.2% of laryngeal cancers. HPV 18 was next most common but found in only 1% of oropharyngeal, 8.0% of oral and 3.9% of laryngeal cancers. A more recent meta-analysis by Termine et al 2008 (Termine et al. 2008), estimated that from studies utilising only FFPE samples, the pooled prevalence of HPV detected in these HNSCC (defined as SCCs originating in the oral, pharyngeal and laryngeal cavities only) was 34.5% (Goon et al. 2009).

3.2 HPV and NPC

NPC is one of the most striking examples of human malignancies that have been found strongly associated with the EBV, and interest in HPV as a cofactor in NPC occurrences has emerged over the last few years (Lin 2009). EBV has been detected in a large proportion of patients with WHO-II/III NPC, but a significant subset of patients with WHO-I NPC are EBV negative (Hording et al. 1994; Rassekh et al. 1998; Tsai et al. 1998). High-risk HPV may contribute to the development of NPC, given HPV's acknowledged role in the pathogenesis of oropharyngeal carcinomas.

Furthermore, it has been suggested that normal human oral epithelial cells, especially nasopharyngeal cells, could be very susceptible to persistent HPV and EBV co-infections and that EBV and high-risk HPV co-infections may play an important role in the initiation of a neoplastic transformation of human oral epithelial cells (Al Moustafa et al. 2009). To date, different degrees of associations between HPV and NPC have been described, yet no conclusive data have been obtained.

Coinfection by HPV and EBV has not been well documented and the significance of the presence of both viruses in nasopharyngeal cells has not been determined. In a recent study, coinfection with both viruses was observed in 34% of patients in Morocco. Tung et al. showed that among 88 fresh NPC specimens from Chinese population, coexistence of EBV and HPV DNA was observed in 42% of samples (Tung et al. 1999).

These results are in agreement with other studies reporting the same prevalence of HPV DNA in NPC cases. In fact, using the same consensus primers, HPV DNA was detected in 31 of 103 NPC samples (30%). Moreover, Krishna et al. have shown that HPV DNA was detected in 38.8% of 36 southern Indian NPC cases (Krishna et al. 2004). Tung et al. in Eighty-eight fresh tissue samples of NPC showed that HPV DNA was detected in 51% of the specimens (Tung et al. 1999).

With regard to HPV genotypes, HPV31 was the most frequent genotype in Moroccan NPC patients (20.8 %). The same genotype was also frequently found in tonsils and nasopharyngeal cells in western Mexico NPC cases (Lopez-Lizarraga et al. 2000). The second prevalent HPV type detected in Moroccan NPC biopsies is HPV59 (16,7%). Of interest, HPV-16 and -18, which are the most virulent genotypes associated with CC in Moroccan woman (35% to 45 %) (Khair et al. 2009), were detected in very few NPC cases (8.3 %), and similar data were reported in an Iranian study (Mirzamani et al. 2006). However, a recent study suggests that WHO-I NPC may be associated with oncogenic HPV. Oncogenic HPV was detected by in situ hybridization in half of the WHO-I NPCs but only 5% of the WHO-II/III NPCs. In addition in a HPV genotyping cohort study, oncogenic HPVs were detected equally in WHO-II/III NPCs (31%, 13/42) and nasopharyngeal controls (35%, 14/40). Tumour high-risk HPV status did not correlate with the prognosis of patients with NPC. In the high-risk HPV in situ hybridisation cohort, 14 (88%) of the 16 oncogenic HPV-positive WHO-II/III NPCs showed a unique cytoplasmic/perinuclear staining pattern, which is distinct from the typical dot/punctate nuclear staining pattern indicating HPV genome integration. In addition, oncogenic HPVs were not always retained in NPC cells during the process of metastasis (Lo et al. 2010). Therefore, considering the fact that oncogenic HPV has not been consistently detected in NPC specimens from different endemic regions, it is likely that HPV infection may not be essential in the carcinogenesis of EBV-associated WHO-II/III NPCs in areas endemic for NPC.

3.3 Insights into the molecular mechanisms of HPV carcinogenesis

These inconsistent results are likely to reflect a difference in life cycles of the different HPV subtypes in different mucosal locations, with an associated difference in mucosal immune responses. The high risk subtypes of HPV involved in cervical carcinogenesis have been defined (Munoz et al. 2003). We speculate the HPV subtypes associated with NPC are broadly similar (but not identical) (figure 2) with those seen in cervical carcinoma. Briefly, through wounds or abrasions, the papillomaviruses infect basal epithelial cells, which are the only actively dividing cells in the epithelial layer. The viral DNA is maintained in the nuclei of infected basal epithelial cells as a low-copy-number plasmid (Stubenrauch & Laimins 1999). Squamous epithelial cells normally undergo differentiation as they move from the basement membrane towards the surface epithelium, and HPV-DNA replicates to a high copy number only in terminally differentiated cells near the epithelial surface (Stubenrauch & Laimins 1999). Similarly, the late viral genes, which encode the L1 and L2 proteins that constitute the virus particle, are expressed only in the highly differentiated cells, where infectious progeny virus is produced and released. Three critical steps can be discriminated in this model (figure 2): the conversion of a single mutated stem cell in a patch into a group of stem cells without proper growth control (field); the eventual transforming event, which turns a field into an overt carcinoma showing invasive growth and metastasis; and the development of metastasis. Both aneuploidy and the accumulation of cancer-associated genetic changes in fields are linked to the risk of malignant progression.

It has been shown that these subtypes (particularly 16) are able to transform and immortalise cells in vitro. These effects are predominantly due to the E6 and E7 oncogenes, which bind and enhance degradation of p53 and Rb tumour suppressor genes respectively. There is evidence that immortalisation of oral keratinocytes and epithelial cells occur quite readily (Park et al. 1991).

HPV integration usually leads to disruption and/or deletion of HPV E1 or E2 open reading frame (ORF), which are important for viral replication and transcription. E2 functions also as a repressor of E6 and E7 and disruption of E2 activity allows increased E6 and E7 expression, thus maintaining the immortalised phenotype (zur Hausen 2009). Integration of HPV 16 DNA also correlates with a selective growth advantage and may allow the cancerous cell to outgrow its rivals; this may be an important step in the pathway of oncogenesis (Jeon, Allen-Hoffmann & Lambert 1995). However, despite the dominance of the integrated HPV genome in terms of cervical carcinogenesis, 15-30% of cervical cancer contains HPV only in the episomal form (Watts et al. 2002). In some of these cases, investigators have found deletions in the YY1-binding sites of the LCR (long control region) of HPV 16 episomal DNA which may allow elevated activity of the E6/ E7 promoter (Dong et al. 1994). It is clear that the actual molecular pathway to cervical carcinogenesis is far from homogeneous. The situation in head and neck cancers is less than clear but heterogeneity and the existence of multiple pathways to carcinogenesis is highly likely. Koskinen et al (2003) reported that in their series of head and neck cancers, 61% were HPV DNA positive. HPV 16 was the dominant subtype, and found in 84% of HPV+ cancers. Tonsillar carcinomas have been reported to have the highest prevalence rate of HPV DNA contained within cancerous cells (51%) of all the forms of head and neck cancers (Syrjanen, S. 2004). Mellin et al 2002 reported that all 11 cases of HPV+ tonsillar carcinomas in their series contained HPV DNA in episomal form (Mellin et al. 2002). Another study in 1992 reported two HPV 16+ tonsillar carcinomas which contained episomal HPV DNA, and two HPV 33+ tonsillar carcinomas in which one was integrated and the other had mixed forms (Snijders et al. 1992). It is unclear why tonsillar carcinomas appear to have a higher predominance of episomal HPV DNA than other types of head and neck cancer. It is likely though, that these various observations suggest a high heterogeneity and variation in the oncogenic pathways among these tumours.

3.4 Similarities between HPV and ZEBRA

HPV and EBV co-infections have not been well documented and the significance of the presence of both viruses in nasopharyngeal cells has not been determined. It has been shown that ZEBRA, an EBV immediate early protein expressed during lytic replication that activates early EBV genes, binds to p53 (Quinlivan et al. 1993). The physical interaction of the ZEBRA and p53 protein prevents p53 from activating p53-responsive promoters (MauserSaito, et al. 2002). Similarly, HPV has been found to interact with p53, suggesting that this interaction promotes cell growth and thereby enhance viral replication (Levine

1990). Targeting p53 may be a common requirement for the replication of many types of DNA viruses (Prayitno 2006). In addition, B cells transfected with EBV latent membrane protein lost the regulatory effects of the retinoblastoma (RB) protein, and the HPV E7 transcript has been shown to immunoprecipitate the RB protein (Giovannelli et al. 2002). Thus, the functional loss of the RB protein might be one event common to both the HPV and EBV carcinogenic pathways.

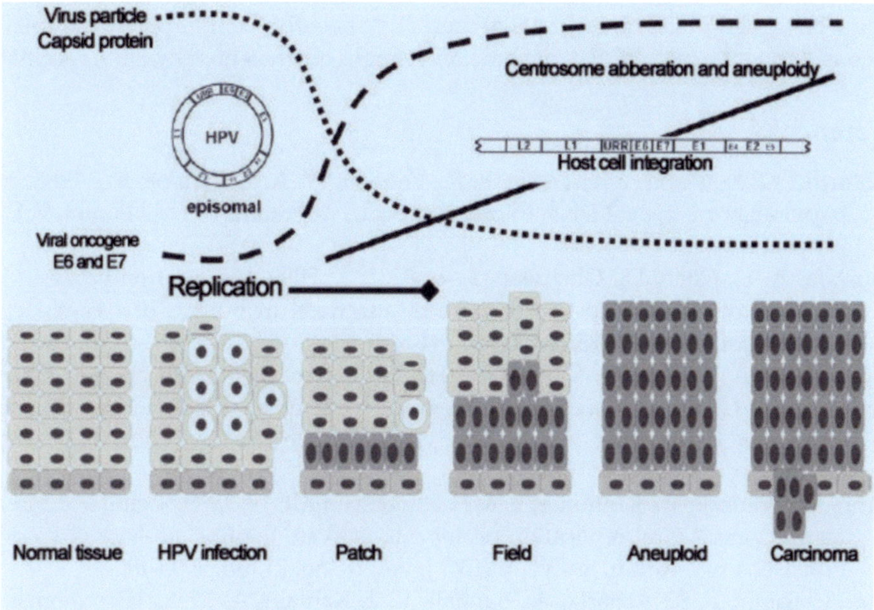

Fig. 2. A hypothetical model of HPV-associated NPC development. Most information has been deciphered from oral carcinogenesis; there are fewer data on the other subsites of NPC. Light cells: Normal epithelium. Cells with a white ring: Koilocytes, as a result of an active viral replication. Dark cells: Dysplastic epithelium with increased chromosomal instability reflected by increasing aneuploidy of the cells and leading to progression to high grade dysplasia and invasive carcinoma.

4. Conclusion

EBV is associated with the development of both B-cell and epithelial cell malignancies. The capacity of EBV to transform B lymphocytes has been well documented. EBV latent proteins are known to contribute to cellular transformation. Several lines of evidence demonstrated that reactivation of the latent viral genome in EBV associated cancers can cause cancer cell death. However, the underlying molecular mechanisms are unclear. Although ZEBRA plays an important role in immunomodulation, its capacity to reprogram the hosT-cell cycle control machinery is also notified in some tumour cell lines. Therefore, gene delivery techniques might be a novel therapeutic strategy for treating EBV positive malignancies especially NPC, via the induction of lytic viral transcription in certain tumour cells.

HPV-associated nasopharyngeal carcinoma represents a distinct clinical and biological entity with many unresolved issues that will be studied in future translational, clinical research. We need to further investigate. It is possible that HPV-associated nasopharyngeal carcinoma arises by a different mechanism from that involved in the pathogenesis of HPV-associated cervical carcinoma. Still that the association between some NPC and HPV infection appears to be not firmly established, and the question that arises is whether there is any need for screening for NPC HPV infection in high-risk groups. Moreover, we need to examine how to treat HPV-positive intraepithelial neoplastic lesions, which are cancer precursor lesions, in the head and neck region. Should HPV-associated nasopharyngeal carcinoma be treated in the same way that their HPV-negative counterpart? And finally, it is worth considering the possibility that some NPC might be prevented by HPV vaccination.

5. References

Adler-Storthz, K., Newland, J. R., Tessin, B. A., Yeudall, W. A. & Shillitoe, E. J. 1986, 'Human papillomavirus type 2 DNA in oral verrucous carcinoma', J Oral Pathol, vol. 15, no. 9, pp. 472-5.

Al Moustafa, A. E., Chen, D., Ghabreau, L. & Akil, N. 2009, 'Association between human papillomavirus and Epstein-Barr virus infections in human oral carcinogenesis', Med Hypotheses, vol. 73, no. 2, pp. 184-6.

Baer, R., Bankier, A. T., Biggin, M. D., Deininger, P. L., Farrell, P. J., Gibson, T. J., Hatfull, G., Hudson, G. S., Satchwell, S. C., Seguin, C. & et al. 1984, 'DNA sequence and expression of the B95-8 Epstein-Barr virus genome', Nature, vol. 310, no. 5974, pp. 207-11.

Baumann, M., Feederle, R., Kremmer, E. & Hammerschmidt, W. 1999, 'Cellular transcription factors recruit viral replication proteins to activate the Epstein-Barr virus origin of lytic DNA replication, oriLyt', EMBO J, vol. 18, no. 21, pp. 6095-105.

Benider, A., Sahraoui, S., Acharki, A., Samlali, R. & Kahlain, A. 1995, '[Carcinomas of the nasopharynx in children. Analysis of 50 cases]', Bull Cancer, vol. 82, no. 2, pp. 155-61.

Busch, S. J. & Sassone-Corsi, P. 1990, 'Dimers, leucine zippers and DNA-binding domains', Trends Genet, vol. 6, no. 2, pp. 36-40.

Cayrol, C. & Flemington, E. 1996, 'G0/G1 growth arrest mediated by a region encompassing the basic leucine zipper (bZIP) domain of the Epstein-Barr virus transactivator Zta', J Biol Chem, vol. 271, no. 50, pp. 31799-802.

Cayrol, C. & Flemington, E. K. 1995, 'Identification of cellular target genes of the Epstein-Barr virus transactivator Zta: activation of transforming growth factor beta igh3 (TGF-beta igh3) and TGF-beta 1', J Virol, vol. 69, no. 7, pp. 4206-12.

Chen, C., Li, D. & Guo, N. 2009, 'Regulation of cellular and viral protein expression by the Epstein-Barr virus transcriptional regulator Zta: implications for therapy of EBV associated tumors', Cancer Biol Ther, vol. 8, no. 11, pp. 987-95.

Chen, Y. F., Tung, C. L., Chang, Y., Hsiao, W. C., Su, L. J. & Sun, H. S. 2011, 'Analysis of global methylation using a Zta-expressing nasopharyngeal carcinoma cell line', Genomics, vol. 97, no. 4, pp. 205-13.

Chien, Y. C., Chen, J. Y., Liu, M. Y., Yang, H. I., Hsu, M. M., Chen, C. J. & Yang, C. S. 2001, 'Serologic markers of Epstein-Barr virus infection and nasopharyngeal carcinoma in Taiwanese men', N Engl J Med, vol. 345, no. 26, pp. 1877-82.

Cohen, J. I. 2000, 'Epstein-Barr virus infection', N Engl J Med, vol. 343, no. 7, pp. 481-92.

Cox, M. A., Leahy, J. & Hardwick, J. M. 1990, 'An enhancer within the divergent promoter of Epstein-Barr virus responds synergistically to the R and Z transactivators', J Virol, vol. 64, no. 1, pp. 313-21.

Dardari, R., Menezes, J., Drouet, E., Joab, I., Benider, A., Bakkali, H., Kanouni, L., Jouhadi, H., Benjaafar, N., El Gueddari, B., Hassar, M. & Khyatti, M. 2008, 'Analyses of the prognostic significance of the Epstein-Barr virus transactivator ZEBRA protein and diagnostic value of its two synthetic peptides in nasopharyngeal carcinoma', J Clin Virol, vol. 41, no. 2, pp. 96-103.

Dolcetti, L., Peranzoni, E., Ugel, S., Marigo, I., Fernandez Gomez, A., Mesa, C., Geilich, M., Winkels, G., Traggiai, E., Casati, A., Grassi, F. & Bronte, V. 2010, 'Hierarchy of immunosuppressive strength among myeloid-derived suppressor cell subsets is determined by GM-CSF', Eur J Immunol, vol. 40, no. 1, pp. 22-35.

Dong, X. P., Stubenrauch, F., Beyer-Finkler, E. & Pfister, H. 1994, 'Prevalence of deletions of YY1-binding sites in episomal HPV 16 DNA from cervical cancers', Int J Cancer, vol. 58, no. 6, pp. 803-8.

El-Guindy, A., Heston, L. & Miller, G. 2010, 'A subset of replication proteins enhances origin recognition and lytic replication by the Epstein-Barr virus ZEBRA protein', PLoS Pathog, vol. 6, no. 8.

Feederle, R. & Delecluse, H. J. 2004, 'Low level of lytic replication in a recombinant Epstein-Barr virus carrying an origin of replication devoid of BZLF1-binding sites', J Virol, vol. 78, no. 21, pp. 12082-4.

Feng, B. J., Jalbout, M., Ayoub, W. B., Khyatti, M., Dahmoul, S., Ayad, M., Maachi, F., Bedadra, W., Abdoun, M., Mesli, S., Hamdi-Cherif, M., Boualga, K., Bouaouina, N., Chouchane, L., Benider, A., Ben Ayed, F., Goldgar, D. & Corbex, M. 2007, 'Dietary risk factors for nasopharyngeal carcinoma in Maghrebian countries', Int J Cancer, vol. 121, no. 7, pp. 1550-5.

Fixman, E. D., Hayward, G. S. & Hayward, S. D. 1995, 'Replication of Epstein-Barr virus oriLyt: lack of a dedicated virally encoded origin-binding protein and dependence on Zta in cotransfection assays', J Virol, vol. 69, no. 5, pp. 2998-3006.

Flemington, E. & Speck, S. H. 1990, 'Autoregulation of Epstein-Barr virus putative lytic switch gene BZLF1', J Virol, vol. 64, no. 3, pp. 1227-32.

Frithiof, L. & Wersall, J. 1967, 'Virus-like particles in papillomas of the human oral cavity', Arch Gesamte Virusforsch, vol. 21, no. 1, pp. 31-44.

Gillison, M. L. & Shah, K. V. 2001, 'Human papillomavirus-associated head and neck squamous cell carcinoma: mounting evidence for an etiologic role for human papillomavirus in a subset of head and neck cancers', Curr Opin Oncol, vol. 13, no. 3, pp. 183-8.

Giovannelli, L., Campisi, G., Lama, A., Giambalvo, O., Osborn, J., Margiotta, V. & Ammatuna, P. 2002, 'Human papillomavirus DNA in oral mucosal lesions', J Infect Dis, vol. 185, no. 6, pp. 833-6.

Goon, P. K., Stanley, M. A., Ebmeyer, J., Steinstrasser, L., Upile, T., Jerjes, W., Bernal-Sprekelsen, M., Gorner, M. & Sudhoff, H. H. 2009, 'HPV & head and neck cancer: a descriptive update', Head Neck Oncol, vol. 1, p. 36.

Gross, G., Pfister, H., Hagedorn, M. & Gissmann, L. 1982, 'Correlation between human papillomavirus (HPV) type and histology of warts', J Invest Dermatol, vol. 78, no. 2, pp. 160-4.

Gutierrez, J., Rodriguez, M., Soto, M. J., Suarez, S., Morales, P., Piedrola, G. & Maroto, M. C. 2001, 'An evaluation of a polyantigenic ELISA to detect Epstein-Barr virus reactivation', Microbios, vol. 106, no. 413, pp. 49-54.

Hammerschmidt, W. & Sugden, B. 1988, 'Identification and characterization of oriLyt, a lytic origin of DNA replication of Epstein-Barr virus', Cell, vol. 55, no. 3, pp. 427-33.

Hicks, M. R., Balesaria, S., Medina-Palazon, C., Pandya, M. J., Woolfson, D. N. & Sinclair, A. J. 2001, 'Biophysical analysis of natural variants of the multimerization region of Epstein-Barr virus lytic-switch protein BZLF1', J Virol, vol. 75, no. 11, pp. 5381-4.

Hildesheim, A. & Levine, P. H. 1993, 'Etiology of nasopharyngeal carcinoma: a review', Epidemiol Rev, vol. 15, no. 2, pp. 466-85.

Hording, U., Nielsen, H. W., Daugaard, S. & Albeck, H. 1994, 'Human papillomavirus types 11 and 16 detected in nasopharyngeal carcinomas by the polymerase chain reaction', Laryngoscope, vol. 104, no. 1 Pt 1, pp. 99-102.

Hsu, M., Wu, S. Y., Chang, S. S., Su, I. J., Tsai, C. H., Lai, S. J., Shiau, A. L., Takada, K. & Chang, Y. 2008, 'Epstein-Barr virus lytic transactivator Zta enhances chemotactic activity through induction of interleukin-8 in nasopharyngeal carcinoma cells', J Virol, vol. 82, no. 7, pp. 3679-88.

Jenkins, P. J., Binne, U. K. & Farrell, P. J. 2000, 'Histone acetylation and reactivation of Epstein-Barr virus from latency', J Virol, vol. 74, no. 2, pp. 710-20.

Jenson, A. B., Lancaster, W. D., Hartmann, D. P. & Shaffer, E. L., Jr. 1982, 'Frequency and distribution of papillomavirus structural antigens in verrucae, multiple papillomas, and condylomata of the oral cavity', Am J Pathol, vol. 107, no. 2, pp. 212-8.

Jeon, S., Allen-Hoffmann, B. L. & Lambert, P. F. 1995, 'Integration of human papillomavirus type 16 into the human genome correlates with a selective growth advantage of cells', J Virol, vol. 69, no. 5, pp. 2989-97.

Joab, I., Nicolas, J. C., Schwaab, G., de-The, G., Clausse, B., Perricaudet, M. & Zeng, Y. 1991, 'Detection of anti-Epstein-Barr-virus transactivator (ZEBRA) antibodies in sera from patients with nasopharyngeal carcinoma', Int J Cancer, vol. 48, no. 5, pp. 647-9.

Kared, H., Leforban, B., Montandon, R., Renand, A., Layseca Espinosa, E., Chatenoud, L., Rosenstein, Y., Schneider, E., Dy, M. & Zavala, F. 2008, 'Role of GM-CSF in tolerance induction by mobilized hematopoietic progenitors', Blood, vol. 112, no. 6, pp. 2575-8.

Khair, M. M., Mzibri, M. E., Mhand, R. A., Benider, A., Benchekroun, N., Fahime, E. M., Benchekroun, M. N. & Ennaji, M. M. 2009, 'Molecular detection and genotyping of human papillomavirus in cervical carcinoma biopsies in an area of high incidence of cancer from Moroccan women', J Med Virol, vol. 81, no. 4, pp. 678-84.

Koutsky, L. A., Galloway, D. A. & Holmes, K. K. 1988, 'Epidemiology of genital human papillomavirus infection', Epidemiol Rev, vol. 10, pp. 122-63.

Kreimer, A. R., Clifford, G. M., Boyle, P. & Franceschi, S. 2005, 'Human papillomavirus types in head and neck squamous cell carcinomas worldwide: a systematic review', Cancer Epidemiol Biomarkers Prev, vol. 14, no. 2, pp. 467-75.

Krishna, S. M., James, S., Kattoor, J. & Balaram, P. 2004, 'Human papilloma virus infection in Indian nasopharyngeal carcinomas in relation to the histology of tumour', Indian J Pathol Microbiol, vol. 47, no. 2, pp. 181-5.

Lee, C. H., Yeh, T. H., Lai, H. C., Wu, S. Y., Su, I. J., Takada, K. & Chang, Y. 2011, 'Epstein-Barr virus Zta-induced immunomodulators from nasopharyngeal carcinoma cells upregulate interleukin-10 production from monocytes', J Virol, vol. 85, no. 14, pp. 7333-42.

Levine, A. J. 1990, 'The p53 protein and its interactions with the oncogene products of the small DNA tumor viruses', Virology, vol. 177, no. 2, pp. 419-26.

Liao, G., Huang, J., Fixman, E. D. & Hayward, S. D. 2005, 'The Epstein-Barr virus replication protein BBLF2/3 provides an origin-tethering function through interaction with the zinc finger DNA binding protein ZBRK1 and the KAP-1 corepressor', J Virol, vol. 79, no. 1, pp. 245-56.

Lieberman, P. M., Hardwick, J. M., Sample, J., Hayward, G. S. & Hayward, S. D. 1990, 'The zta transactivator involved in induction of lytic cycle gene expression in Epstein-Barr virus-infected lymphocytes binds to both AP-1 and ZRE sites in target promoter and enhancer regions', J Virol, vol. 64, no. 3, pp. 1143-55.

Lin, C. T. 2009, 'Relationship between Epstein-Barr virus infection and nasopharyngeal carcinoma pathogenesis', Ai Zheng, vol. 28, no. 8, pp. 791-804.

Lo, E. J., Bell, D., Woo, J. S., Li, G., Hanna, E. Y., El-Naggar, A. K. & Sturgis, E. M. 2010, 'Human papillomavirus and WHO type I nasopharyngeal carcinoma', Laryngoscope, vol. 120, no. 10, pp. 1990-7.

Loning, T., Reichart, P., Staquet, M. J., Becker, J. & Thivolet, J. 1984, 'Occurrence of papillomavirus structural antigens in oral papillomas and leukoplakias', J Oral Pathol, vol. 13, no. 2, pp. 155-65.

Lopez-Lizarraga, E., Sanchez-Corona, J., Montoya-Fuentes, H., Bravo-Cuellar, A., Campollo-Rivas, O., Lopez-Demerutis, E., Morgan-Villela, G., Arcaute-Velazquez, F., Monreal-Martinez, J. A. & Troyo, R. 2000, 'Human papillomavirus in tonsillar and nasopharyngeal carcinoma: isolation of HPV subtype 31', Ear Nose Throat J, vol. 79, no. 12, pp. 942-4.

Lu, H., Ouyang, W. & Huang, C. 2006, 'Inflammation, a key event in cancer development', Mol Cancer Res, vol. 4, no. 4, pp. 221-33.

Lu, J., Chen, S. Y., Chua, H. H., Liu, Y. S., Huang, Y. T., Chang, Y., Chen, J. Y., Sheen, T. S. & Tsai, C. H. 2000, 'Upregulation of tyrosine kinase TKT by the Epstein-Barr virus transactivator Zta', J Virol, vol. 74, no. 16, pp. 7391-9.

Mahot, S., Sergeant, A., Drouet, E. & Gruffat, H. 2003, 'A novel function for the Epstein-Barr virus transcription factor EB1/Zta: induction of transcription of the hIL-10 gene', J Gen Virol, vol. 84, no. Pt 4, pp. 965-74.

Marshall, W. L., Yim, C., Gustafson, E., Graf, T., Sage, D. R., Hanify, K., Williams, L., Fingeroth, J. & Finberg, R. W. 1999, 'Epstein-Barr virus encodes a novel homolog of the bcl-2 oncogene that inhibits apoptosis and associates with Bax and Bak', J Virol, vol. 73, no. 6, pp. 5181-5.

Mauser, A., Holley-Guthrie, E., Zanation, A., Yarborough, W., Kaufmann, W., Klingelhutz, A., Seaman, W. T. & Kenney, S. 2002, 'The Epstein-Barr virus immediate-early protein BZLF1 induces expression of E2F-1 and other proteins involved in cell cycle progression in primary keratinocytes and gastric carcinoma cells', J Virol, vol. 76, no. 24, pp. 12543-52.

Mauser, A., Saito, S., Appella, E., Anderson, C. W., Seaman, W. T. & Kenney, S. 2002, 'The Epstein-Barr virus immediate-early protein BZLF1 regulates p53 function through multiple mechanisms', J Virol, vol. 76, no. 24, pp. 12503-12.
McGlennen, R. C. 2000, 'Human papillomavirus oncogenesis', Clin Lab Med, vol. 20, no. 2, pp. 383-406.
Mellin, H., Dahlgren, L., Munck-Wikland, E., Lindholm, J., Rabbani, H., Kalantari, M. & Dalianis, T. 2002, 'Human papillomavirus type 16 is episomal and a high viral load may be correlated to better prognosis in tonsillar cancer', Int J Cancer, vol. 102, no. 2, pp. 152-8.
Mirzamani, N., Salehian, P., Farhadi, M. & Tehran, E. A. 2006, 'Detection of EBV and HPV in nasopharyngeal carcinoma by in situ hybridization', Exp Mol Pathol, vol. 81, no. 3, pp. 231-4.
Morrison, T. E., Mauser, A., Wong, A., Ting, J. P. & Kenney, S. C. 2001, 'Inhibition of IFN-gamma signaling by an Epstein-Barr virus immediate-early protein', Immunity, vol. 15, no. 5, pp. 787-99.
Munoz, N., Bosch, F. X., de Sanjose, S., Herrero, R., Castellsague, X., Shah, K. V., Snijders, P. J. & Meijer, C. J. 2003, 'Epidemiologic classification of human papillomavirus types associated with cervical cancer', N Engl J Med, vol. 348, no. 6, pp. 518-27.
Niller, H. H., Wolf, H. & Minarovits, J. 2009, 'Epigenetic dysregulation of the host cell genome in Epstein-Barr virus-associated neoplasia', Semin Cancer Biol, vol. 19, no. 3, pp. 158-64.
Park, N. H., Min, B. M., Li, S. L., Huang, M. Z., Cherick, H. M. & Doniger, J. 1991, 'Immortalization of normal human oral keratinocytes with type 16 human papillomavirus', Carcinogenesis, vol. 12, no. 9, pp. 1627-31.
Parkin, D. M. & Muir, C. S. 1992, 'Cancer Incidence in Five Continents. Comparability and quality of data', IARC Sci Publ, no. 120, pp. 45-173.
Pathmanathan, R., Prasad, U., Chandrika, G., Sadler, R., Flynn, K. & Raab-Traub, N. 1995, 'Undifferentiated, nonkeratinizing, and squamous cell carcinoma of the nasopharynx. Variants of Epstein-Barr virus-infected neoplasia', Am J Pathol, vol. 146, no. 6, pp. 1355-67.
Prayitno, A. 2006, 'Cervical cancer with human papilloma virus and Epstein Barr virus positive', J Carcinog, vol. 5, p. 13.
Punwaney, R., Brandwein, M. S., Zhang, D. Y., Urken, M. L., Cheng, R., Park, C. S., Li, H. B. & Li, X. 1999, 'Human papillomavirus may be common within nasopharyngeal carcinoma of Caucasian Americans: investigation of Epstein-Barr virus and human papillomavirus in eastern and western nasopharyngeal carcinoma using ligation-dependent polymerase chain reaction', Head Neck, vol. 21, no. 1, pp. 21-9.
Quinlivan, E. B., Holley-Guthrie, E. A., Norris, M., Gutsch, D., Bachenheimer, S. L. & Kenney, S. C. 1993, 'Direct BRLF1 binding is required for cooperative BZLF1/BRLF1 activation of the Epstein-Barr virus early promoter, BMRF1', Nucleic Acids Res, vol. 21, no. 14, pp. 1999-2007.
Raab-Traub, N. 1996, 'Pathogenesis of Epstein-Barr virus and its associated malignancies', Seminars in Virology, vol. 7, no. 5, pp. 315-23.
Rassekh, C. H., Rady, P. L., Arany, I., Tyring, S. K., Knudsen, S., Calhoun, K. H., Seikaly, H. & Bailey, B. J. 1998, 'Combined Epstein-Barr virus and human papillomavirus infection in nasopharyngeal carcinoma', Laryngoscope, vol. 108, no. 3, pp. 362-7.

Rennekamp, A. J., Wang, P. & Lieberman, P. M. 2010, 'Evidence for DNA hairpin recognition by Zta at the Epstein-Barr virus origin of lytic replication', J Virol, vol. 84, no. 14, pp. 7073-82.

Rickinson, A. 2002, 'Epstein-Barr virus', Virus Res, vol. 82, no. 1-2, pp. 109-13.

Rosenquist, K., Wennerberg, J., Schildt, E. B., Bladstrom, A., Goran Hansson, B. & Andersson, G. 2005, 'Oral status, oral infections and some lifestyle factors as risk factors for oral and oropharyngeal squamous cell carcinoma. A population-based case-control study in southern Sweden', Acta Otolaryngol, vol. 125, no. 12, pp. 1327-36.

Sbih-Lammali, F., Clausse, B., Ardila-Osorio, H., Guerry, R., Talbot, M., Havouis, S., Ferradini, L., Bosq, J., Tursz, T. & Busson, P. 1999, 'Control of apoptosis in Epstein Barr virus-positive nasopharyngeal carcinoma cells: opposite effects of CD95 and CD40 stimulation', Cancer Res, vol. 59, no. 4, pp. 924-30.

Schaade, L., Kleines, M. & Hausler, M. 2001, 'Application of virus-specific immunoglobulin M (IgM), IgG, and IgA antibody detection with a polyantigenic enzyme-linked immunosorbent assay for diagnosis of Epstein-Barr virus infections in childhood', J Clin Microbiol, vol. 39, no. 11, pp. 3902-5.

Schepers, A., Pich, D. & Hammerschmidt, W. 1993, 'A transcription factor with homology to the AP-1 family links RNA transcription and DNA replication in the lytic cycle of Epstein-Barr virus', EMBO J, vol. 12, no. 10, pp. 3921-9.

---- 1996, 'Activation of oriLyt, the lytic origin of DNA replication of Epstein-Barr virus, by BZLF1', Virology, vol. 220, no. 2, pp. 367-76.

Schwartz, S. M., Daling, J. R., Doody, D. R., Wipf, G. C., Carter, J. J., Madeleine, M. M., Mao, E. J., Fitzgibbons, E. D., Huang, S., Beckmann, A. M., McDougall, J. K. & Galloway, D. A. 1998, 'Oral cancer risk in relation to sexual history and evidence of human papillomavirus infection', J Natl Cancer Inst, vol. 90, no. 21, pp. 1626-36.

Shaffer, E. L., Jr., Reimann, B. E. & Gysland, W. B. 1980, 'Oral condyloma acuminatum. A case report with light microscopic and ultrastructural features', J Oral Pathol, vol. 9, no. 3, pp. 163-73.

Sinclair, A. J. 2003, 'bZIP proteins of human gammaherpesviruses', Journal of General Virology, vol. 84, no. 8, pp. 1941-9.

---- 2006, 'Unexpected structure of Epstein-Barr virus lytic cycle activator Zta', Trends Microbiol, vol. 14, no. 7, pp. 289-91.

Sinclair, A. J. & Farrell, P. J. 1992, 'Epstein-Barr virus transcription factors', Cell Growth Differ, vol. 3, no. 8, pp. 557-63.

Snijders, P. J., Meijer, C. J., van den Brule, A. J., Schrijnemakers, H. F., Snow, G. B. & Walboomers, J. M. 1992, 'Human papillomavirus (HPV) type 16 and 33 E6/E7 region transcripts in tonsillar carcinomas can originate from integrated and episomal HPV DNA', J Gen Virol, vol. 73 (Pt 8), pp. 2059-66.

Stubenrauch, F. & Laimins, L. A. 1999, 'Human papillomavirus life cycle: active and latent phases', Semin Cancer Biol, vol. 9, no. 6, pp. 379-86.

Syrjanen, K., Syrjanen, S. & Pyrhonen, S. 1982, 'Human papilloma virus (HPV) antigens in lesions of laryngeal squamous cell carcinomas', ORL J Otorhinolaryngol Relat Spec, vol. 44, no. 6, pp. 323-34.

Syrjanen, K. J. & Surjanen, S. M. 1981, 'Histological evidence for the presence of condylomatous epithelial lesions in association with laryngeal squamous cell carcinoma', ORL J Otorhinolaryngol Relat Spec, vol. 43, no. 4, pp. 181-94.

Syrjanen, S. 2004, 'HPV infections and tonsillar carcinoma', J Clin Pathol, vol. 57, no. 5, pp. 449-55.

Syrjanen, S. M. 1990, 'Basic concepts and practical applications of recombinant DNA techniques in detection of human papillomavirus (HPV) infection. Review article', APMIS, vol. 98, no. 2, pp. 95-110.

Takimoto, T., Ishiguro, H., Umeda, R., Ogura, H. & Hatano, M. 1984, 'Effects of chemical inducers on the Epstein-Barr virus cycle in epithelial/nasopharyngeal carcinoma hybrid cell line', ORL J Otorhinolaryngol Relat Spec, vol. 46, no. 4, pp. 192-4.

Termine, N., Panzarella, V., Falaschini, S., Russo, A., Matranga, D., Lo Muzio, L. & Campisi, G. 2008, 'HPV in oral squamous cell carcinoma vs head and neck squamous cell carcinoma biopsies: a meta-analysis (1988-2007)', Ann Oncol, vol. 19, no. 10, pp. 1681-90.

Tsai, S. T., Jin, Y. T., Mann, R. B. & Ambinder, R. F. 1998, 'Epstein-Barr virus detection in nasopharyngeal tissues of patients with suspected nasopharyngeal carcinoma', Cancer, vol. 82, no. 8, pp. 1449-53.

Tung, Y. C., Lin, K. H., Chu, P. Y., Hsu, C. C. & Kuo, W. R. 1999, 'Detection of human papilloma virus and Epstein-Barr virus DNA in nasopharyngeal carcinoma by polymerase chain reaction', Kaohsiung J Med Sci, vol. 15, no. 5, pp. 256-62.

Watts, K. J., Thompson, C. H., Cossart, Y. E. & Rose, B. R. 2002, 'Sequence variation and physical state of human papillomavirus type 16 cervical cancer isolates from Australia and New Caledonia', Int J Cancer, vol. 97, no. 6, pp. 868-74.

Wu, F. Y., Chen, H., Wang, S. E., ApRhys, C. M., Liao, G., Fujimuro, M., Farrell, C. J., Huang, J., Hayward, S. D. & Hayward, G. S. 2003, 'CCAAT/enhancer binding protein alpha interacts with ZTA and mediates ZTA-induced p21(CIP-1) accumulation and G(1) cell cycle arrest during the Epstein-Barr virus lytic cycle', J Virol, vol. 77, no. 2, pp. 1481-500.

Yip, T. T., Ngan, R. K., Lau, W. H., Poon, Y. F., Joab, I., Cochet, C. & Cheng, A. K. 1994, 'A possible prognostic role of immunoglobulin-G antibody against recombinant Epstein-Barr virus BZLF-1 transactivator protein ZEBRA in patients with nasopharyngeal carcinoma', Cancer, vol. 74, no. 9, pp. 2414-24.

Young, L. S. & Rickinson, A. B. 2004, 'Epstein-Barr virus: 40 years on', Nat Rev Cancer, vol. 4, no. 10, pp. 757-68.

Yu, M. C. 1991, 'Nasopharyngeal carcinoma: epidemiology and dietary factors', IARC Sci Publ, no. 105, pp. 39-47.

Zhang, Q., Holley-Guthrie, E., Ge, J. Q., Dorsky, D. & Kenney, S. 1997, 'The Epstein-Barr virus (EBV) DNA polymerase accessory protein, BMRF1, activates the essential downstream component of the EBV oriLyt', Virology, vol. 230, no. 1, pp. 22-34.

zur Hausen, H. 1999, 'Papillomaviruses in human cancers', Proc Assoc Am Physicians, vol. 111, no. 6, pp. 581-7.

4

Chemical Carcinogenesis and Nasopharyngeal Carcinoma

Faqing Tang[1], Xiaowei Tang[2], Daofa Tian[3] and Ya Cao[4]
[1]Zhuhai Hospital, Jinan University, Guang Dong,
[2]Metallurgical Science and Engineering, Central South University, Changsha, Hunan,
[3]The First Affiliated Hospital, The Hunan University of Traditional- Chinese, Changsha, Hunan,
[4]Cancer Research Institute of Xiangya School of Medicine, Central South University, Changsha, Hunan,
P.R. China

1. Introduction

1.1 Epidemiology of nasopharyngeal carcinoma

The non-viral exposure that is most consistently and strongly associated with risk of nasopharyngeal carcinoma (NPC) is the consumption of salt-preserved fish, a traditional staple food in several NPC-endemic areas [1]. In studies of the Chinese population, the relative risk of NPC associated with weekly consumption of salt-preserved fish generally ranges from 1.4 to 3.2, whereas the risk for daily consumption ranges from 1.8 to 7.5 [2-7]. This indicates that consumption frequency of salt-preserved fish is associated with the risk of NPC. However, elevated NPC risk is also associated with other preserved food items, including meats, eggs, fruits, and vegetables [4-15].

In southern China, intake of salted and other preserved foods is particularly high among boat-dwelling fishermen and their families, this is also the population subgroup at highest risk of developing NPC [16]. Salt-preserved foods are a dietary staple in all NPC-endemic populations [14, 17]. Furthermore, salted fish is a traditional weaning food and is fed early and frequently to infants, especially in the Cantonese population [4, 14] and in families of lower socioeconomic status [3, 18]. Childhood exposure, especially at weaning, appears to be more strongly related to NPC risk than exposure during adulthood [3, 4, 14, 15, 17, 19-21]. This dietary association may partly explain the international distribution of NPC incidence.

The carcinogenic potential of salt-preserved fish is supported by experiments in rats, which develop malignant nasal and nasopharyngeal carcinoma [22-24]. The process of salt preservation is inefficient, allowing fish and other foods to become partially putrefied [25, 26]. As a result, these foods accumulate significant levels of nitrosamines, which are known carcinogens [25, 27-29]. Consumption of salted fish is a significant source of nitrosamines. Total volatile N-nitrosamines, consisting of N-dimethylnitrosamine, N-diethylnitrosamine, N-nitrosopyrrolidine, and N-nitrosopiperidine, are present in salted fish at concentrations of

0.028 to 4.54 mg/kg [25] and are converted into carcinogenic N-nitrosocompounds including N,N′-dinitrosopiperazine after food intake [26]. N-nitrosodimethylamine is the predominant volatile nitrosamine in salted fish. In addition, some bacteria can also induce conversion of nitrate to nitrite, which forms important carcinogenic N-nitroso compounds [26]. Experiments in rats have demonstrated the carcinogenicity of nitrosamines and N-nitroso compounds such as diethylnitrosamine (DEN), dimethlbenzanthracene anthracene (DMBA), and Dinitrosopiperazine (DNP) [6, 15, 30].

2. Carcinogens related to the etiology of human NPC

NPC occurs most frequently in Southeast Asia and Africa. The highest incidence rate is reported to be in the southern provinces of China, and NPC contributes to a high mortality rate among Chinese people [31]. There are many articles and publications focusing on the viral and hereditary factors associated with NPC but few on chemical factors such as environmental carcinogens. The importance of each factor may vary between different tumors and in different areas of the world [32]. Moreover, it appears that a multiple-factor concept of cancer etiology may be relevant to human NPC and chemical carcinogens should be taken into consideration within this context. Although numerous chemical agents are suspected to be related to human tumors, the discussion here will be limited to certain polycyclic hydrocarbons, nitrosamines, and some related compounds that might play a more intimate role in the etiology of human NPC [33].

2.1 Polycyclic aromatic hydrocarbons

Since Pott's [34] observation on scrotal cancer and the first demonstration of the induction of cancer in animals by painting coal tar on the skin, the importance of hydrocarbons in human carcinogenesis has been extended to include a possible role as a risk factor in human NPC.

Some clinicians have paid attention to hydrocarbon as one of the etiological factors of human NPC due to the continued exposure of their patients to coal dust. Furthermore, Schoental et al [35] reported that the incidence rate of NPC was higher among the inhabitants of the mountainous district than in those living at low altitude in the flatlands. It was subsequently found that the inhabitants of districts with a higher incidence of NPC warmed themselves by burning firewood. In low and poorly ventilated living rooms, the accumulation of sooty fumes results in environmental pollution. In the high incidence region, studies found that the benzo(a)pyrene concentration reached a level of 85-29 $\mu g/1{,}000\ m^3$, and that of benzanthrene reached 79-515 $\mu g/1{,}000\ m^3$, so it was believed that NPC in this district is related to exposure to polycyclic aromatic hydrocarbons [36].

Fong YY et al [37] tried to instill the oil extraction of soot obtained from the houses of NPC patients into the nasal cavities of the mice three times a week, but this did not induce NPC. The control group was treated with methylcholanthrene and developed nasal cavity tumors but not NPC. He concluded that nasopharyngeal mucosa is not sensitive to chemical carcinogens. Similarly, Lo et al [38] injected carcinogenic agents methylcholanthrene and benzo(a)pyrene into the nasopharyngeal region of rabbits, rats, mice, and dogs, and did not observe any positive results. In contrast, Pan et al [72, 73] inserted DMBA crystals into ectopically implanted nasopharyngeal tissues of homologous mice, and two cases of squamous carcinoma were induced in 20 mice. This result implied that nasopharyngeal epithelium could be induced to develop carcinoma, and was not insusceptible to these carcinogens.

Toth B et al [39] injected benzo(a)pyrene and dimethylbenzanthrere into AKR mice through the posterior nasal orifice. The induced tumors were mainly located at the hard palate and nasal cavity. Pan et al [72] developed a method for inducing NPC in rats. Long thin polyethylene tubes loaded with benzo(a)pyrene, DMBA, or 3-methylcholanthrene (MC) were inserted into the nasopharyngeal cavities of rats under anesthesia, resulting in squamous carcinoma of the nasopharynx. One animal developed a cancerous ulcer on the mucosa of the nasopharynx. This nasopharynx cancer was a grade III squamous cell carcinoma, which malignant cells grew upwards protruding into the cavity or downwards into the stroma. The incidence rates of the respective groups were as high as those in the group of rats treated with DMBA or DEN.

2.2 Nitrosamines

Since Magee [40] first described the toxicity and carcinogenicity of dimethylnitrosamine in rats, the carcinogenicity of nitroso-compounds in different animals has aroused increasing interest and received intensive investigation. A series of reports confirmed that nitroso-compounds could induce a variety of malignant tumors in a great number of different animal species [41-44]. Moreover, nitroso-compounds may result from the interaction of nitrites and secondary amines. These precursors are produced from nitrosamines by bacterial action in the acidic environment of stomach or alkaline intestinal contents [45, 46]. The putative role of nitroso-compounds in the induction of NPC has fascinated many researchers. Ho [47] raised the tentative assumption that the high incidence of NPC in Hong Kong was due to the ingestion of salted fish as main protein source. An appreciable amount of dimethylnitrosamine was reportedly detected in salted fish in the markets of Hong Kong [48]. However, a control survey carried out in Guangzhou demonstrated no such relationship between NPC and the intake of salted fish [4].

Generally, the saliva of NPC patients has a higher nitrite content and lower nitrate content than that of normal individuals. In addition, the urinary nitrite content of NPC patients was higher than those of normal controls. These differences were statistically significant in Sihui County [49]. It was suggested that nitrate content of saliva from NPC patients might be reduced by microorganisms in oral cavity; however, the precise mechanism needs to be further investigated. Yi Z et al [50] analyzed nitrate levels in saliva and urine samples collected from 75 NPC patients. The nitrate content in the urine sample of these patients was considerably lower than that of normal subjects, whereas the nitrite content was significantly higher in the urine samples of NPC patients. It was proposed that NPC patients might possess certain reduction mechanisms that could reduce nitrates into nitrites, thus resulting in increased urinary excretion of nitrites and enhanced endogenous synthesis of nitroso-compounds.

There were no reports on experimental nasopharyngeal carcinoma induced by nitroso - compounds as carcinogens until 1972. Huang et al [24] reported that out of 22 white rats fed with salted fish, four developed nasal tumors but none developed nasopharyngeal cancer. However, in 1972, Pan et al [72, 73] successfully induced NPC in rats using nitroso-compounds, thus providing new clues in the investigation of the cause of NPC.

3. Establishment of an animal model of NPC with chemical carcinogens

3.1 General principles of establishing a NPC animal model

An important approach in studying the etiology and pathogenesis of malignant tumors is to establish various animal models. As it is impossible to carry out experiments directly on patients, a simple method to induce tumor in animals with high incidence provides a valuable research tool to simulate the human cancer. The following is a discussion on the general principles of establishing a NPC animal model.

3.1.1 Animal selection

There is a great variation in the susceptibility of different animal species to carcinogens. It is better to choose animals with a low incidence of spontaneous tumors and a predicted high incidence of induced tumor. Some scholars originally believed that animal nasopharyngeal epithelium was not susceptible to aromatic hydrocarbons. Nonetheless, Wang successfully induced experimental "NPC in situ" in mice [51]. However, because rat nasopharynx is analogous to that of humans and rats are readily available, the rat is the preferred model animal. The rats used in these experiments were of mixed breeds, but they very rarely suffered from spontaneous tumors.

As a preferred model animal, the anatomical and histological characteristics of rat nasopharyngeal organs were studied in detail. The anatomical location of rat nasopharynx has been clearly defined [52], but some confusing terms are used in these reports to describe the same structure. For example, rat's nasopharynx is tubular, and some authors called it a nasopharyngeal duct. Actually, rat's nasopharynx is histologically similar to that of humans; both are lined with two kinds of epithelia, stratified squamous epithelium and pseudostratified ciliated columnar epithelium, and have orifices of Eustachian tubes near otopharyngeal end. The term "nasopharyngeal duct" may be confused with another tubular structure lying above the hard palate between the nasopharynx and posterior naris, which is lined completely with ciliated columnar epithelium. This structure is often called the nasopharyngeal tube, and is in fact in the posterior part of nasal cavity. Therefore, if the induced tumor was located above the hard palate, it should be classified as a nasal tumor rather than a nasopharyngeal tumor. Certain terms used in these reports, such as "cancer of nasal cavities," "cancer of nasal turbinates," "ethmoid cancer," and "cancer of nasal sinuses," actually describe malignant tumors developed from nasal turbinates, which are often different from NPC in histological appearance.

Leaton-Jones P et al [52] described histology of normal rat nasopharyngeal epithelium in 1971. Subsequently, Albin N et al [53] have systematically studied serial sections of rat nasopharynxes at different ages. They demonstrated that nasopharyngeal epithelium consists of three different kinds of epithelium: pseudostratified ciliated columnar epithelium, stratified squamous epithelium, and transitional epithelium. In adult rats approximately two-thirds of nasopharynx towards cephalic end is lined with ciliated columnar epithelium. The third near oropharyngeal end is a mixed-type epithelium, with increasing abundance of stratified squamous epithelium towards oropharyngeal end. The cover epithelium on roof and lateral sides of nasopharynx is mainly ciliated columnar epithelial cells, with predominantly continuous stratified squamous epithelium at bottom. The nasopharynx of newborn rats is mainly lined with ciliated columnar epithelium, which is poorly differentiated. Stratified squamous epithelium appears 10 days after birth. The nasopharyngeal epithelium of 60-day-old rats is similar to that of adult rats.

3.1.2 Selection of carcinogens and induction methods

Generally, potent carcinogen with short induction time is chosen as tumor-inducing agent, for example, benzo(a)pyrene for lung cancer induction [54] and aflatoxin for liver cancer [55]. Human NPC is too complicated to determine one or two factors because there are many factors involved in NPC development, such as viral and genetic factors, chemical carcinogens in the environment [56]. Moreover, the etiology of human cancers can be complicated, and might not be attributed to a single factor or initiation event [2]. The combined action of chemical carcinogens, viruses, and genetic factor, and also co-carcinogens should be discussed.

3.2 Establishment of experimental NPC and further studies

3.2.1 Establishment of the NPC animal model

After establishing the optimal carcinogens and method of administration, we succeeded in the induction of experimental NPC in rats using DNP [57]. This suggests that chemical carcinogens might be among etiologic factors of NPC. Furthermore, subcutaneous injection of DNP could induce NPC without complications of liver cancer. Therefore, DNP showed organ specificity for nasopharyngeal epithelium. Moreover, DNP-induced NPC exhibited a consistently high incidence rate, thereby paving the way for a subsequent study of DNP in which the carcinogenesis of experimental NPC in rats was further investigated, including atypical cytokinetics in carcinogenesis of the nasopharyngeal epithelium, DNA damage and repair of the nasopharyngeal epithelium by DNP and its relation to tissue specificity, and changes in enzyme activities during carcinogenesis. The results of these studies are discussed below.

3.2.2 Susceptibility of rat nasopharyngeal epithelium to the carcinogens DEN and DMBA

The induction of NPC in rats by treatment with DEN and DMBA is summarized in Table 1 [72, 73]. These studies showed that the highest incidence of NPC was achieved in the DEN instillation group, and that NPC with less differentiated cells at early stages developed in the rats receiving DEN instillation and DMBA insertion. Occasional lymphatic emboli and multiple metastases to lung were observed. The data suggest some synergic effect between these chemical compounds.

Incidence of NPC in the DEN instillation group was higher than that of the group treated with *s.c.* injection of DEN and empty plastic tube insertion. This suggested that DNE was most effective on nasopharyngeal epithelium. The group with empty tube insertion was examined to exclude any possible carcinogenic action of the polyvinyl chloride tube. The empty tube itself occasionally induced NPC (two cases of NPC in 23 rats). Incidence of NPC in this group was quite lower than other groups [72, 73]. Therefore, it was suggested that NPC development in these groups was mainly caused by the action of carcinogens.

Group	Administration route	Examined animals	Number of tumors	Incidence of NPC (%)
Saline	Subcutaneous	10	0	0
DEN	Instillation	27	17	63
DMBA	Loaded-tube insertion	45	18	40
DEN+DMBA	DEN:subcutaneous DMBA: loaded-tube insertion	27	16	59

Table 1. NPC induced in rats by DEN and DMBA

The induced tumors resembled human nasopharyngeal cancers but were of a well-differentiated type, including squamous cell carcinoma (Grade I and II), occasional multiform cell type, and papillary or basal cell carcinomas [57, 72, 73]. The serial sections of nasopharynx enabled us to trace number, sites, and distribution, as well as histogenesis of experimental NPC. This model could be helpful in further study on nasopharyngeal carcinogenesis. The finding that chemical carcinogens such as nitrosamine and aromatic hydrocarbon compounds are capable of inducing nasopharyngeal carcinoma in rats suggests that chemical carcinogens might be one of the etiological factors of human nasopharyngeal carcinoma.

3.2.3 Induction of nasopharyngeal carcinoma by nitroso-compounds

DEN, DNP, and cyclic nitrosocompounds including nitrosomorpholin could induce NPC. The next step was to facilitate studies on pathomorphology, histogenesis, and carcinogenesis of experimental NPC. Two methods were used to minimize the occurrence of hepatoma in DEN-treated rats: the rats were injected intramuscularly with vitamin B_{12} twice a week and given glucose in their drinking water at the time of DEN administration. DEN was sometimes given through rectal instillation because it causes little damage to this organ. Rats were treated with cyclic nitroso-compounds by two treatment methods, *s.c.* injection and nasopharyngeal instillation. The results of these studies are shown in Table 2 [72, 73].

Groups	n	NPC			animals	incidence
		In situ	Early invasive	Invasive	tumor	of NPC (%)
Saline	30	0	0	0	0	0
DEN Inst.	98	11	37	21	69	70
DEN Inj.	16	1	3	0	4	25
DEN Rectal Adm.	23	1	5	0	6	26
DEN Nasal Inst. +Vit.B12-glucose	42	4	24	11	39	93

Inst, instillation; Inj, injection; Adm, administration; Vit, vitamin

Table 2. Induction of NPC by DEN administered by various routes

The data showed that DEN instillation resulted in the highest incidence of NPC. The highest incidence of tumor was in the group treated with DEN and vitamin B_{12}, followed by the group given nitrosomorpholin carcinogen. Two tumors with a nodular and ulcerated appearance were visible to the naked eye, one in DEN group and one in nitrosomorpholin group. Both cases were squamous cell carcinomas, partly involving or arising from the soft palate. These tumors invaded surrounding stroma, nerve bundles, and salivary glands without lymph node metastasis.

A few other points were of interest: (a) many squamous carcinomas occurred in neighborhood of auditory pharyngeal tubes or extended along tube walls, indicating that pathological lesions occurred in nasopharyngeal cavity. (b) In nasal cavities of some rats with extensive tumor, the tumor was found only in nasopharyngeal region without invasion of the nasal cavities or the base of the skull. Under naked-eye examination, no tumor was visible in the esophagus or other organs except the liver. (c) Subcutaneous injection of cyclic nitrosamines induced a considerably high incidence of nasopharyngeal tumors, providing some clues to organ specificity of carcinogens. (d) It is worth noting that administration of vitamin B_{12} markedly increased the incidence of nasopharyngeal cancer ($p<0.01$), but significantly decreased the incidence of hepatoma. Poirier et al [58] observed that vitamin B_{12} enhanced hepatic carcinogenesis and shortened the animals' lives. In the present experiments, vitamin B_{12} increased the incidence of NPC in the DEN group but had the opposite effect in the DNP group. The precise mechanism of this complicated relationship between the carcinogen and nutritional factors needs further study. (e) Vitamin B_{12}, piperazine, and morpholin are usually used in clinics or in pharmaceutical chemistry. Some of them are precursors of the carcinogenic substance and some have an enhancing effect on the development of cancer.

Further investigation into experimental induction of NPC showed that N-nitrosomorpholin and DNP could induce NPC in rats, and subcutaneous injection of DNP could induce NPC without complications of liver cancer. These results are summarized in Table 3 [72, 73].

Group	n	Sex	NPC	Nasal cavity	Esophageal	Other
1	12	M	8	6	3	Soft palate 1
2	13	F	10	8	5	Tongue root 1, soft palate2
3	18	M	18	11	10	Tongue root1,soft palate 4, maxilla1
4	20	M	18	14	14	Tongue root 1, soft palate 5

M, male; F, female

Table 3. Types and site distribution of tumors induced by DNP

A total of 54 rats developed NPC in this experiment. In addition, 39 cancers of the nasal cavities, 32 esophageal tumors, and a few other tumors were observed. Upon postmortem examination, six rats were found to have gross tumor masses in nasopharynx, and two of these had a cauliflower-like tumor mass on the soft palate, representing co-existing squamous cell carcinoma of the soft palate. The induced nasopharyngeal tumors were all squamous cell carcinomas, most of which were well-differentiated (Fig. 1). The cancer pattern observed in this experiment was somewhat different from that of NPC induced by diethylnitrosamine. The cancer cells invaded the stroma in trabecular or branched cords, but more frequently grew intraepithelially to form patches of masses before invading the stroma. A lymphatic cancer embolus consisting of poorly differentiated cancer cells was found in a case of invasive NPC. No metastatic foci could be found in the lymph nodes of this animal [72, 73].

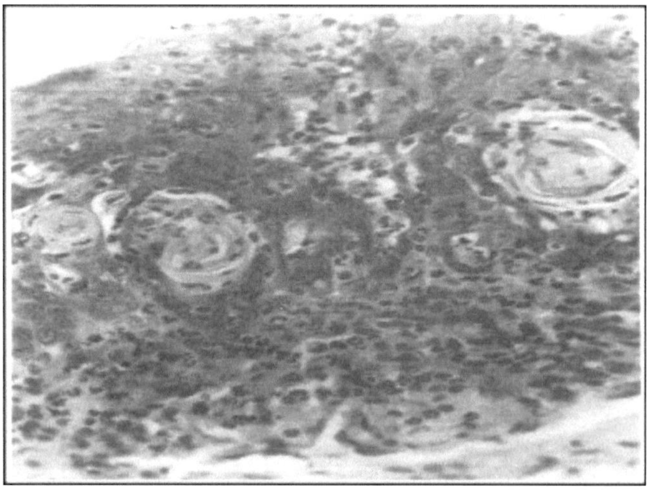

Fig. 1. DNP- induced early nasopharyngeal cancer **(**Original magnification, ×200**).** Wistar rats were injected subcutaneously with DNP in a stumped needle at a dosage of 40 mg/kg, twice a week and 38 times in total to accumulation dose of 99.5–122 mg per rat. The rats were sacrificed to collect nasopharyngeal samples at 308 days after DNP injections. Nasopharyngeal samples were histopathologically examined under microscope 200.

Most of nasal cavity tumors developed from nasal turbinates. Occasionally, tumors destroyed nasal bone and bulged out as a local prominence. The soft tumor mass with a pink-grey tint frequently destroyed cribriform plate and invaded or replaced olfactory bulb, but it was well demarcated from brain tissue. The tumors of nasal cavity were of different histological types, including squamous cell carcinoma, adenocarcinoma, and the so-called "olfactory neuroepithelial tumor." The olfactory neuroepithelial tumors had a pleomorphic histology that suggested that these tumors originated from epithelia. On gross examination, most of esophageal tumors were multiple papillomas, that developed mainly from the upper and middle parts of esophagus; these papillomas were histologically confirmed as squamous cell carcinoma [73].

Some remaining points need to be clarified: (a) the induced rat NPC was of a squamous cell type. Most of tumors were well-differentiated and developed from base and lateral side of nasopharynx, and some co-existed with squamous carcinoma of soft palate mucosa. There was rarely distant metastasis; in this regard NPC induced by nitroso-compounds was somewhat different from human NPC. (b) DNP-induced NPC and cancer of nasal cavities and esophagus in rats resulted from a subcutanrouic effect. (c) Nitroso-compounds often exist as cis- and trans-isomers, and rapid axial-equatorial conversion of dinitrospiperazin and the respective carcinogenicity of these isomers should be explored in the future.

4. Morphologic and histogenetic studies of experimental NPC

In the normal rat, cephalic and middle portion of nasopharyngeal cavity is covered by ciliated columnar epithelium, while caudal portion is covered by squamous and columnar epithelium.

4.1 Pathology of the experimental NPC

In the soft palates of tumor-bearing rats, nodules ranging from1-2 mm to 1cm in diameter were observed by palpation. Some of the invasive tumors were ulcerative cauliflowerlike or nodular in appearance when the soft palate was cut open, cancerous ulcer with elevated irregular edge was observed when cancerous ulcer with elevated irregular edge was cut open [24]. Under the microscope, cancer cell foci in different stages of differentiation could be found in many serial sections, indicating the multiple growth pattern of malignancy (Fig.1. DNP- induced early nasopharyngeal cancer. Wistar rats were injected subcutaneously with DNP in a stumped needle at a dosage of 40 mg/kg, twice a week and 38 times in total to accumulation dose of 99.5–122 mg per rat. The rats were sacrificed to collect nasopharyngeal samples at 308 days after DNP injections. Nasopharyngeal samples were histopathologically examined under microscope 200). A localized solitary malignancy was observed in rats that received carcinogen for a short period. Tumors often developed at the base of nasopharynx or at the junction of the base and lateral side of nasopharyngeal wall. Carcinomas in situ, and early invasive or infiltrative carcinomas were observed, and were of a well-differentiated squamous cell type [73].

The diagnostic criterion of experimental NPC is generally that of human nasopharyngeal cancer, but the structural characteristics of rat nasopharynx must also be taken into consideration. For example, the epithelium at nasopharynx base, especially at nasopharynx roof next to skull base, consists of two or three layers of cells surrounded by bony plates[59]. The observed malignancy may be composed of basal cells with thin solid strands of cancer cells.

Carcinoma in situ, early invasive carcinoma, and infiltrative carcinoma were observed in tumor-bearing rats. Carcinoma in situ might arise from epithelium of normal thickness, or from highly hyperplastic or atrophic epithelium (Fig.2. DEN- induced nasopharyngeal cancer. Wistar rats were injected subcutaneously with DEN in a stumped needle at a dosage of 40 mg/kg, twice a week and 38 times in total to accumulation dose of 89.8–119.3 mg per rat. The rats were sacrificed to collect nasopharyngeal samples at 365 days after DEN injections. Nasopharyngeal samples were histopathologically examined under microscope). It often originates from columnar epithelium and evolves through squamous cell metaplasia, atypical hyperplasia, and Grade I and II anaplasia. The early invasive lesions were of two types: arising from basal layer with normal looking superficial layers, or extending into stroma (primarily seen in the DEN group). Downward growth of the lesion, which formed trabecular, branching, rounded, or small square nests, infiltrated into the stroma. The neoplasms were usually moderately or even poorly differentiated squamous carcinomas. This downward growth of neoplasms, which often occurs in human NPC, may cause difficulty in early detection or in producing a good smear of exfoliative cells for cytological diagnosis [57,72,73].

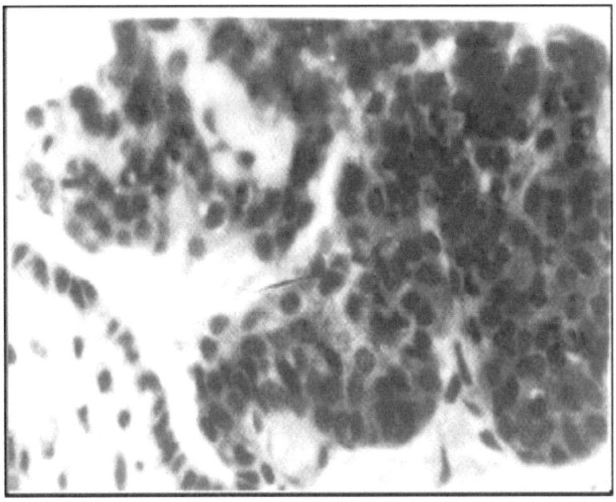

Fig. 2. DEN- induced nasopharyngeal cancer (Original magnification, ×400). Wistar rats were injected subcutaneously with DEN in a stumped needle at a dosage of 40 mg/kg, twice a week and 38 times in total to accumulation dose of 89.8–119.3 mg per rat. The rats were sacrificed to collect nasopharyngeal samples at 365 days after DEN injections. Nasopharyngeal samples were histopathologically examined under microscope 400.

Arising from a dyaplasitc squamous epithelium, cancer protruded into nasopharyngeal cavity at the one hand and invaded the stroma at the other. This growth pattern occurred more frequently in the DNP group, and sometimes formed papillary carcinomas [57,72,73]. The infiltrative carcinomas were usually of a squamous cell type, although basal cell carcinoma was observed occasionally. This kind of tumor growth could be seen in many serial sections. The cancer cells forming trabecular, solid masses, or patches were not well differentiated at the periphery but had cornified cells in the central portion. Cancer cells invaded salivary glands, muscle, and nerve bundles with occasional lymphatic emboli but without widespread metastases to the lymph nodes. The primary site or origin of the infiltrative tumor was usually difficult to recognize, but could occasionally be traced by serial sectioning.

4.2 The histogenesis of experimental NPC

In early lesions, dysplasia occurred in the ciliated columnar, transitional, or squamous epithelium, and was possibly preceded or accompanied by squamous metaplasia. ^{3}H-thymidine autoradiography showed that a single dose of dinitrospiperazine could cause DNA damage of the squamous or transitional cells followed by unscheduled DNA synthesis [74]. This may give some clues to NPC carcinogenesis. Hyperplastic, dysplastic, and neoplastic foci often co-existed without sharp demarcation. The cancer cell population was more localized and clearly demarcated from the surrounding normal epithelium or stromal tissues. Inflammatory infiltration into the surrounding normal stroma was rarely found except in ulcerative carcinomas.

NPC was present in multiple serial sections due to the extension of a large tumor mass or multiple diffusely scattered lesions. Some of the irregular cords or trabeculae of tumor cells, arising from different portions of the epithelium, might finally fuse together to form a large solid mass of tumor [57, 72, 73]. It was evident that most of the lesions were multicentric rather than unicentric in origin. Sometimes the same cancer cell focus contained not only undifferentiated fusiform cells and small cornified epithelial pearls, but also small cysts containing mucinous material. These kinds of lesions may be seen in human NPC and are considered to represent the biphasic differentiation of nasopharyngeal epithelium.

4.3 Statistical analysis of NPC carcinogenesis

The well-known two-stage concept suggested by Berenblum et al [60] was developed from experimental study of carcinogenesis. They proposed that carcinogenesis might be divided into two different but related stages, a stage of specific initiation and a stage of relatively non-specific promotion. However, on the basis of epidemiological data and statistical studies of human cancer, carcinogenesis is generally considered a multi-hit/multi-step process. The multistage theory of carcinogenesis proposed by Amitage and Dell is representative of this concept [61]. Therefore, it is interesting to analyze the carcinogenesis of experimental NPC by means of mathematical statistics.

Yao et al [73] reported the results of statistical analysis of experimental NPC induced by DNP. The corrected cumulative percentage of dead rats with NPC was calculated and fitted with Weibull and lognormal distributions. The data fitted both distributions well as verified by χ^2-test, but the value of χ^2 was smaller in the Wieibull distribution than in the lognormal distribution. The mathematical expression of NPC carcinogenesis in rats according to Weibull distribution was as follows:

$$G=1-e^{-2.55\times10^{-4}(t-192)^{1.69}}$$

G, corrected cumulative percentage of the dead rats bearing NPC; t, time in days

Peto [62] and Emmelot et al[63] suggested that Weibull's distribution represents the number of "hits" or "stages" in cancer development. Therefore, the above mathematical expression seems to indicate that rat NPC development experienced two hits. Using retrospective survey data of cancer mortalities in Hunan Province, Yao [73] analyzed the age distribution of NPC mortality and proposed that the development of NPC needs three hits. Hence, the relationship and differences between carcinogenesis in experimental NPC and human NPC need to be explored further.

4.4 Carcinogenesis mechanism of experimental NPC

4.4.1 Atypical cytokinetics of nasopharyngeal epithelium in rats treated with DNP

Cytokinetic studies may be helpful in elucidating the mechanism of carcinogenesis and providing important data for improving chemotherapeutic regimens for malignancies. In 1981, Chen et al [74] studied the cytokinetics of nasopharyngeal epithelium of rats treated with DNP using stathmokinetic and autoradiographic techniques. The mitotic blocking agent selected was vincristine, which had an optimal dose of 0.83 mg/kg body weight and a blocking effect that lasted 10 to 12 h. The metaphase chromosomes of mitotic cells appeared as deeply stained rosette-like structures under the microscope. The cytokinetic parameters of normal and DNP-treated rats were measured *in vivo* using ^{3}H-TdR labeling in combination with stathmokinetics. After DNP treatment there were many hyperplastic foci in nasopharyngeal squamous epithelium. Within the hyperplastic foci and apparently normal nasopharyngeal epithelium there was a significant increase in the number of labeled basal cells, but no change in labeling index (LI) of the transitional epithelium lining the lateral side of nasopharynx.

In normal rats, LI was highest in the squamous epithelium lining nasopharynx lateral side, followed by the base and then the transitional epithelium. The differences between these were highly significant. After DNP treatment, LI of both the lateral and base side increased, and there was no difference between them. This suggested that LI of the bottom side increased more significantly than that of the lateral side. In the normal rats, ^{3}H-TdR labeled cells in nasopharyngeal squamous epithelium were confined to the basal layer (Fig.3. Autoradiograph of nasopharyngeal squamous epithelium of normal rat, showing labeled cells in basal cell layer. Rats were treated with vincristine at 0.83 mg/kg body weight for 12 h, and then ^{3}H-TdR was injected for 1 h. The rats were sacrificed to collect nasopharyngeal samples. The nasopharyngeal samples were histopathologically examined. Cells with ^{3}H-TdR labeling were observed under microscope.). After DNP treatment, there was a significant increase in the number of labeled basal cells. Moreover, a few cells in the prickle cell layer were found to be labeled, indicating that the proliferation compartment had expanded. This phenomenon suggested that stem cells in the G0 stage might enter the proliferation stage and the two daughter cells of mitosis had proliferative ability. S phase of nasopharyngeal epithelium located at the lateral bottom side was prolonged from 6.7 to 9 h after DNP treatment. The time of cell cycle can be calculated according to the formula if the proliferation of nasopharyngeal epithelium in normal and DNP-treated rats remains in steady state.

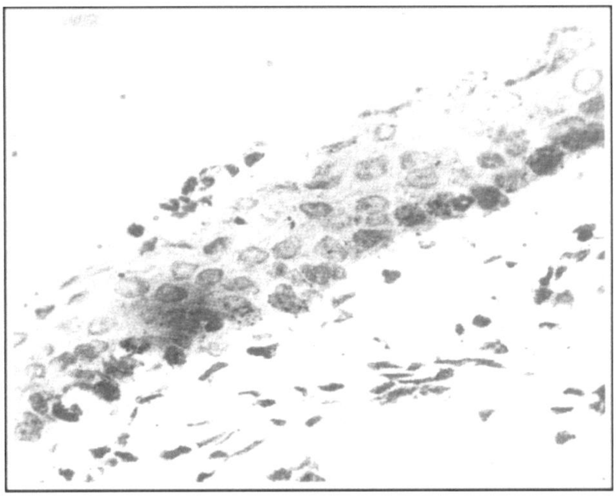

Fig. 3. Autoradiograph of nasopharyngeal squamous epithelium of normal rat, showing labeled cells in basal cell layer (Original magnification, ×400). For mitotic blocking of nasopharyngeal epithelium, rats were treated with vincristine at 0.83 mg/kg body weight for 12 h. ^{3}H-TdR (0.5 mCi/kg bodyweight) was intraperitoneally injected into the rats for 1 h. The rats were sacrificed to collect nasopharyngeal samples. The nasopharyngeal samples were histopathologically examined. Cells with ^{3}H-TdR labeling were observed under microscope 400

Carcinogenesis is a multistep process. Cytokinetic parameters may be changed with morphological progression from normal epithelium, hyperplasia, atypical hyperplasia, to carcinoma. Atypical cytokinetics, increased LI, expansion of the proliferation compartment, and prolongation of S phase were observed in nasopharyngeal epithelium after DNP treatment.

4.4.2 Effect of DNP on ^{3}H-thymidine incorporation into DNA of rat nasopharyngeal epithelium

The adult rats were sacrificed at 4 hrs after a single injection of DNP intramuscularly, and then the tissue fragments of nasopharynx, esophayus, kidney and liver were cultured in ^{3}H - thymidine - 199 medium for 10 hrs. Autoradiography was performed to examine ^{3}H - thymidine labeled epithelial cells. The experimental data indicated that LI of nasopharyngeal epithelium markedly decreased to 2.40% in the experimental group with DNP treatment compared with the saline control, which suggested that a single dose of DNP inhibits DNA synthesis of nasopharyngeal epithelium. This inhibition may be result of DNA damage, providing a key link in carcinogenesis process of experimental nasopharyngeal cancer [73].

4.4.3 Organotropic action of nitroso-compound carcinogensis

Le et al [75] injected 0.25% DNP solution (15 mg/kg bodyweight) into the dorsum of rats. Animals were sacrificed by cervical dislocation at 4 h, 79 h, and 124 h after injection. ^{3}H-TdR (0.5 mCi/kg bodyweight) was injected intraperitoneally 1 h before the animals were sacrificed. The nasopharynx, esophagus, and forestomach were sectioned and processed histologically and autoradiographically. A count of 1,000 consecutive basal cells was performed in the epithelia of nasopharynx, esophagus, and fore stomach of each animal. The labeled cells (>5 silver grains/nucleus) were scored and the LIs were expressed as percentages of the mean value for the controls of the same experiment. LI of squamous epithelia in the base of nasopharynx and esophagus significantly decreased 4 h after DNP injection and recovered gradually by the 3rd and 5th days; the LI of squamous epithelium in nasopharynx base was actually significantly higher than that of the control at 5 days after DNP injection. LI in the squamous epithelium of forestomach did not significantly change at 4 h or on the 3rd day, but declined significantly 5 days after DNP treatment.

4.4.4 Unscheduled DNA Synthesis (UDS)

UDS was detected autoradiographically. 30, 50 or 80 mg/kg in 0.5% DNP was injected subcutaneously into the dorsum of rats [64] and an equivalent amount of saline was injected into rats of the control group. The rats were sacrificed 2 h after injection and small epithelial tissue fragments of the nasal concha, soft palate, esophagus, and forestomach, as well as the basal and lateral side of nasopharynx, were removed immediately. The tissues were processed histologically and autoradiographically. It is easy to identify the nuclei of S phase cells by their extremely heavy labeling. UDS was considered present if there were at least nuclei, each covered by 5-20 silver grains, in a cluster and the number of grains covering the nuclei was no more than that of the background (Fig.4. UDS autoradiograph of nasopharyngeal squamous epithelium. DNP was injected subcutaneously into the dorsum of rats at 80 mg/kg. The rats were sacrificed 2 h after injection, and the epithelial tissue fragments of nasal concha were immediately removed. The tissues samples were processed histologically and autoradiographically). The results showed that at 4 h after subcutaneous injection of DNP (30 mg/kg), DNA synthesis was inhibited in the squamous epithelia of nasopharynx base and esophagus, both of which are tumor prone [75]. This finding is in agreement with reports of Mirvish [65] et al that some carcinogens inhibited DNA synthesis in their respective target organs. While UDS induction was not detected in the forestomach, there are no references indicating that carcinoma of the stomach was induced by DNP. It was also noted that UDS was autoradiographically present only in the epithelia of organs prone to develop cancer after DNP treatment whereas no fibroblasts in the stroma were positive for UDS. These findings suggest that DNP fails to induce any local and distant sarcoma in the rats, and may be related to selective activation of carcinogens in the target organs epithelia with subsequent DNA damage and repair.

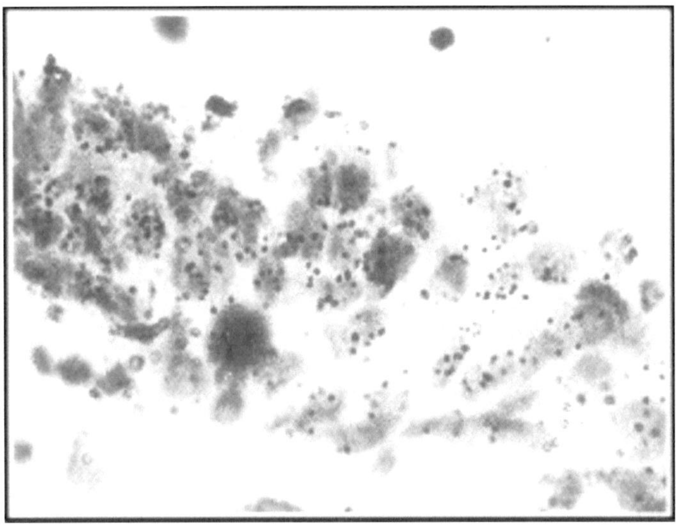

Fig. 4. UDS autoradiograph of nasopharyngeal squamous epithelium. DNP was injected subcutaneously into the dorsum of rats at 80 mg/kg. The rats were sacrificed 2 h after injection, and the epithelial tissue fragments of nasal concha were immediately removed. The tissues samples were processed histologically and autoradiographically. UDS was considered present when nuclei with 5-20 silver grains UDS positive (Original magnification, ×1000)

4.4.5 Induction of lactic dehydrogenase, its isozymes, and acid esterase in NPC by DNP

To investigate enzymatic and isozymatic changes in NPC development, concentrations of urea and pyruvate for the demonstration of H-type and M-type isozymes were determined [76]. The reaction intensity was scored as grade 0-4, depending on the size and color of the formazan granules. The data were statistically analyzed by the ranked data method. There was no significant difference in total activity between squamous and ciliated columnar epithelium, but the reaction in transitional epithelium was more intense. All normal epithelia were mainly of the M-type. In the late embryonic stage, nasopharynx was well developed but covered with less differentiated epithelium. In the medial stage, undifferentiated flat cuboid cells located below brain vesicle between the optic cups on both sides of bony plate were designated as primordial respiratory epithelium. The activity of lactic dehydrogenase and its isozymes in nasopharynx during the embryonic and neonatal stages was as follows: In the medial stage, enzymatic activity of the undifferentiated epithelium was clearly higher than that of the late embryonic stage and neonatal rats, but no significant difference was found between the latter two groups. In the nasopharyngeal epithelium of medial, late embryonic, or neonatal stages, the isozymes were mainly of M-type.

After DNP treatment for 7 months, different kinds of lesions were present in the nasopharyngeal epithelium, such as hyperplasia, dysplasia, carcinoma in situ, and early invasive growth. There were 14 cases of NPC in 24 rats, and some of these had more than one lesion, a total of 22 cancer foci composed of three carcinomas in situ, 14 early infiltrative lesions, and five papillary carcinomas. The histochemical results demonstrated that there was no difference in enzymatic activity of squamous epithelium in normal and experimental groups, while hyperplastic and dysplastic squamous epithelium showed higher enzymatic activity than the normal cells. During these stages, the increased isozymes were mainly of the M-type. In the 22 cancer foci, total activity of lactic dehydrogenase and isozymes (including both M- and H-types) increased to a much higher level than that of the normal tissue, and total activity and isozyme types resembled the undifferentiated cells of the 14- to 17-day-old embryos. At this stage there was also a high level of H-type isozyme activity. Nasopharyngeal epithelium in hyperplastic, dysplastic, or neoplastic stages showed an appreciable increase in the enzymes activity. During the first and second stages, the isozyme was initially mainly M-type, and then H-type isozymes. Since the lactic dehydrogenase in normal nasopharyngeal epithelium was mainly of M-type, the increase in H-type isozyme activity might represent abnormal gene expression during the course of carcinogenesis.

There were two different types of enzymatic change in carcinogenesis course induced by DNP. Lactic dehydrogenase activity increased throughout the stages from hyperplasia and dysplasia up to neoplasia, while acid nonspecific esterase activity significantly increased in the hyperplastic stage, and then decreased or even disappeared in the neoplastic lesions. This suggests that nonspecific esterase is related to the development, diagnosis, and prognosis of carcinoma.

Esterase activity was histochemically detected in the different sites of nasopharynx, with stronger activity in the base wall than in other sites. The activity was different in various types of nasopharyngeal epithelia; stronger activity was observed in the stratified squamous and transitional epithelium than in the ciliated columnar epithelium, but the intensity was similar in the squamous and transitional epithelium. The deposits of esterase in squamous epithelium were diffusely distributed in the cytoplasm of basal and spinous cells, which were mainly localized at the margin of cilia and cytoplasm of cells. The former were distributed diffusely, while the latter took the shape of dot-like granules. Very weak activity was observed in the goblet cells and the reaction in transitional epithelium was similar to that in the squamous epithelium.

There were hyperplastic lesions in the squamous epithelium of all animals treated with DNP for 7 months. The enzymatic activity was markedly decreased compared with the surrounding epithelia, squamous epithelium of the control animals, or hyperplasic lesions. No difference was found between dysplasia and neoplasia. In short, enzymatic activity increased in hyperplasia but was decreased in dysplasia and neoplasia, and sometimes even totally disappeared. Similarly, the esterase activity of human NPC was markedly decreased compared with the surrounding epithelia of the cancer foci and the squamous or ciliated columnar epithelia of the nasopharynx in the control cases, and decreased to varying extents in different cancer cells of various cases or in different foci of the same case. The reactivity remained in well-differentiated cancer cells, but entirely disappeared in poorly differentiated cancer cells.

5. Molecular and signal transduction activated by chemical carcinogens

5.1 Biomolecular and signal pathways activated by DEN

Activation of β-catenin is the central effector of canonical Wnt pathway. DEN-induced tumorigenesis was examined in hepatic β-catenin conditional knockout (β-cat KO) mice. β-cat KO mice show a paradoxical increase in susceptibility to DEN-induced tumorigenesis. This accelerated tumorigenesis is due to increased injury and inflammation, unrestricted oxidative stress, fibrosis, and a compensatory increase in hepatocyte proliferation secondary to PDGFRα/phosphoinositide 3-kinase (PIK3CA)/Akt activation and c-Myc overexpression. Loss of β-catenin impairs the ability of liver to counteract DEN-induced oxidative stress and enhances tumorigenesis through PDGFRα/PIK3CA/Akt signaling. [66].

C/EBPα is a transcription factor that regulates liver quiescence. Phosphorylation of C/EBPα at serine 193 (S193-ph) is upregulated in older mice and is thought to contribute to age-associated liver dysfunction. DEN treatment of knock-in mice expressing a phospho-mimetic aspartic acid residue in place of serine at position 193 (S193D) of C/EBPα induces the formation of liver cancer, and actually results in earlier development of liver tumors. DEN/phenobarbital treatment is associated with specific degradation of both the S193-ph and S193D isoforms of C/EBPα through activation of the ubiquitin-proteasome system (UPS) [66].

The role of PBP/MED1 [peroxisome proliferator-activated receptor-binding protein (PBP)/mediator subunit 1 (MED1)] in DEN-induced hepatocarcinogenesis was also examined. The carcinogenic process of PBP/MED1D mice was initiated by injection of DEN and initiated cells were promoted with phenobarbital. These mice revealed a striking proliferative response in the few residual PBP/MED1-positive hepatocytes that escaped Cre-mediated deletion of the PBP/MED1 gene. No proliferative expansion of PBP/MED1 null hepatocytes was noted in the PBP/MED1DLiv mouse livers. Multiple hepatocellular carcinomas developed in the DEN-initiated PBP/MED1fl/fl and PBP/MED1DLiv mice [67].

DEN may activate PDGFRα/PIK3CA/Akt signaling through β-Catenin, and mediate C/EBPα phosphorylation through the ubiquitin-proteasome system (UPS), and regulate PBP/MED1, and involve nasopharyngeal carcinogenesis.

5.2 Biomolecular and signal pathways activated by DMAB

When K5-protein kinase C-alpha (PKCA) mice (transgenic mice that overexpress PKCA in the epidermis) were initiated with DMBA and promoted with a low dose of 12-O-tetradecanoylphorbol-13-acetate (TPA), 58% of the mice developed skin papillomas that progressed to carcinoma. CXCR2 is expressed by keratinocytes and transformation by oncogenic ras (a hallmark of DMBA initiation) or TPA exposure induced all CXCR2 ligands. Ras induction of CXCR2 ligands was mediated by autocrine activation of epidermal growth factor receptor and nuclear factor-KB, and potentiated by PKCA. Oncogenic ras also induced CXCR2 ligands in keratinocytes that were genetically ablated for CXCR2. *In vitro*, CXCR2 was found to be essential for CXCR2 ligand-stimulated migration of ras-transformed keratinocytes and for ligand activation of the extracellular signal-regulated kinase (ERK) and Akt pathways. Both cell migration and activation of ERK and Akt were restored by CXCR2 reconstitution of CXCR2 null keratinocytes [68].

Constitutive activation of signal transducer and activator of transcription 3 (Stat3) has been described in a variety of human malignancies and has been suggested to play an important role in carcinogenesis. The epidermis of inducible Stat3-deficient mice treated with 4-hytroxytamoxifen (TM) showed a significant increase in apoptosis induced by DMBA and reduced proliferation following exposure to TPA. In two-stage skin carcinogenesis assays, inducible Stat3-deficient mice treated with TM during the promotion stage showed a significant delay in tumor development and a significantly reduced number of tumors compared with control groups. Inducible Stat3-deficient mice treated with TM before initiation with DMBA also showed a significant delay in tumor development and a significantly reduced number of tumors compared with control groups [69]

5.3 Biomolecular and signal transduction targeted by DNP

DNP displays some degree of organ specificity for nasopharyngeal epithelium in inducing rat NPC. To clarify the mechanism underlying this DNP organotropic action, a rat NPC model was constructed using DNP, and atypical hyperplasic nasopharyngeal and NPC tissue was obtained from rats at different stages of tumorigenesis. Differential protein expression was screened using proteome analysis and further confirmed by immunoblotting. Expression of heat shock protein 70 (HSP70) and Mucin was increased in the atypical hyperplasia and NPC cells, and we therefore postulated that DNP might up-regulate these genes. In further studies to determine whether DNP does regulate HSP70 and Mucin, we treated HENE cells (cultured from biopsies of normal nasopharyngeal tissue) with 2μM and 4μM DNP and showed that expression of HSP70 and Mucin increased in dose-dependent manner. To confirm the specificity of DNP, we used arsenite as a control because its carcinogenicity has previously been proven [70]. Expression of HSP70 and Mucin was not induced by arsenite. We therefore think that HSP70 and Mucin might be specific and important targets of DNP [57].

DNP induced expression of phosphorylated ezrin at threonine 567 (phos-ezrin Thr567) in a dose- and time-dependent manner in 6-10B nasopharyngeal carcinoma cells (Fig.5 Effects of DNP on ezrin phosphorylation at Thr 567. 6-10B cells were treated with 2 or 4 μM DNP for 24 h (A), and treated with 4μM DNP for 12 or 24 h (B), and ezrin and phos-ezrin expression were assayed with immunoblotting). Furthermore, DNP-induced expression of phos-ezrin Thr567 was dependent on increased Rho kinase and PKC activity. The activation of Rho kinase and PKC occurred through binding to Rho kinase pleckstrin-homology (PH) and promotion of PKC translocation to the plasma membrane. Ezrin is associated with induction of filopodia growth in 6-10B cells, and further studies showed that DNP induces filopodia formation in 6-10B NPC cells and also increases invasion and motility of these cells. This indicated that DNP is involved in NPC metastasis, and DNP-mediated NPC metastasis was indeed confirmed in nude mice. However, DNP did not effectively induce motility and invasion of DNP-treated NPC cells containing ezrin mutated at Thr 567. Similarly, motility and invasion were not induced in DNP-treated NPC cells transfected with si-RNAs against Rho or PKC. These findings indicate that DNP induces ezrin phosphorylation at Thr567, increases motility and invasion of cells, and promotes tumor metastasis. DNP may therefore be involved in NPC metastasis through regulation of ezrin phosphorylation at Thr567 [71].

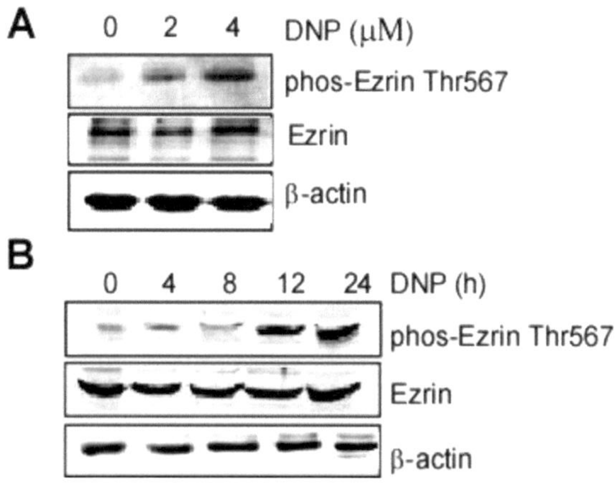

Fig. 5. Effects of DNP on ezrin phosphorylation at Thr 567. 6-10B cells were treated with 2 or 4 μM DNP for 24 h (A), and treated with 4μM DNP for 12 or 24 h (B), and ezrin and phos-ezrin expression were assayed with immunoblotting.

6. Acknowledgment

This work was in part supported by National Natural Science Foundation of China (81071718, 81000881), Program for New Century Excellent Talents in University, NCET (NCET-06-0685), the Fundamental Research Funds for the Central Universities

7. References

[1] West S, Hildesheim A, Dosemeci M: Non-viral risk factors for nasopharyngeal carcinoma in the Philippines: results from a case-control study. *Int J Cancer* 1993, 55(5):722-727.

[2] Henderson BE, Louie E: Discussion of risk factors for nasopharyngeal carcinoma. *IARC Sci Publ* 1978(20):251-260.

[3] Yu MC, Ho JH, Lai SH, Henderson BE: Cantonese-style salted fish as a cause of nasopharyngeal carcinoma: report of a case-control study in Hong Kong. *Cancer Res* 1986, 46(2):956-961.

[4] Yu MC, Huang TB, Henderson BE: Diet and nasopharyngeal carcinoma: a case-control study in Guangzhou, China. *Int J Cancer* 1989, 43(6):1077-1082.

[5] Armstrong RW, Imrey PB, Lye MS, Armstrong MJ, Yu MC, Sani S: Nasopharyngeal carcinoma in Malaysian Chinese: salted fish and other dietary exposures. *Int J Cancer* 1998, 77(2):228-235.

[6] Yuan JM, Wang XL, Xiang YB, Gao YT, Ross RK, Yu MC: Preserved foods in relation to risk of nasopharyngeal carcinoma in Shanghai, China. *Int J Cancer* 2000, 85(3):358-363.

[7] Zou J, Sun Q, Akiba S, Yuan Y, Zha Y, Tao Z, Wei L, Sugahara T: A case-control study of nasopharyngeal carcinoma in the high background radiation areas of Yangjiang, China. *J Radiat Res (Tokyo)* 2000, 41 Suppl:53-62.

[8] Jeannel D, Hubert A, de Vathaire F, Ellouz R, Camoun M, Ben Salem M, Sancho-Garnier H, de-The G: Diet, living conditions and nasopharyngeal carcinoma in Tunisia--a case-control study. *Int J Cancer* 1990, 46(3):421-425.

[9] Sriamporn S, Vatanasapt V, Pisani P, Yongchaiyudha S, Rungpitarangsri V: Environmental risk factors for nasopharyngeal carcinoma: a case-control study in northeastern Thailand. *Cancer Epidemiol Biomarkers Prev* 1992, 1(5):345-348.

[10] Lanier A, Bender T, Talbot M, Wilmeth S, Tschopp C, Henle W, Henle G, Ritter D, Terasaki P: Nasopharyngeal carcinoma in Alaskan Eskimos Indians, and Aleuts: a review of cases and study of Epstein-Barr virus, HLA, and environmental risk factors. *Cancer* 1980, 46(9):2100-2106.

[11] Armstrong RW, Kutty MK, Armstrong MJ: Self-specific environments associated with nasopharyngeal carcinoma in Selangor, Malaysia. *Soc Sci Med* 1978, 12(3D-4D):149-156.

[12] Lee HP, Gourley L, Duffy SW, Esteve J, Lee J, Day NE: Preserved foods and nasopharyngeal carcinoma: a case-control study among Singapore Chinese. *Int J Cancer* 1994, 59(5):585-590.

[13] Laouamri S, Hamdi-Cherif M, Sekfali N, Mokhtari L, Kharchi R: [Dietary risk factors of nasopharyngeal carcinoma in the Setif area in Algeria]. *Rev Epidemiol Sante Publique* 2001, 49(2):145-156.

[14] Yu MC, Mo CC, Chong WX, Yeh FS, Henderson BE: Preserved foods and nasopharyngeal carcinoma: a case-control study in Guangxi, China. *Cancer Res* 1988, 48(7):1954-1959.

[15] Gallicchio L, Matanoski G, Tao XG, Chen L, Lam TK, Boyd K, Robinson KA, Balick L, Mickelson S, Caulfield LE *et al*: Adulthood consumption of preserved and nonpreserved vegetables and the risk of nasopharyngeal carcinoma: a systematic review. *Int J Cancer* 2006, 119(5):1125-1135.

[16] Yu MC: Diet and nasopharyngeal carcinoma. *FEMS Microbiol Immunol* 1990, 2(4):235-242.

[17] Yang XR, Diehl S, Pfeiffer R, Chen CJ, Hsu WL, Dosemeci M, Cheng YJ, Sun B, Goldstein AM, Hildesheim A: Evaluation of risk factors for nasopharyngeal carcinoma in high-risk nasopharyngeal carcinoma families in Taiwan. *Cancer Epidemiol Biomarkers Prev* 2005, 14(4):900-905.

[18] Armstrong RW, Eng AC: Salted fish and nasopharyngeal carcinoma in Malaysia. *Soc Sci Med* 1983, 17(20):1559-1567.

[19] Ning JP, Yu MC, Wang QS, Henderson BE: Consumption of salted fish and other risk factors for nasopharyngeal carcinoma (NPC) in Tianjin, a low-risk region for NPC in the People's Republic of China. *J Natl Cancer Inst* 1990, 82(4):291-296.

[20] Armstrong RW, Armstrong MJ, Yu MC, Henderson BE: Salted fish and inhalants as risk factors for nasopharyngeal carcinoma in Malaysian Chinese. *Cancer Res* 1983, 43(6):2967-2970.

[21] Ward MH, Pan WH, Cheng YJ, Li FH, Brinton LA, Chen CJ, Hsu MM, Chen IH, Levine PH, Yang CS *et al*: Dietary exposure to nitrite and nitrosamines and risk of nasopharyngeal carcinoma in Taiwan. *Int J Cancer* 2000, 86(5):603-609.
[22] Zheng X, Luo Y, Christensson B, Drettner B: Induction of nasal and nasopharyngeal tumours in Sprague-Dawley rats fed with Chinese salted fish. *Acta Otolaryngol* 1994, 114(1):98-104.
[23] Yu MC, Nichols PW, Zou XN, Estes J, Henderson BE: Induction of malignant nasal cavity tumours in Wistar rats fed Chinese salted fish. *Br J Cancer* 1989, 60(2):198-201.
[24] Huang DP, Ho JH, Saw D, Teoh TB: Carcinoma of the nasal and paranasal regions in rats fed Cantonese salted marine fish. *IARC Sci Publ* 1978(20):315-328.
[25] Zou XN, Lu SH, Liu B: Volatile N-nitrosamines and their precursors in Chinese salted fish--a possible etological factor for NPC in china. *Int J Cancer* 1994, 59(2):155-158.
[26] Bartsch H, Ohshima H, Pignatelli B, Calmels S: Endogenously formed N-nitroso compounds and nitrosating agents in human cancer etiology. *Pharmacogenetics* 1992, 2(6):272-277.
[27] Preston-Martin S, Correa P: Epidemiological evidence for the role of nitroso compounds in human cancer. *Cancer Surv* 1989, 8(2):459-473.
[28] Jakszyn P, Gonzalez CA: Nitrosamine and related food intake and gastric and oesophageal cancer risk: a systematic review of the epidemiological evidence. *World J Gastroenterol* 2006, 12(27):4296-4303.
[29] Poirier S, Hubert A, de-The G, Ohshima H, Bourgade MC, Bartsch H: Occurrence of volatile nitrosamines in food samples collected in three high-risk areas for nasopharyngeal carcinoma. *IARC Sci Publ* 1987(84):415-419.
[30] Chen ZC, Pan SC, Yao KT: Chemical transformation of human embryonic nasopharyngeal epithelial cells in vitro. *IARC Sci Publ* 1991(105):434-438.
[31] Huang DP: Epidemiology of nasopharyngeal carcinoma. *Ear Nose Throat J* 1990, 69(4):222-225.
[32] Marsh GM, Youk AO, Morfeld P: Mis-specified and non-robust mortality risk models for nasopharyngeal cancer in the National Cancer Institute formaldehyde worker cohort study. *Regul Toxicol Pharmacol* 2007, 47(1):59-67.
[33] Eichholzer M, Gutzwiller F: Dietary nitrates, nitrites, and N-nitroso compounds and cancer risk: a review of the epidemiologic evidence. *Nutr Rev* 1998, 56(4 Pt 1):95-105.
[34] Pott P: [The first description of an occupational cancer in 1777 (scrotal cancer, cancer of chimney sweeps)]. *Bull Soc Liban Hist Med* 1993(4):98-101.
[35] Schoental R, Magee PN: Induction of squamous carcinoma of the lung and of the stomach and oesophagus by diazomethane and N-methyl-N-nitroso-urethane, respectively. *Br J Cancer* 1962, 16:92-100.
[36] Ball JK: Immunosuppression and carcinogenesis: contrasting effects with 7,12-dimethylbenz[a]anthracene, benz[a]pyrene, and 3-methylcholanthrene. *J Natl Cancer Inst* 1970, 44(1):1-10.
[37] Fong YY, Walsh EO: Carcinogenic nitrosamines in Cantonese salt-dried fish. *Lancet* 1971, 2(7732):1032.
[38] Lo NM: [Effect of neuroticism on the pathogenesis and development of induced mammary gland tumors in rats]. *Fiziol Zh* 1962, 8:664-670.
[39] Toth B, Shubik P: Carcinogenesis in AKR mice injected at birth with benzo(a)pyrene and dimethylnitrosamine. *Cancer Res* 1967, 27(1):43-51.

[40] Magee PN, Barnes JM: The production of malignant primary hepatic tumours in the rat by feeding dimethylnitrosamine. *Br J Cancer* 1956, 10(1):114-122.
[41] Schoental R: Induction of Tumours of the Stomach in Rats and Mice by N-Nitroso-Nalkylurethanes. *Nature* 1963, 199:190.
[42] Thomas C, Schmaehl D: [on the Morphology of Diethylnitrosamine-Induced Liver Tumors in Mice and Guinea Pigs]. *Z Krebsforsch* 1963, 65:531-536.
[43] Shvemberger IN: [On histogenesis of anaplastic tumors induced in rats by nitrosamines]. *Tsitologiia* 1965, 7(3):365-372.
[44] Schoental R: Carcinogenic activity of N-methyl-N-nitroso-N'-nitroguanidine. *Nature* 1966, 209(5024):726-727.
[45] Fiddler W, Pensabene JW, Doerr RC, Wasserman AE: Formation of N-nitrosodimethylamine from naturally occurring quaternary ammonium compounds and tertiary amines. *Nature* 1972, 236(5345):307.
[46] Sen NP, Smith DC, Schwinghamer L: Formation of N-nitrosamines from secondary amines and nitrite in human and animal gastric juice. *Food Cosmet Toxicol* 1969, 7(4):301-307.
[47] Ho JH: Nasopharyngeal carcinoma (NPC). *Adv Cancer Res* 1972, 15:57-92.
[48] Weng YM, Hotchkiss JH, Babish JG: N-nitrosamine and mutagenicity formation in Chinese salted fish after digestion. *Food Addit Contam* 1992, 9(1):29-37.
[49] Zou X, Li J, Lu S, Song X, Wang X, Guo L, Lin Q, Ye J: Volatile N-nitrosamines in salted fish samples from high- and low-risk areas for NPC in China. *Chin Med Sci J* 1992, 7(4):201-204.
[50] Yi Z, Ohshima H, Bouvier G, Roy P, Zhong J, Li B, Brouet I, de The G, Bartsch H: Urinary excretion of nitrosamino acids and nitrate by inhabitants of high- and low-risk areas for nasopharyngeal carcinoma in southern China. *Cancer Epidemiol Biomarkers Prev* 1993, 2(3):195-200.
[51] Wang HW, Chiang FL: [Studies on the chemical induction of in-situ masopharyngeal carcinoma in the mouse]. *Shi Yan Sheng Wu Xue Bao* 1965, 10(3):190-204.
[52] Cleaton-Jones P: Histological observations in the soft palate of the albino rat. *J Anat* 1971, 110(Pt 1):39-47.
[53] Albiin N, Hellstrom S, Salen B, Stenfors LE, Soderberg O: The anatomy of the eustachian tube in the rat: a macro- and microscopical study. *Anat Rec* 1983, 207(3):513-521.
[54] Yoshimoto T, Hirao F, Sakatani M, Nishikawa H, Ogura T: Induction of squamous cell carcinoma in the lung of C57BL/6 mice by intratracheal instillation of benzo[a]pyrene with charcoal powder. *Gann* 1977, 68(3):343-352.
[55] Linsell CA, Peers FG: The aflatoxins and human liver cancer. *Recent Results Cancer Res* 1972, 39:125-129.
[56] Chu EA, Wu JM, Tunkel DE, Ishman SL: Nasopharyngeal carcinoma: the role of the Epstein-Barr virus. *Medscape J Med* 2008, 10(7):165.
[57] Tang FQ, Duan CJ, Huang DM, Wang WW, Xie CL, Meng JJ, Wang L, Jiang HY, Feng DY, Wu SH *et al*: HSP70 and mucin 5B: novel protein targets of N,N'-dinitrosopiperazine-induced nasopharyngeal tumorigenesis. *Cancer Sci* 2009, 100(2):216-224.
[58] Poirier LA: Hepatocarcinogenesis by diethylnitrosamine in rats fed high dietary levels of lipotropes. *J Natl Cancer Inst* 1975, 54(1):137-140.
[59] Cammoun M, Ellouz R, Behi J, Attia RB: Histological types of nasopharyngeal carcinoma in an intermediate risk area. *IARC Sci Publ* 1978(20):13-26.

[60] Berenblum I, Armuth V: Two independent aspects of tumor promotion. *Biochim Biophys Acta* 1981, 651(1):51-63.
[61] Cook PJ, Doll R, Fellingham SA: A mathematical model for the age distribution of cancer in man. *Int J Cancer* 1969, 4(1):93-112.
[62] Armitage P, Doll R: The age distribution of cancer and a multi-stage theory of carcinogenesis. *Br J Cancer* 1954, 8(1):1-12.
[63] Hirayama T: Descriptive and analytical epidemiology of nasopharyngeal cancer. *IARC Sci Publ* 1978(20):167-189.
[64] Stich HF, Kieser D: Use of DNA repair synthesis in detecting organotropic actions of chemical carcinogens. *Proc Soc Exp Biol Med* 1974, 145(4):1339-1342.
[65] Mirvish SS, Chu C, Clayson DB: Inhibition of [3H]thymidine incorporation into DNA of rat esophageal epithelium and related tissues by carcinogenic N-nitroso compounds. *Cancer Res* 1978, 38(2):458-466.
[66] Zhang XF, Tan X, Zeng G, Misse A, Singh S, Kim Y, Klaunig JE, Monga SP: Conditional beta-catenin loss in mice promotes chemical hepatocarcinogenesis: role of oxidative stress and platelet-derived growth factor receptor alpha/phosphoinositide 3-kinase signaling. *Hepatology* 2010, 52(3):954-965.
[67] Matsumoto K, Huang J, Viswakarma N, Bai L, Jia Y, Zhu YT, Yang G, Borensztajn J, Rao MS, Zhu YJ *et al*: Transcription coactivator PBP/MED1-deficient hepatocytes are not susceptible to diethylnitrosamine-induced hepatocarcinogenesis in the mouse. *Carcinogenesis* 2010, 31(2):318-325.
[68] Cataisson C, Ohman R, Patel G, Pearson A, Tsien M, Jay S, Wright L, Hennings H, Yuspa SH: Inducible cutaneous inflammation reveals a protumorigenic role for keratinocyte CXCR2 in skin carcinogenesis. *Cancer Res* 2009, 69(1):319-328.
[69] Kataoka K, Kim DJ, Carbajal S, Clifford JL, DiGiovanni J: Stage-specific disruption of Stat3 demonstrates a direct requirement during both the initiation and promotion stages of mouse skin tumorigenesis. *Carcinogenesis* 2008, 29(6):1108-1114.
[70] Waalkes MP, Ward JM, Diwan BA: Induction of tumors of the liver, lung, ovary and adrenal in adult mice after brief maternal gestational exposure to inorganic arsenic: promotional effects of postnatal phorbol ester exposure on hepatic and pulmonary, but not dermal cancers. *Carcinogenesis* 2004, 25(1):133-141.
[71] Tang F, Zou F, Peng Z, Huang D, Wu Y, Chen Y, Duan C, Cao Y, Mei W, Tang X *et al*: N,N'-Dinitrosopiperazine-mediated ezrin phosphorylation via activating Rho kinase and protein kinase C involves in metastasis of nasopharyngeal carcinoma 6-10B cells. *J Biol Chem* 2011.
[72] Pan S, Sun Q, Wang J, Wen D, Peng X. Induction of rat nasopharyngeal carcinoma with Nitrosamine compound in lab research. *Chinese Sci Bullet*,1978; 28: 756–9.
[73] Yao K, Pan S, Huang J, Wen D. Further investigation of experimental induction of nasopharyngeal carcinoma in rats by N,N′-Dinitrosopiperazine. Bulletin of Hunan Medical College, 1981,6(11)1-6
[74] Chen Z, Pan S, Sun Q, Yao K. Renewal of nasopharyngeal squamous epithelium of rats treated with N,N′-Dinitrosopiperazine. Bulletin of Hunan Medical College, 1984,9(4)317-323
[75] Le J, Pan S, Yao S. The mechanism of organ specific carcinogenicity of N,N′-Dinitrosopiperazine in rats. Bulletin of Hunan Medical College, 1982,7(2)129-135
[76] Wen D, Pan S, Yao K. Histochemistry investigation of non-specific acid esterase during carcinogenesis of rat nasopharyngeal epithelium and human nasopharyngeal carcinoma. Bulletin of Hunan Medical College, 1982,7(1)18-2

5

Epstein-Barr Virus Serology in the Detection and Screening of Nasopharyngeal Carcinoma

Li-Jen Liao[1,2] and Mei-Shu Lai[2]
[1]*Department of Otolaryngology, Far Eastern Memorial Hospital, New Taipei City,*
[2]*Graduate Institute of Epidemiology and Preventive Medicine, College of Public Health, National Taiwan University, Taipei,*
Taiwan

1. Introduction

Nasopharyngeal carcinoma (NPC) is a common cancer among Southern Chinese with a male dominance of about 3:1. The age-adjusted incidence for both sexes is less than one per 100, 000 population worldwide. The reported incidence of NPC among men and women in Hong Kong is 20–30 per 100, 000 and 15–20 per 100, 000.(Wei and Sham, 2005) The reported incidence of NPC among men and women in Taiwan is 8.3 per 100 000 and 2.8 per 100 000, respectively.(Bureau of health promotion, Taiwan, 2010) It mainly afflicts people in mid-life. There is now compelling evidences to suggest that Epstein-Barr virus (EBV) is associated with the development of NPC and is most likely to be involved in the multi-step and multi-factorial carcinogenesis of NPC. In this chapter, the role of EBV in pathogenesis of NPC is reviewed briefly, and principle applications of EBV antibodies and circulating EBV DNA as markers of NPC are outlined. Based on current knowledge of EBV antibody responses by NPC and taking available testing technologies into account, serologic screening strategy to facilitate efficient early detection of NPC is formulated.

2. EBV related pathogenesis of NPC

The pathogenesis of NPC includes multi-stepped process that leads to the development of NPC **(Fig. 1.)**. EBV infection alone cannot drive normal cells towards carcinoma development. It is thought that loss of heterozygosity (LOH on chromosome 3p and 9p, which are the location of some tumor suppressor genes), possibly as a result of inherited traits (Chinese ethnicity) as well as exposure to dietary factors (salted fish) and other environmental cofactors (Formaldehyde), is an early stage event in the pathogenesis of this disease. EBV is infected within these low-grade pre-invasive lesions, subsequent to further genetic and epigenetic alterations.

EBV was first suspected to be linked with NPC on the basis of the serological observations by Old and colleagues (Old et al., 1966) in 1966. This link was formally demonstrated later by in situ hybridization of the viral DNA in the nuclei of epithelial cells (zur Hausen et al., 1970). The full length EBV genome is contained in all malignant epithelial cells, but not in most infiltrating lymphocytes. The association with EBV is constant, regardless of the patient's geographical origin and is observed in World Health Organization (WHO) types II and III. However, the association of NPC type I with EBV has long been a matter of controversy. It is now clear that WHO type I tumors are frequently associated with EBV in endemic regions, but not in non-endemic regions, where they often result from tobacco and alcohol abuse (Nicholls et al., 1997). Types II and III may be accompanied by an inflammatory infiltrate of lymphocytes, plasma cells, and eosinophils.

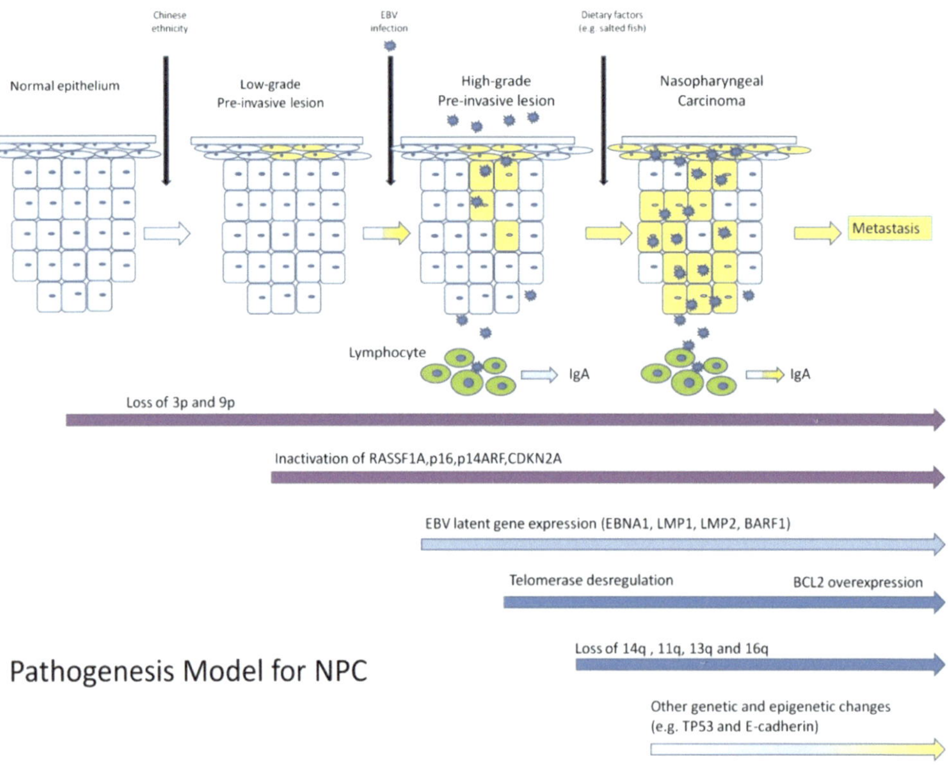

Fig. 1. EBV in the pathogenesis model for nasopharyngeal carcinoma

More than 95% adults in all ethnic groups across the world are healthy carriers of EBV (Ooka et al., 1991). This means that NPC oncogenesis is not simply a consequence of EBV infection. It probably results from a form of viral reactivation in combination with other events, such as cellular genetic lesions due to environmental carcinogens and/or some form of immune defects. EBV-encoded RNA signal (EBER) has been shown, by in-situ hybridization, to be present in nearly all tumor cells, whereas EBV-encoded RNA is absent from the adjacent normal tissue, except perhaps for a few scattered lymphoid cells. Premalignant lesions of the nasopharyngeal epithelium have also been shown to harbor EBV, which suggests that the infection occurs in the early phases of carcinogenesis (Gulley, 2001). Consistent with this hypothesis, is the fact that NPC generally occur several years after EBV primary infection. The expression of EBV latent genes provides growth and survival advantages to these infected cells, ultimately leading to the development of NPC. Further genetic and epigenetic alterations post-NPC development can occur, which may result in a more metastatic disease. Because of it takes years for premalignant lesion after

EBV infection to NPC formation(Choi et al., 2011; Ji et al., 2007; Ng et al., 2010; Ng et al., 2005), the long period of pre-clinical detectable phase (PCDP) offer the opportunity for screening and early diagnosis of NPC.

3. Applications of EBV antibodies and EBV DNA as markers of NPC in population

3.1 Plasma EBV protein in the diagnosis of NPC

Serological studies have shown that the clinical onset of NPC is preceded by the appearance of a high titer of various EBV antibodies such as viral capsid antigens (VCA) IgA(Li et al., 2010; Ng et al., 2010; O et al., 2007), anti-EBV DNase(Chien et al., 2001) and combined EBV EA(early antigen) + EBNA-1 (Nuclear antigen 1) IgA test(Chang et al., 2008)(**Table 1.**).

Study type	Author	Marker	Results of the utility
Case-control study	O *et al.* (O et al., 2007)	VCA IgA (ELISA)	Sensitivity 90.6% Specificity 93.5%
	Ng *et al.* (2010) (Ng et al., 2010)	VCA IgA (ELISA and IF)	Sensitivity 83.3% Specificity 87.0%
	Chang *et al.* (2008) (Chang et al., 2008)	EA+EBNA1 IgA (ELISA)	Sensitivity 94.2% Specificity 82.6%
Meta-analysis	Li *et al.* (2010) (Li et al., 2010)	VCA IgA (ELISA and IF)	Sensitivity 92% Specificity 98%
Cohort study	Chien *et al.* (2001) (Chien et al., 2001)	VCA IgA(IF) and anti-DNase (enzyme neutralization assay)	Rate ratio VCA IgA 22.0 (7.3-66.9) anti-DNase 3.5 (1.4-8.7)
	Yu *at al.* (2011) (Yu et al., 2011).	EBNA1 IgA (ELISA)	Rate ratio 4.7 (1.4-16)

IF: immunofluorescent assay; ELISA: enzyme-linked immunosorbent assay

Table 1. Reported plasma EBV antibody in NPC diagnosis and risk assessment of NPC

For NPC serodiagnosis, cell-based indirect immunofluorescent assay (IF) methods are widely considered the gold standard (Paramita et al., 2009). IF involves the separate analysis of antibody responses to VCA, EA, and EBNA, and requiring different cell lines for specific analysis. However, this method shows considerable variation among laboratories and is time-consuming, subjective, and not suitable for large-scale automatic handling. Enzyme-linked immunosorbent assay (ELISA) techniques are increasingly used recently and have shown a better sensitivity and specificity compared to IFA and which are suitable for large-scale application. Stage is one of the most important prognostic predictors of NPC. NPC in its early stages are highly curable with radiotherapy. Screening may change the distribution of stage and prognosis. In a cohort study undertaken in Wuzhou (Guangxi province, China) in the early 1980s (Zeng et al., 1985), total 1136 individuals identified as positive for Ig A against VCA received regular clinical examinations of the nasopharynx and neck for 4 years. During this follow-up period, 35 cases of NPC were detected, most of which (92%) were diagnosed early at either stage I or stage II. The annual detection rate of NPC for this group was 31·7 times higher than for the population as a whole. Distribution of different stages of screen-detected and symptomatic NPC in Hong Kong (Ng et al., 2010) also revealed early diagnosis of NPC in screen-detected patients, comparing to symptomatic NPC (**Table 2.**).

	Stage I	Stage II	Stage III	Stage IV
Screen-detected	41.2%	17.6%	35.3%	5.9%
Clinically detected	0.7%	23.2%	36.3%	39.5%

Table 2. The comparison of the stage distribution between screen-detected and clinically detected based on published data on NPC screening during 1979-1992 (Ng et al., 2010).

Li conducted a systematic review of studies in Chinese on the accuracy of VCA-IgA concentrations in the diagnosis of NPC using random effects models (Li et al., 2010). Twenty studies met the inclusion criteria for the meta-analysis. The summary estimates (**Fig. 2.**) for VCA-IgA in the diagnosis of NPC were: sensitivity 0.92 (95% confidence interval (CI): 0.89–0.95), specificity 0.98 (95% CI: 0.95–0.99), positive likelihood ratio 38.5 (95% CI: 19.0–78.0), negative likelihood ratio 0.08 (95% CI: 0.05–0.12) and diagnostic odds ratio 487 (95% CI: 224–1059). The area under the summary receiver operating characteristic curves was 0.98(95%

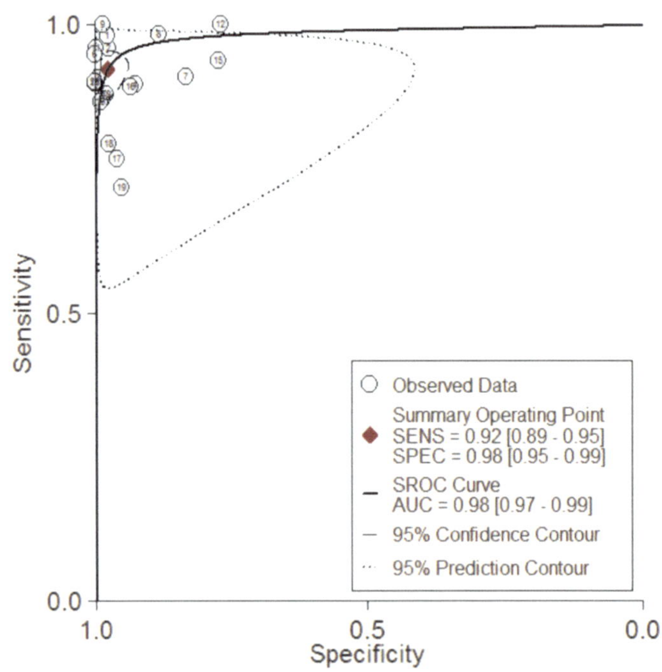

Fig. 2. Summary receiver operating characteristic curves for VCA-IgA in the diagnosis of NPC. Each solid circle represents each study in the meta-analysis.

CI: 0.97–0.99, **Fig. 3.**). There are limitations of this meta-analysis: (1) All of the included studies were Chinese articles, which would lead to language bias. (2) Significant heterogeneity exists in this metaanalysis, even with random effect model, pooling is not a proper method.

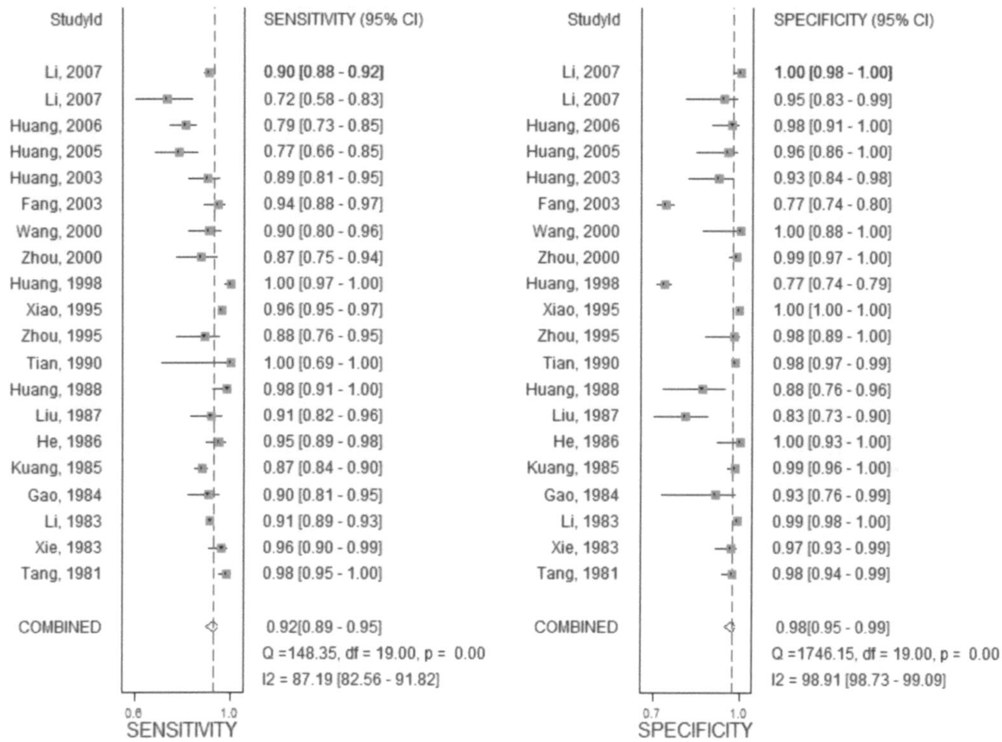

Fig. 3. Forest plot of estimates of sensitivity and specificity for VCA-IgA in the diagnosis of NPC. The point estimates of sensitivity from each study are shown as solid squares. Error bars are 95% *CI*.

Sustained elevation of EBV antibody had a high possibility of NPC formation. Ji monitored serologically and clinically 39 cases for different periods of up to 15 years before NPC was diagnosed, and assessed the preclinical serologic status of another 68 cases(Ji et al., 2007). The results identify a serologic window preceding diagnosis when antibody levels are raised and sustained. This window can persist for as long as 10 years, with a mean duration estimated to as 37 months.

3.2 Circulating EBV DNA in the diagnosis of NPC

The presence of circulating DNA was first reported by Mandel and Metais in 1948 (Chan and Lo, 2002). They demonstrated that extracellular DNA and RNA could be detected from the blood of healthy as well as sick individuals. The blood plasma EBV DNA load was shown to be proportionately related to the presence of malignant disease (Tan et al., 2006). While the EBV copy number in untreated NPC patients had a median of 2,043 copies/ml, viral load in plasma of healthy controls was significantly lower (median of 0 copy/ml). The demonstration of EBV DNA in the plasma/serum of patients suffering from NPC has provided us with a new tool for NPC detection and monitoring.

Liu reported a systematic review of 15 studies in English on the accuracy of EBV-DNA in the diagnosis of NPC (Liu et al., 2011). NPC could be diagnosed by detecting plasma or serum EBV DNA. Pooling using random effects models showed that EBV DNA detection was also highly sensitive and specific for cancer detection, and can possibly help the clinician to diagnose NPC. The summary estimates (**Fig. 4.**) for DNA in the diagnosis of NPC were: sensitivity 0.92 (95% confidence interval (CI): 0.82–0.96), specificity 0.88 (95% CI: 0.78–0.94), positive likelihood ratio 7.7 (95% CI: 4.1–14.6), negative likelihood ratio 0.09 (95% CI: 0.05–0.15) and diagnostic odds ratio 89 (95% CI: 44–181). The area under the summary receiver operating characteristic curves was 0.96(95% CI: 0.94–0.97, **Fig. 5.**).

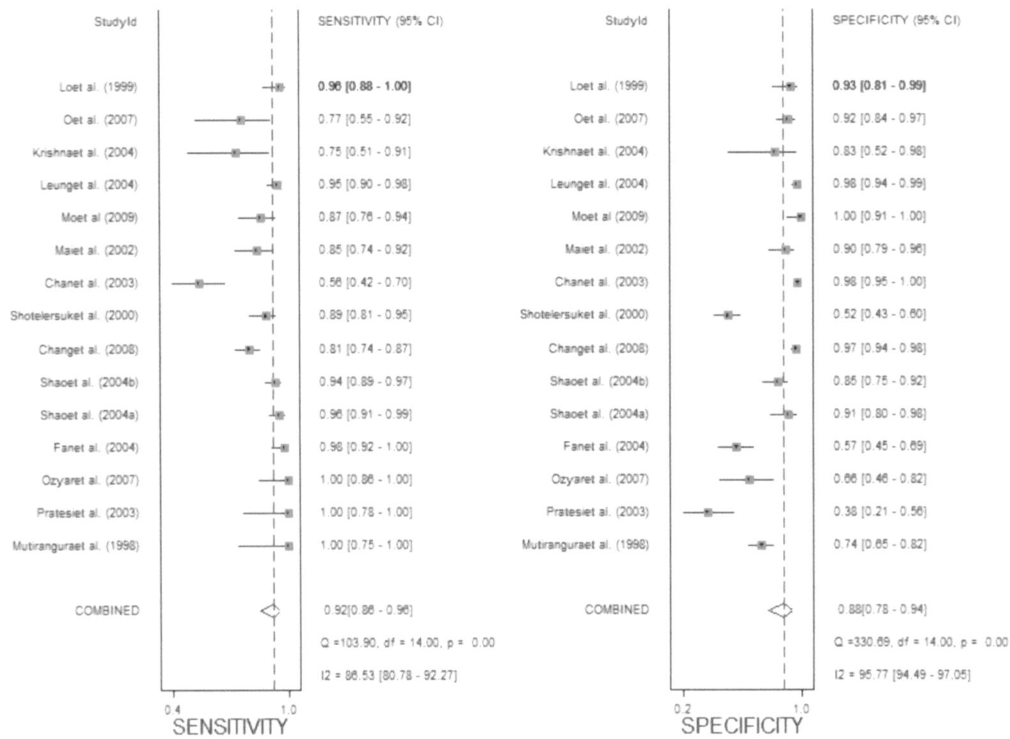

Fig. 4. Forest plot of estimates of sensitivity and specificity for EBV DNA in the diagnosis of NPC. The point estimates of sensitivity from each study are shown as solid squares. Error bars are 95% CI.

The presentation with "occult primary" of NPC is a diagnostic challenge for the clinician. Detection of EBV DNA by PCR in metastatic neck nodes has a good diagnostic rate (97.1%) (Yap et al., 2007). PCR is an ideal tool for suggesting occult primary NPC and guiding the diagnostic workup, facilitating earlier diagnosis and reducing morbidity and mortality. It is, therefore, expected that this promising molecular tumor marker would soon be incorporated into routine clinical use.

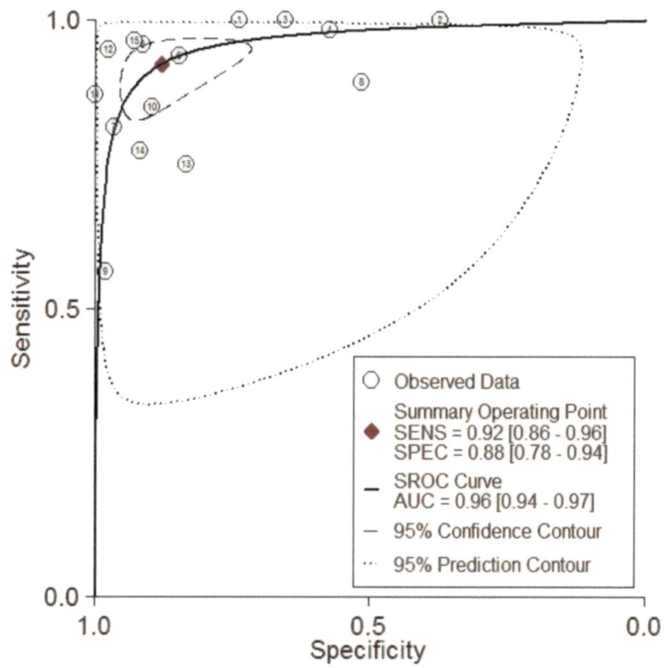

Fig. 5. Summary receiver operating characteristic curves for VCA-IgA in the diagnosis of NPC. Each solid circle represents each study in the meta-analysis.

3.3 EBV DNA in the monitoring of NPC

With the demonstration of the presence of extracellular EBV DNA in the circulation of NPC patients and its disappearance following radiotherapy, the levels of plasma/serum EBV DNA in patients with NPC recurrence were much higher than the levels of those who remained in continuous clinical remission. A significant decrease in EBV load was observed in patients who had undergone radiotherapy while a high viral load indicated in patients correlated to tumor relapse and presence of distant metastasis upon clinical investigation(Lo et al., 1999; Tan et al., 2006). The median EBV DNA concentration in the relapsed patients was 32, 350 copies/ml, whereas that in patients in remission was 0 copy/ml (Lo et al., 1999). Plasma EBV DNA is superior to serum EBV VCA antibodies in prognostic predictions and monitoring for NPC (Twu et al., 2007). Relapsed patients had significantly higher pretreatment EBV DNA concentration than patients without relapse ($p<0.05$). No associations of VCA-IgA ($p = 0.97$) or VCA-IgG ($p=0.61$) were observed between patients with and without relapse (Twu et al., 2007).

3.4 Comparison of DNA and serology in the diagnosis and follow-up of NPC

Plasma EBV DNA detection has a similar sensitive and specific as the serum IgA antibody titer for the diagnosis of patients with NPC. In terms of real costs, however, the IgA test costs approximately $20, whereas the DNA test ranges from $100 to $200 (5-10 times more)(O et al., 2007). For screening purposes, the serologic assays may be made first, so that more patients can be evaluated. If a patient is assessed to be at high risk, then EBV DNA

PCR can be performed in a series fashion (O et al., 2007). If this work-up is positive; then the patient should be referred to a specialist for further work-up including fiberoptic nasopharyngoscopy or MRI examination. The economic cost of providing this screening is reduce by prescreening to exclude the low-risk patients and performing series testing on the at-risk patients.

4. Applications of EBV antibodies and EBV DNA as markers of NPC among individual from high risk NPC families

4.1 Screening in high risk group with positive family history

The incidence of NPC is relative low through most of the world (less 1/100,000). However, familial clustering of NPC has been widely documented in Chinese population (Chen and Huang, 1997) and individual with family history are at a high risk of developing the disease. Both family history and anti-EBV seropositivity are determinants in subsequent NPC development. Based on mass screening with positive family history conducted in Taiwan and Hong-Kong (Choi et al., 2011; Hsu et al., 2011; Ng et al., 2010; Yu et al., 2011), subjected with positive family history will increase risk of subsequent NPC development. Screening this high risk group significantly shifted to earlier stage (Ng et al., 2010), which mean it is a screening modality to be worth.

The etiology of NPC is not completely understood now; approaches to primary prevention of NPC remain inconclusive. This situation highlights the need of secondary prevention for early detection, diagnosis, and treatment of NPC. The effectiveness of a screening program rests on several key factors: "the importance of the disease; a well-defined population at risk; the availability of noninvasive, low-cost screening tests that can detect disease at an early stage; and effective treatments resulting in long term survival."(Choi et al., 2011) Screening for NPC for positive family history with EBV serology meets all of these criteria.

Chen first reported an evaluation of screening for NPC using Markov chain models (Chen et al., 1999). Average duration of the PCDP is estimated as 3.1 years was estimated; therefore it is possible for massive screening in NPC. The stage distribution for EBV-IgA antibodies is higher (68.7%) than in the non-screened (25%) group for stage I and II. Based on these findings, they suggest design a randomized trial in a high incidence area such as Hong Kong.

In another cohort study from Taiwan (Hsu et al., 2011) comparing different covariates, the authors compared the long-term risk NPC of male participants in a NPC cohort after adjusting for anti- EBV seromarkers and cigarette smoking. The adjusted hazard ratio was 6.8 (95% CI: 2.3, 20.1) for the multiplex family cohort compared with the community cohort. In the evaluation of anti-EBV VCA IgA and anti-EBV DNase, the adjusted hazard ratios were 2.8 (95% CI: 1.3, 6.0) and 15.1 (95% CI: 4.2, 54.1) for those positive for 1 EBV seromarker and positive for both seromarkers, respectively, compared with those negative for both EBV seromarkers. The adjusted hazard ratio was 31.0 (95% CI: 9.7, 98.7) for participants who reported a family history of NPC and who were anti-EBV-seropositive compared with individuals without such a history who were anti-EBV-seronegative. These findings suggest that both family history of NPC and anti-EBV seropositivity are important determinants of subsequent NPC development. Screening for high risk multiplex family may be more cost-effective.

Screening in Hong-Kong with positive NPC family history was conducted since 1994 (Lee et al., 2005; Ng et al., 2010; Ng et al., 2005). Participants in this screening program for NPC were all first degree relatives of patients with NPC and they were all 18 years of age or older. Participants were offered annual assessment serological test of EBV and endoscopic examination of the nasopharynx. Between 1994 and 2005, total 1,199 asymptomatic family members of NPC patients were recruited and reported (Ng et al., 2010). Eighteen participants of the screening program developed NPC; 16 of them were detected in the screening. Stage distributions and survival outcomes of the 17 cases were compared with that of 1,185 consecutive symptomatic patients diagnosed in the same period through general referral. It was found that the screening program resulted in early detection of cancer (Table 2), with 59% presenting at early stage (stage I: 41%, stage II: 18%) compared to 24% (stage I: 1%, stage II: 23%) of symptomatic cancers (P=0.001), and a significant improvement in disease-free survival (P = 0.04). The cancer specific survival and overall survival rate at 5-year are also higher (92 vs. 77% and 92 vs. 70%, respectively).

4.2 Screening strategies of NPC among individual from high risk NPC families

The efficacy of any screening strategy should be evaluated before putting it into practice. Based on Markov chain models, Choi simulated and compared the outcomes of 4 screening strategies over a period of 12 years: (A) Annual screening, (B) biennial screening, (C) triennial screening, and (D) triennial screening for participants tested EBV negative and annual screening once the participants are tested EBV positive (Choi et al., 2011) . The result is summarized at **Table 3**, strategy A (screening annually) yields the maximum disease pick-up rate, but strategy D (triennial screening for participants tested EBV negative and annual screening once the participants are tested EBV positive) offered the highest efficacy for NPC screening of family members of NPC patients.

	Strategy A	Strategy B	Strategy C	Strategy D	No screening
Total screens	77,652	41,837	29,898	44,618	-
Positive EBV test	14,962	8,071	5,772	11,413	-
Screen detected case	47	42	38	47	-
Disease pick up rate	88.2%	78.6%	70.8%	87.4%	-
Reduction in disease pick up rate*	-	9.6%	17.3%	0.8%	-
Screen missed cases	7	12	16	7	-
5-year overall survival	80.1%	78.8%	77.7%	80.0%	67.9%

* Relative to strategy A
Strategy A. Annual screening
Strategy B. Biennial screening
Strategy C. Triennial screening
Strategy D. Triennial screening for participants tested EBV negative and annual screening once the participants are tested EBV positive

Table 3. Simulated screening result with the four strategies based on an imaginary population of 6,000 participants follow up for 12 years with family history of NPC (Choi et al., 2011).

Various EBV screening seromarkers were ever been reported for massive screening in high risk group with positive family NPC history (**Table 4.**) (Ng et al., 2010; Yu et al., 2011). The positive predicative value (PPV) of EBV seromarkers was below 10% and the negative predicative value (NPV) was higher than 99%. Because the average duration of the preclinical screen-detectable phase is estimated as 3.1 years, annual check-up once the participants are tested EBV positive is necessary. For the high NPV, triennial screening is reasonable for NPC family history with negative EBV seromarkers.

Author	Journal	Modality	Sensitivity/ Specificity	Positive%	NPV	PPV
Wai *el al.* (Ng et al., 2010) (Hong-Kong)	Fam Cancer (2010)	Anti-EBV VCA IgA	83.3%/87.0%	14.0%	99.7%	8.9%
		Annual anti-EBV serology and nasopharyngoscopy	88.9%/87.0%	15.1%	99.8%	9.5%
Yu *et al.* *(Yu et al., 2011)* (Taiwan)	Clin Cancer Res (2011)	VCA IgA (IF) Positive (>1:10 dilution of serum)	36.4%/73.8%	26.2%	99.5%	0.8%
		VCA IgA (ELISA) Positive (OD405 > 0.50)	7.1%/95.7%	4.3%	99.4%	1.0%
		VCA IgA (ELISA) Positive (OD405 > 0.10)	92.9%/16.0%	84.0%	99.7%	0.6%
		EBNA1 IgA Positive (OD405 > 0.20)	50.0%/84.3%	15.9%	99.7%	1.8%
		EBNA1 IgA Positive (OD405 > 0.10)	85.7%/51.2%	49.0%	99.8%	1.0%
		Dnase Positive (>400 neutralizing units)	23.1%/88.1%	12.0%	99.5%	1.1%
		Dnase Positive (>160 neutralizing units)	84.6%/92.3%	8.1%	99.9%	5.6%

Table 4. Comparing different screening seromarkers in high risk NPC screening with positive family history.

5. Conclusion

EBV is associated with the development of NPC and the infection occurs in the early phases of carcinogenesis. A long period of pre-clinical detectable phase offers the opportunity for screening and early diagnosis of NPC. EBV antibodies and EBV DNA have the potential for screening, diagnosis, monitoring and prognosis of NPC. NPC screening in a high-risk, endemic population using EBV-specific serologic markers seems effective. Conduction of prospective randomized controlled screening trials is necessary to validate the cost-effectiveness.

6. Acknowledgment

I am heartily thankful for Miss Wan-Lun Hsu and Miss Yu-Ping Cheng for data collection, manuscript reviewing and modification.

7. References

Bureau of health promotion, Executive Yuan, Taiwan, (2010). *Cancer registry annual report.* 28.

Chan, K. C., and Lo, Y. M. (2002). Circulating EBV DNA as a tumor marker for nasopharyngeal carcinoma. *Semin Cancer Biol* 12, 489-496.

Chang, K. P., Hsu, C. L., Chang, Y. L., Tsang, N. M., Chen, C. K., Lee, T. J., Tsao, K. C., Huang, C. G., Chang, Y. S., Yu, J. S., and Hao, S. P. (2008). Complementary serum test of antibodies to Epstein-Barr virus nuclear antigen-1 and early antigen: a possible alternative for primary screening of nasopharyngeal carcinoma. *Oral Oncol* 44, 784-792.

Chen, D. L., and Huang, T. B. (1997). A case-control study of risk factors of nasopharyngeal carcinoma. *Cancer Lett* 117, 17-22.

Chen, H. H., Prevost, T. C., and Duffy, S. W. (1999). Evaluation of screening for nasopharyngeal carcinoma: trial design using Markov chain models. *Br J Cancer* 79, 1894-1900.

Chien, Y. C., Chen, J. Y., Liu, M. Y., Yang, H. I., Hsu, M. M., Chen, C. J., and Yang, C. S. (2001). Serologic markers of Epstein-Barr virus infection and nasopharyngeal carcinoma in Taiwanese men. *N Engl J Med* 345, 1877-1882.

Choi, C. W., Lee, M. C., Ng, W. T., Law, L. Y., Yau, T. K., and Lee, A. W. (2011). An analysis of the efficacy of serial screening for familial nasopharyngeal carcinoma based on Markov chain models. *Fam Cancer* 10, 133-139.

Gulley, M. L. (2001). Molecular diagnosis of Epstein-Barr virus-related diseases. J Mol Diagn 3, 1-10.

Hsu, W. L., Yu, K. J., Chien, Y. C., Chiang, C. J., Cheng, Y. J., Chen, J. Y., Liu, M. Y., Chou, S. P., You, S. L., Hsu, M. M., et al. (2011). Familial tendency and risk of nasopharyngeal carcinoma in taiwan: effects of covariates on risk. *Am J Epidemiol* 173, 292-299.

Ji, M. F., Wang, D. K., Yu, Y. L., Guo, Y. Q., Liang, J. S., Cheng, W. M., Zong, Y. S., Chan, K. H., Ng, S. P., Wei, W. I., et al. (2007). Sustained elevation of Epstein-Barr virus antibody levels preceding clinical onset of nasopharyngeal carcinoma. *Br J Cancer* 96, 623-630.

Lee, A. W., Sze, W. M., Au, J. S., Leung, S. F., Leung, T. W., Chua, D. T., Zee, B. C., Law, S. C., Teo, P. M., Tung, S. Y., et al. (2005). Treatment results for nasopharyngeal carcinoma in the modern era: the Hong Kong experience. *Int J Radiat Oncol Biol Phys* 61, 1107-1116.

Li, S., Deng, Y., Li, X., Chen, Q. P., Liao, X. C., and Qin, X. (2010). Diagnostic value of Epstein-Barr virus capsid antigen-IgA in nasopharyngeal carcinoma: a meta-analysis. *Chin Med J* 123, 1201-1205.

Liu, Y., Fang, Z., Liu, L., Yang, S., and Zhang, L. (2011). Detection of epstein-barr virus DNA in serum or plasma for nasopharyngeal cancer: a meta-analysis. *Genet Test Mol Biomarkers* 15, 495-502.

Lo, Y. M., Chan, L. Y., Chan, A. T., Leung, S. F., Lo, K. W., Zhang, J., Lee, J. C., Hjelm, N. M., Johnson, P. J., and Huang, D. P. (1999). Quantitative and temporal correlation between circulating cell-free Epstein-Barr virus DNA and tumor recurrence in nasopharyngeal carcinoma. *Cancer Res* 59, 5452-5455.

Ng, W. T., Choi, C. W., Lee, M. C., Law, L. Y., Yau, T. K., and Lee, A. W. (2010). Outcomes of nasopharyngeal carcinoma screening for high risk family members in Hong Kong. *Fam Cancer* 9, 221-228.

Ng, W. T., Yau, T. K., Yung, R. W., Sze, W. M., Tsang, A. H., Law, A. L., and Lee, A. W. (2005). Screening for family members of patients with nasopharyngeal carcinoma. *Int J Cancer* 113, 998-1001.

Nicholls, J. M., Agathanggelou, A., Fung, K., Zeng, X., and Niedobitek, G. (1997). The association of squamous cell carcinomas of the nasopharynx with Epstein-Barr virus shows geographical variation reminiscent of Burkitt's lymphoma. *J Pathol* 183, 164-168.

O, T. M., Yu, G., Hu, K., and Li, J. C. (2007). Plasma Epstein-Barr virus immunoglobulin A and DNA for nasopharyngeal carcinoma screening in the United States. *Otolaryngol Head Neck Surg* 136, 992-997.

Old, L. J., Boyse, E. A., Oettgen, H. F., Harven, E. D., Geering, G., Williamson, B., and Clifford, P. (1966). Precipitating antibody in human serum to an antigen present in cultured burkitt's lymphoma cells. *Proc Natl Acad Sci U S A* 56, 1699-1704.

Ooka, T., de Turenne-Tessier, M., and Stolzenberg, M. C. (1991). Relationship between antibody production to Epstein-Barr virus (EBV) early antigens and various EBV-related diseases. *Springer Semin Immunopathol* 13, 233-247.

Paramita, D. K., Fachiroh, J., Haryana, S. M., and Middeldorp, J. M. (2009). Two-step Epstein-Barr virus immunoglobulin A enzyme-linked immunosorbent assay system for serological screening and confirmation of nasopharyngeal carcinoma. *Clin Vaccine Immunol* 16, 706-711.

Tan, E. L., Looi, L. M., and Sam, C. K. (2006). Evaluation of plasma Epstein-Barr virus DNA load as a prognostic marker for nasopharyngeal carcinoma. *Singapore Med J* 47, 803-807.

Twu, C. W., Wang, W. Y., Liang, W. M., Jan, J. S., Jiang, R. S., Chao, J., Jin, Y. T., and Lin, J. C. (2007). Comparison of the prognostic impact of serum anti-EBV antibody and plasma EBV DNA assays in nasopharyngeal carcinoma. *Int J Radiat Oncol Biol Phys* 67, 130-137.

Wei, W. I., and Sham, J. S. (2005). Nasopharyngeal carcinoma. Lancet 365, 2041-2054.

Yap, Y. Y., Hassan, S., Chan, M., Choo, P. K., and Ravichandran, M. (2007). Epstein-Barr virus DNA detection in the diagnosis of nasopharyngeal carcinoma. *Otolaryngol Head Neck Surg* 136, 986-991.

Yu, K. J., Hsu, W. L., Pfeiffer, R. M., Chiang, C. J., Wang, C. P., Lou, P. J., Cheng, Y. J., Gravitt, P., Diehl, S. R., Goldstein, A. M., et al. (2011). Prognostic utility of anti-EBV antibody testing for defining NPC risk among individuals from high-risk NPC families. *Clin Cancer Res* 17, 1906-1914.

Zeng, Y., Zhang, L., Wu, Y., Huang, Y., Huang, N., Li, J., Wang, Y., Jiang, M., Fang, Z., and Meng, N. (1985). Prospective studies on nasopharyngeal carcinoma in epstein barr virus IgA/VCA antibody positne persons in Wuzhou city, china. *International journal of cancer* 36, 545-547.

zur Hausen, H., Schulte-Holthausen, H., Klein, G., Henle, W., Henle, G., Clifford, P., and Santesson, L. (1970). EBV DNA in biopsies of Burkitt tumours and anaplastic carcinomas of the nasopharynx. *Nature* 228, 1056-1058.

6

Imaging of Nasopharyngeal Carcinoma

Michael Chan[1], Eric Bartlett[2], Arjun Sahgal[3],
Stephen Chan[4] and Eugene Yu[5]
[1]*Faculty of Medicine, University of Toronto*
[2]*Department of Medical Imaging and Otolaryngology-Head and Neck Surgery, University of Toronto*
[3]*Department of Radiation Oncology, University of Toronto*
[4]*Division of Life Sciences, University of Western Ontario*
[5]*Department of Medical Imaging and Otolaryngology-Head and Neck Surgery, University of Toronto*
Canada

1. Introduction

1.1 Imaging of nasopharyngeal carcinoma

Nasopharyngeal carcinoma (NPC) is the most common neoplasm to affect the nasopharynx (NP). Arising from the epithelial lining of the nasopharyngeal mucosa, NPC is distinct from squamous cell carcinoma affecting other sites of the pharyngeal space. NPC typically originates in the lateral wall of the nasopharynx and is noted as a locally aggressive neoplasm with a high incidence of metastases to cervical lymph nodes. The primary tumour can extend within the nasopharynx and/or to the base of the skull, palate, nasal cavity or oropharynx. Distant metastases can arise in bone, lung, mediastinum, and, more rarely, the liver (Brennan, 2006).

The etiology of NPC is multifactorial and involves many environmental and genetic risk factors (Henderson *et al.*, 1976). In particular, diets high in salt-preserved foods - such as salted fish, meat, eggs, fruits and vegetables in the Southern Asian diet - have been identified as possible causative factors acting through the carcinogen, *N*-nitrosodimethylamine (Yu *et al.*, 1988). In contrast, frequent consumption of fresh fruits and/or vegetables - especially during childhood - is associated with a lower risk of NPC. In addition, studies have indicated a causal role for the Epstein-Barr virus (EBV) in the development of NPC (Chang & Adami, 2006). EBV is a DNA virus responsible for infectious mononucleosis, post-transplantation lymphoproliferative disease, and Burkitt's lymphoma. Elevated IgG and IgA antibody titres against viral capsid antigen, early antigen, and latent viral nuclear antigens have been noted in NPC patients. Furthermore, these antibodies have been shown to precede tumour development by several years. EBV DNA, RNA, and gene products have also been detected in tumour cells (Chang & Adami, 2006). EBV serology is currently used as a screening tool for high-risk populations in southern China (Glastonbury, 2007). Certain genetic haplotypes - HLA A2, Bsn 2, B46, and B58 - are also associated with increased risk (Ren & Chan, 1996). Other exposures implicated in NPC include cigarette smoking, other smoke, and occupational exposures including wood dust and industrial heat (Yu *et al.*, 2010).

2. Epidemiology of NPC

NPC is a rare malignancy that exhibits a distinct ethnic and geographic variation (Chang & Adami, 2006). While in most regions of the world, age standardized incidence rates for both males and females are <1 per 100,000 person-years (Chang & Adami, 2006; Chong, 2006)), higher rates are observed in a few well-defined populations. Studies have demonstrated intermediate incidence rates in several indigenous populations in Southeast Asia, the Arctic, and the Middle East/North Africa (ranging from 0.5 to 31.5 per 100,000 person-years in males and 0.1 to 11.8 person-years in females) (Chang & Adami, 2006; Parkin *et al.*, 2002), and endemic rates in the natives of southern China reaching 20-30 per 100,000 person-years and 15-20 per 100,000 person-years amongst males and females, respectively, in the province of Guangdong (Ho, 1978; Yoshizaki *et al.*, 2011). In addition, within geographic regions, a distinct ethnic variation also exists. For example, in the US, rates are highest amongst Chinese Americans, followed by Filipino Americans, Japanese Americans, Blacks, Hispanics, and finally Caucasians (Burt *et al.*, 1992).

Globally, there are more than 80,000 incident cases and 50,000 deaths annually due to NPC (Parkin *et al.*, 2005). NPC shows a male predilection of 2-3:1 (Parkin *et al.*, 2002). In low risk populations, incidence increases with age, while in high risk populations, incidence peaks in the 6th decade of life and declines thereafter. NPC is rare in pediatric populations. Thus, the highest incidence rates are observed in middle-aged men (Chang & Adami, 2006).

3. Histopathology of NPC

Three histologic subtypes are recognized by the World Health Organization (WHO) classification system:

- Type 1 – squamous cell carcinoma; typically found in older adult populations
    - Type 1 is further subdivided into poorly, moderately, and well-differentiated
- Type 2 – non-keratinizing carcinoma
- Type 3 – undifferentiated or poorly differentiated carcinoma, including lymphoepithelioma and anaplastic variants; comprises most cases of childhood and adolescent NPC

In contrast to Type 1, Type 2 and 3 are associated with elevated EBV titres. In addition, Type 2 and 3 may also be accompanied by lymphoepithelioma, which is an inflammatory infiltrate of lymphocytes, plasma cells, and eosinophils. Histopathologic typing has prognostic significance, as Type 2 and Type 3 exhibit a more favourable prognosis and greater radiosensitivity than Type 1. Risk factors for Type 1 include cigarette smoke and ethanol consumption, whereas Type 2 and 3 are the endemic forms (Brennan, 2006).

In NPC, two histological patterns may be recognized: (1) the Regaud type which is a well-defined collection of epithelial cells surrounded by lymphocytes and connective tissue, and (2) the Schmincke type, which appears as diffuse tumours intermingled with inflammatory cells (Brennan, 2006).

4. Presentation of NPC

While some patients are asymptomatic, 50% to 70% of patients initially present with cervical lymphadenopathy in the form of a neck mass and are diagnosed by lymph node biopsy (Glastonbury, 2007). Symptoms at presentation may include trismus, pain, otitis media due to Eustachian tube dysfunction, nasal regurgitation due to paresis of the soft palate, and hearing loss. Depending on the degree of local infiltration, patients may also suffer from cranial nerve dysfunction and headache. Cranial nerve neuropathies (most often CN5 and CN6) are an indication of skull base infiltration. Larger growths may also produce nasal obstruction or bleeding and a "nasal twang". Metastatic spread may result in bone pain or organ dysfunction. Rarely, a paraneoplastic syndrome of osteoarthropathy may occur with widespread disease.

5. Role of imaging in the management of NPC

All stages of NPC patient management, from diagnosis and staging to treatment and follow-up, involve imaging. On presentation, a full diagnostic work-up for NPC involves a physical examination (including neurological examination of the cranial nerves), laboratory testing (including a complete blood count, liver function tests, and alkaline phosphate levels), an endoscopic-guided biopsy, as well as imaging studies. Since 6% of NPC is submucosal and cannot been seen on endoscopy (King *et al.*, 2006), cross-sectional imaging studies, such as magnetic resonance imaging (MRI) or computed tomography (CT), are required to help confirm the diagnosis, as well as accurately demarcate the exact limits of pharyngeal wall involvement and tumour invasion into surrounding structures. Currently, MRI and CT are not routinely used for screening purposes; however, the radiologist should consider NPC whenever head and neck imaging is obtained, especially in high-risk patients - such as those of Asian descent - being evaluated for otitis media or with incidental findings of middle ear opacification.

Early findings of NPC on imaging include asymmetry of the nasopharynx and an obstructed Eustachian tube (ET) **(Figure 1)** (Glastonbury, 2007). Most NPC masses originate in the fossa of Rosenmuller, otherwise known as the lateral pharyngeal recess. Furthermore, involvement of the lateral pharyngeal recess may cause dysfunction of the ET - either directly or indirectly by infiltrating the surrounding musculature - leading to stasis of middle ear secretions and unilateral hearing loss **(Figure 2).** In cases of head and neck imaging for neck masses of "unknown primary," careful attention should be paid to the possibility of NPC since cervical lymphadenopathy is the most common presentation.

Like other neoplasms, a mainstay in NPC treatment is staging. Staging contributes information regarding prognosis and helps guide treatment planning, facilitate stratification of treatment, and coordinate clinical studies (Mao *et al.*, 2009; Yu *et al.*, 2010). While in the past, CT was preferred, MRI is currently the imaging modality of choice for NPC staging using the American Joint Committee on Cancer (AJCC) tumour, node, metastasis (TNM) staging system (King *et al.*, 1999; Liang, 2009; Ng *et al.*, 1997). CT still has a role in the assessment of bony skull base involvement (Olmi, 1995), but MRI is considered superior to CT for assessing primary tumour invasion into surrounding soft tissue and bony structures, pharyngobasilar fascia invasion, invasion into the sinus of Morgagni, skull base invasion, as well as cavernous sinus extension and perineural disease (Liao *et al.*, 2008; Sakata, 1999).

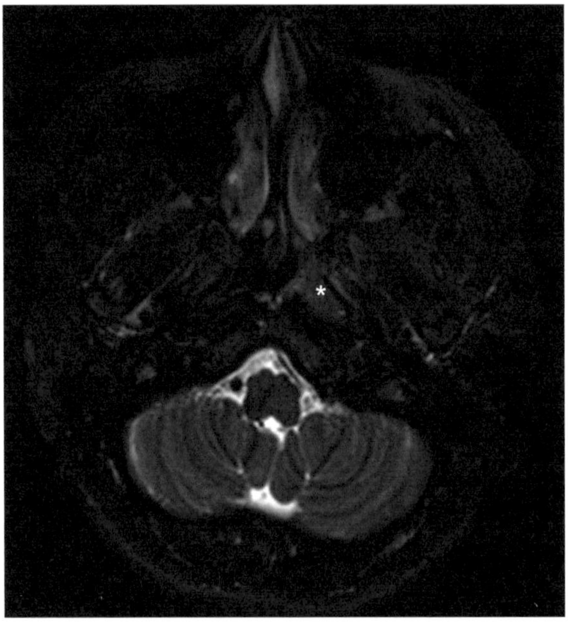

Fig. 1. Axial T2 weighted image shows a mass filling the left fossa of Rosenmuller (*).

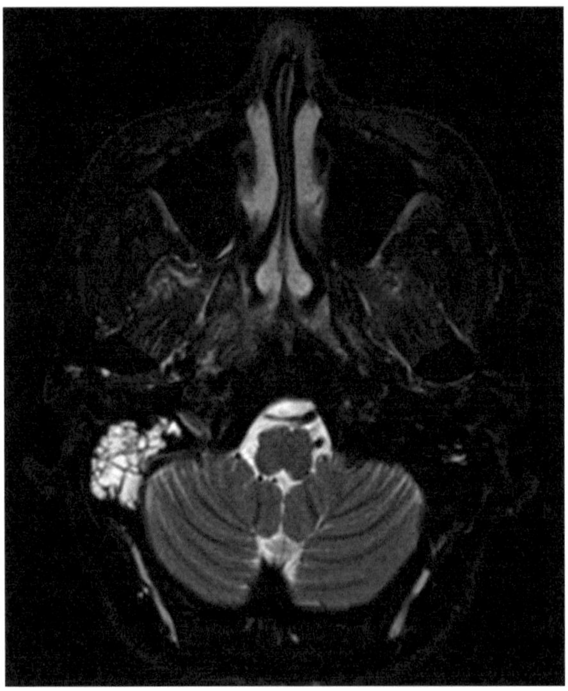

Fig. 2. Axial T2 weighted image shows a right sided NPC that is resulting in right Eustachian tube dysfunction and fluid build up in the right mastoid.

MRI is also more reliable for differentiating between the primary tumor and retropharyngeal adenopathy (Chang, 2005; Chong, 1996; Chung, 2004; King, 2000). For patients with clinical or biochemical evidence of advanced disease, additional investigations - including bone scintigraphy, chest x-ray, CT of thorax, abdomen, and pelvis, and/or fluorodeoxyglucose (FDG)-positron emission tomography (PET)-CT imaging - may be indicated (Caglar, 2003; Chen *et al.*, 2006; Chiesa & De Paoli, 2001; Chua *et al.*, 2009; Comoretto *et al.*, 2008; Lee, 1992).

The mainstay of treatment in NPC is radiation therapy (RT) with the addition of concurrent and/or adjuvant chemotherapy reserved for higher stages of disease. Surgical salvage (nasopharyngectomy) has also been used in cases of recurrent disease (Yu *et al.*, 2010). The goal of treatment is to be curative. To be effective, RT must target the primary lesion as well as any associated neck adenopathy. Thus, cross-sectional imaging, in particular MRI, is needed to determine areas of disease infiltration. NPC has been shown to spread in a step-wise pattern along privileged pathways, such as the neuroforamina (Liang *et al.*, 2009). In addition, involvement of critical structures located near the NP - including the cavernous sinus, pituitary gland, orbit and brainstem - must be evaluated to guide appropriate treatment and to spare these structures of the radiation dose if they are clear of disease (Yu *et al.*, 2010). In the case of intensity-modulated RT (IMRT), CT is also required to correctly calculate dose based on absorption rates (Glastonbury, 2007).

Follow-up evaluation involves a baseline imaging study that is typically performed 2 to 3 months after completion of radiation treatment, followed by imaging every 3 to 6 months for the first 2 post-treatment years (Glastonbury, 2007). Any soft tissue signal abnormalities on MRI in the nasopharynx, deep face, or skull base should remain stable over this period or show further reduction in volume. Recurrent disease is seen as any increase in the bulk of abnormal signal from baseline imaging. Most recurrences, local or systemic, occur within the first 2 years after treatment (Glastonbury, 2007). Of patients with recurrences, 10% to 20% may be curable with additional treatment (Glastonbury, 2007). After 2 years without evidence of recurrence, the imaging interval is typically extended to every 6 to 12 months. Although not yet the mainstay of treatment, one meta-analysis demonstrated that FDG-PET/CT is more sensitive and specific than CT and MRI for the diagnosis of local residual or recurrent NPC (Liu *et al.*, 2007).

5.1 MRI technique

The staging MRI protocol for NPC varies from center to center. In general, the images should cover the area from above the frontal sinuses to the thoracic inlet on axial studies and from the tip of the nose to the fourth ventricle on coronal sequences. At our institution, axial and coronal T1- and T2-weighted images, as well as a sagittal T1 or T2 fat saturation series covering the entire head and neck are obtained. A head and neck imaging coil is routinely used for both the 1.5T and 3.0T MRI scanners. The axial, coronal and sagittal T1 series are performed using a T1-FLAIR technique. Postgadolinium-enhanced axial images with fat saturation and coronal images without fat saturation are also acquired using a conventional spin echo T1 technique. Lau *et al.* found that the axial precontrast and postcontrast series were the most informative MRI sequences for evaluating primary tumour extension and achieved approximately 100% diagnostic accuracy in T-staging of NPC (Lau *et al.*, 2004). We find that axial and coronal noncontrast T1-weighted images are the best for providing detailed views of the local NP anatomy and surrounding structures, whereas postcontrast images allow for accurate assessment of perineural disease along major nerves, such as the maxillary and mandibular divisions of the trigeminal nerve, as well as the cavernous sinus (Yu *et al.*, 2010).

5.2 Comparison of imaging methods

	MRI	CT	PET/CT
Strengths	Superior to CT and PET/CT for assessing primary tumour invasion into surrounding soft tissue and boney structures, pharyngobasilar fascia invasion, invasion into the sinus of Morgagni, skull base invasion, intracranial invasion, as well as cavernous sinus extension and perineural disease (Liao *et al.*, 2008; Ng *et al.*, 2009 Sakata *et al.*, 1999) Superior to CT and PET/CT for evaluating retropharyngeal adenopathy No exposure to ionizing radiation	Relatively inexpensive Rapid image acquisition time Widely available	Superior to MRI and CT for assessing lymph node metastasis, especially cervical nodal metastases, and distant metastases, especially occult metastatic disease (i.e., N- and M-staging of NPC) (Comoretto *et al.*, 2008; King & Bhatia, 2010; King *et al.*, 2008; Lin *et al.*, 2008; Ng *et al.*, 2009, Wang *et al.*, 2007) Screens the entire patient for local recurrence, lymph node metastases and distant metastases during a single whole-body examination using a single injection of FDG Significantly better sensitivity and specificity compared to CT and MRI for diagnosis of local residual or recurrent nasopharyngealcarcinoma (Liu *et al.*, 2007)
Weaknesses	Expensive Long image acquisition times compared to CT Less readily available compared to CT not always reliable in distinguishing between enhancing residual	Less accurate than MRI and PET/CT for evaluating tumour invasion into surrounding tissues (Ng *et al.*, 2009) Exposure to ionizing radiation	Accessibility issues (in some regions) Expensive Exposure to ionizing radiation Compared to MRI, PET/CT undermaps the

	disease versus posttherapy changes due to treatment-related edema, fibrosis, inflammation, and scarring (Comoretto *et al.*, 2008)	Treatment-related edema, fibrosis, inflammation, and scarring limit ability to diagnose residual or recurrent disease	involvement of the nasopharynx, skull base, intracranial disease, perineural spread, parapharyngeal space, and brain (due to high FDG uptake by the brain) (Comoretto *et al.*, 2008; King *et al.*, 2008; Ng *et al.*, 2009) Inferior to MRI for detecting retropharyngeal lymph node metastases (Ng *et al.*, 2009; Ng *et al.*, 2010, Su *et al.*, 2006) False-positive and false-negative related to inflammatory hyperplastic nodes, nodes with large areas of necrosis, small nodes that are beyond the spatial resolution limits of PET (Ng *et al.*, 2009; Zhang *et al.*, 2006)

6. Anatomy of the nasopharynx

The nasopharynx is at the superior and posterior aspect of the aerodigestive tract. The nasopharyngeal mucosa is lined with squamous epithelium and surrounded by a muscular and fascial sling consisting of the superior constrictor muscle and the buccopharyngeal fascia derived from the middle layer of the deep cervical fascia. The space has three walls and a roof. It opens anteriorly to the posterior nasal cavity via the posterior nasal choanae, and inferiorly into the oropharynx at the level of the hard palate. On imaging, the C1/2 junction is also an accepted marker between the nasopharynx and oropharynx (Dubrulle *et al.*, 2007). The roof of the nasopharynx abuts the sphenoid sinus floor, and slopes posteroinferiorly along the clivus/basiocciput to the upper cervical vertebrae. Remains of adenoid tissue may persist into adulthood and exist as tags in the roof of the nasopharynx.

The pharyngobasilar fascia (PBF), a tough aponeurosis connecting the superior constrictor muscles to the skull base, is perhaps the most important structure of the nasopharynx. The tough fibers of the pharyngobasilar fascia create a framework that determines the configuration of the nasopharynx and the support by which the entire pharynx hangs from the skull base (Dillon *et al.*, 1984). The parallel lateral walls of the pharyngobasilar fascia extend from the posterior margin of the medial pterygoid plate anteriorly to the occipital pharyngeal tuber and prevertebral muscles posteriorly. The foramen lacerum, which is within the confines of the pharyngobasilar fascia, is a fibrocartilaginous structure that forms part of the floor of the horizontal carotid canal and roof of the nasopharynx. It provides a route for nasopharyngeal tumors to access the cavernous sinus and intracranial cavity. The pharyngobasilar fascia is a fibrous structure and occasionally can be seen as a thin dark line on T2-weighted axial MR images, deep to the submucosal tissues of the nasopharynx (**Figure 3**).

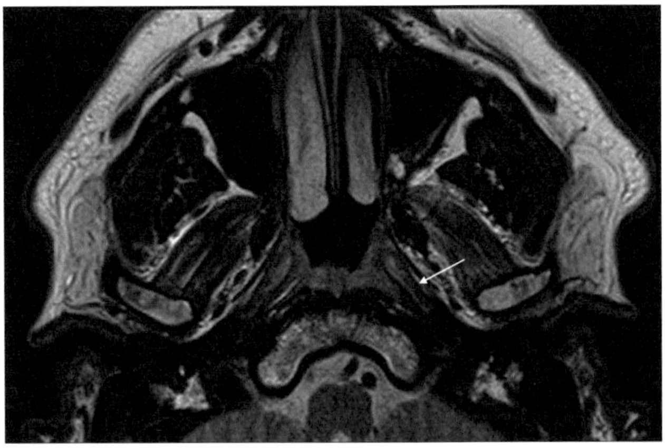

Fig. 3. Axial T2 weighted image at the level of the nasopharynx. The arrow shows the pharyngobasilar fascia on the left side.

The paired Eustachian tubes, along with the medial fibers of the levator veli palatini muscle pass into the nasopharynx via the sinus of Morgagni, a posterolateral defect in the pharyngobasilar fascia. The opening of the Eustachian tube is anterior (on axial images) and inferior (on coronal images) to the torus tubarius, the distal cartilaginous end of the eustachian tube that forms a mucosal-lined structure projecting into the lumen of the nasopharynx from the superior aspect of the posterior lateral nasopharyngeal walls. The fossa of Rosenmüller, otherwise known as the lateral pharyngeal recess, is posterior (on axial images) and superior (on coronal images) to the torus tubarius. The fossa of Rosenmüller is the most common site of origin of NPC (Goh & Lim, 2009) (**Figure 4**). However, asymmetry of the lateral pharyngeal recesses is a common and normal incidental finding, and should not be mistaken as tumours.

Lateral to the nasopharynx is the parapharyngeal space (PPS), a fibrofatty space which separates the nasopharynx from the masticator space (**Figure 4).** Involvement of the parapharyngeal fat serves as an important marker of tumour infiltration used in staging. The posterolateral boundary of the nasopharynx consists of the carotid space (post-styloid parapharyngeal space), which is located posterior to the parapharyngeal space. Located posterior to the nasopharynx, between the nasopharyngeal mucosal space and the prevertebral muscles, is the retropharyngeal space, a potential space that contains the medial and lateral retropharyngeal lymph nodes. The lateral retropharyngeal nodes, also known as the nodes of Röuviere, are the first nodes in the lymphatic drainage of the nasopharynx and, along with the cervical Level II nodes, are reported to be the most common site of nodal metastases (Wang *et al.*, 2009). The lateral retropharyngeal lymph nodes can be identified on MRI from the skull base to the level of C3 (King & Bhatia, 2010). The medial retropharyngeal nodes do not form a discrete nodal chain, and thus, are less often visible on imaging.

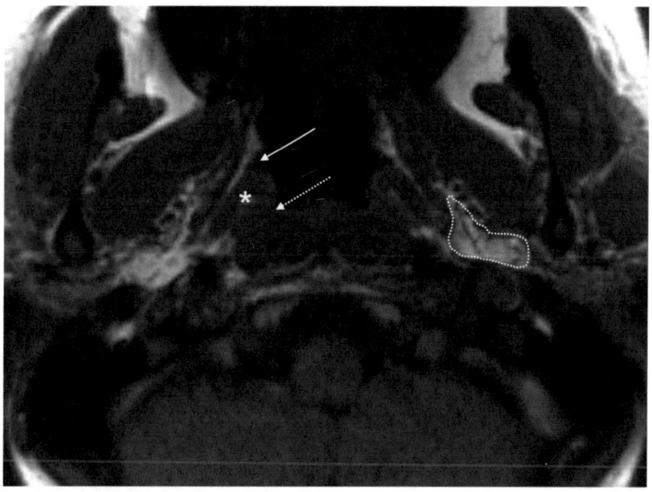

Fig. 4. Axial T1 image shows the torus tubarius (*). The solid arrow points to the opening of the Eustachian tube. Dashed arrow is the fossa of Rosenmuller. The dashed area shows the fat in the left prestyloid parapharyngeal space.

Other important structures include the foramen rotundum and pterygoid (or Vidian) canal, which communicate with the pterygopalatine fossa and are potential routes of tumour spread.

7. Staging of NPC

After the initial diagnosis of NPC is made on history, physical examination, and biopsy, cross-sectional imaging is required for cancer staging. Currently, the 7th edition of the International Union Against Cancer (UICC) and American Joint Committee on Cancer (AJCC) TMN staging system is used, which was recently revised and released on 1 January 2010. As previously described, most cases of NPC originate in the lateral pharyngeal recess and spread submucosally with early infiltration into deeper neck spaces. NPC tends to have well-defined patterns of spread.

TMN Staging of Nasopharyngeal Carcinoma Overview

Primary Tumor (T)

T1	Tumor confined to the nasopharynx, or extends to oropharynx and/or nasal cavity without parapharyngeal extension*
T2	Tumor with parapharyngeal extension*
T3	Tumor involves bony structures of skull base and/or paranasal sinuses
T4	Tumor with intracranial extension and/or involvement of involvement of cranial nerves, hypopharynx, orbit, or with extension to the infratemporal fossa/masticator space

* Parapharyngeal extension denotes posterolateral infiltration of tumor.

Regional Lymph Nodes (N)

NX	Regional lymph nodes cannot be assessed
N0	No regional lymph node metastasis
N1	Unilateral metastasis in lymph node(s), 6 cm or less in greatest dimension, above the supraclavicular fossa, and/or unilateral or bilateral, retropharyngeallymph nodes, 6 cm or less, in greatest dimension*
N2	Bilateral metastasis in lymph node(s), 6 cm or less in greatest dimension, above the supraclavicular fossa*
N3	Metastasis in a lymph node(s)* >6 cm and/or extension to supraclavicular fossa
N3a	Greater than 6 cm in dimension
N3b	Extension to the supraclavicular fossa

* Midline nodes are considered ipsilateral nodes.

Distant Metastasis (M)

MX	Distant metastasis cannot be assessed
M0	No distant metastasis (no pathologic M0; use clinical M to complete stage group)
M1	Distant metastasis

AJCC Stage Groupings

Stage 0	Tis, N0, M0	Stage IVA	T4, N0, M0
Stage I	T1, N0, M0		T4, N1, M0
Stage II	T1, N1, M0		T4, N2, M0
	T2, N0, M0	Stage IVB	Any T, N3, M0
	T2, N1, M0	Stage IVC	Any T, Any N, M1
Stage III	T1, N2, M0		
	T2, N2, M0		
	T3, N0, M0		
	T3, N1, M0		
	T3, N2, M0		

Box 1.

7.1 T1 NPC

Stage T1 refers to disease that is localized to the nasopharynx, as well as disease that has extended inferiorly into the oropharynx or anteriorly into the nasal cavity (Lee,2004; Liu *et al.*, 2008; Yu *et al.*, 2010). Disease that is isolated to the NP is described as being superficial to the pharyngobasilar fascia (PBF). In this case, there is no evidence of tumour breaching or crossing the PBF barrier, which occasionally can be identified on T2-weighted studies as a thin dark curvilinear line running from the medial pterygoid plate laterally and following the contour of the longus musculature along the back wall of the NP **(Figure 3).** The tumour appears as a hypointense to isointense mass on T1-weighted imaging that enhances to a lesser degree than normal mucosa (Chin *et al.*, 2003).

Oropharyngeal extension is readily noted on coronal or sagittal MR imaging as tumour that has extended inferiorly past the plane of palate (**Figure 5**). On axial sections, the oropharynx is considered involved when tumour is seen inferior to the C1/C2 junction.

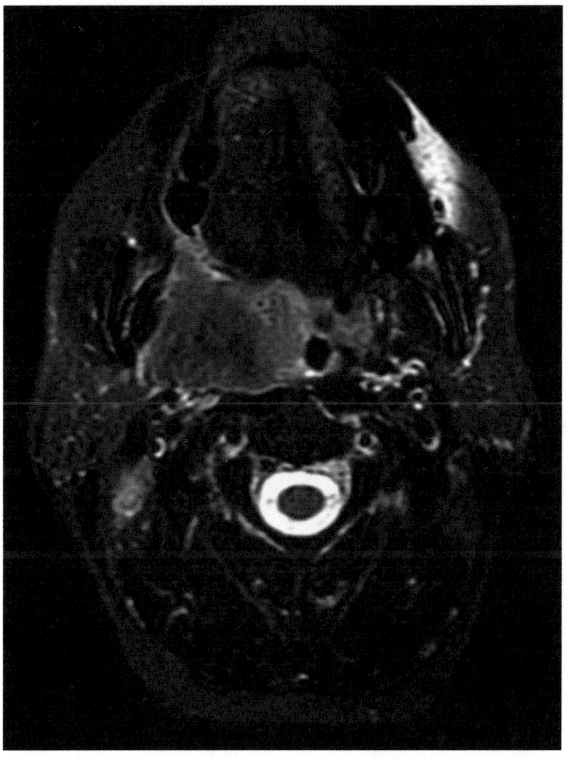

Fig. 5. Axial image of a patient with NPC that shows disease that has extended down to the level of the right oropharynx.

In addition, stage T1 disease comprises anterior extension past the plane of the posterior choana into the nasal cavity (**Figure 6**). From the nasal cavity, NPC can invade through the sphenopalatine foramen into the pterygopalatine fossa (stage T3 disease), resulting in obliteration of the normal fat content in this fossa (**Figure 7**). Direct extension from the nasal cavity is the most common route of NPC invasion into the pterygopalatine fossa, followed by extension from the ethmoid and/or sphenoid sinuses. The significance of pterygopalatine fossa involvement is described later (T3 NPC).

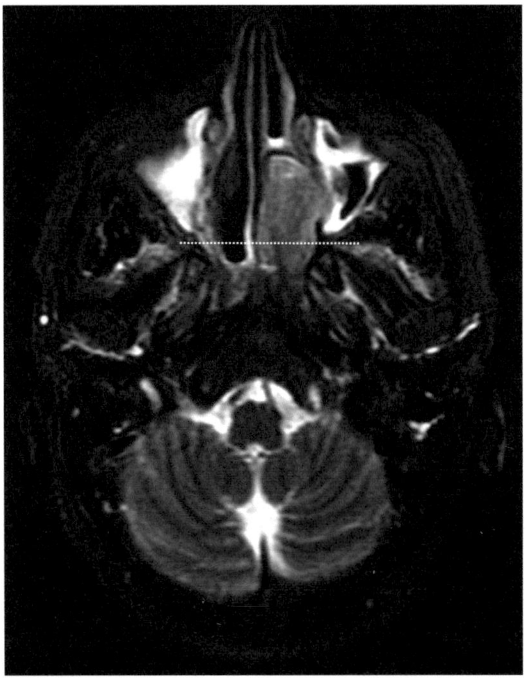

Fig. 6. NPC which has extended beyond the plane of the posterior choana (dashed line) into the nasal cavity.

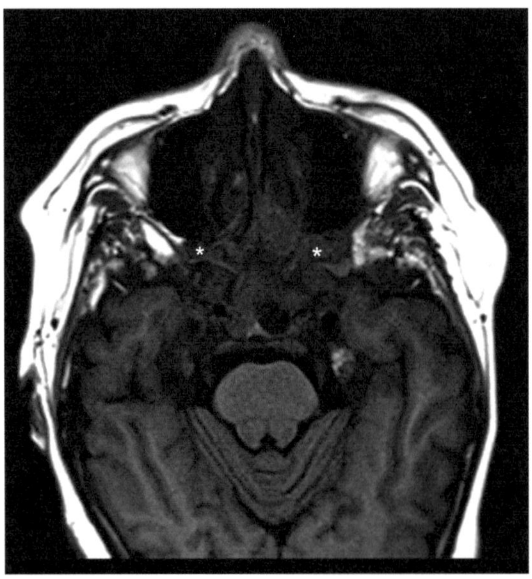

Fig. 7. Axial T1 weighted image shows abnormal soft tissue filling the right and left pterygopalatine fossae (*).

7.2 T2 NPC

Disease that has spread beyond the PBF and infiltrated posterolaterally into the parapharyngeal space (PPS) is considered stage T2. This can lead to compression of the Eustachian tube, resulting in middle ear and mastoid effusion (King & Bhatia, 2010). PPS invasion is associated with worse disease control and survival rates, as well as increased rate of distant metastases compared to stage T1 (Cheng *et al.*, 2005; Chua *et al.*, 1996; Ho *et al.*, 2008; Teo *et al.*, 1996). On imaging, key components of the PPS include the tensor veli palatini and levator palatine muscles. PPS involvement is recognized as a disruption or attenuation of the PBF, infiltration of the tensor veli palatini, or breach of the intrapharyngeal portion of the levator veli palatini muscle.

Infiltration of the fatty component of the PPS is visible on T1-weighted imaging as an intermediate signal mass invading into the hyperintense fat of the PPS (**Figure 8**). As the disease progresses, the full thickness of the intrapharyngeal portion of the levator veli muscle and the tensor veli palatini muscle (appearing as a thin strip of muscle just lateral to the levator veli palatini) may also become involved, followed by infiltration of the normally pristine fat of the prestyloid PPS, which is located deep to the tensor muscle. With further posterolateral spread, the poststyloid PPS structures, such as the carotid sheath, also become vulnerable to disease (**Figure 9**).

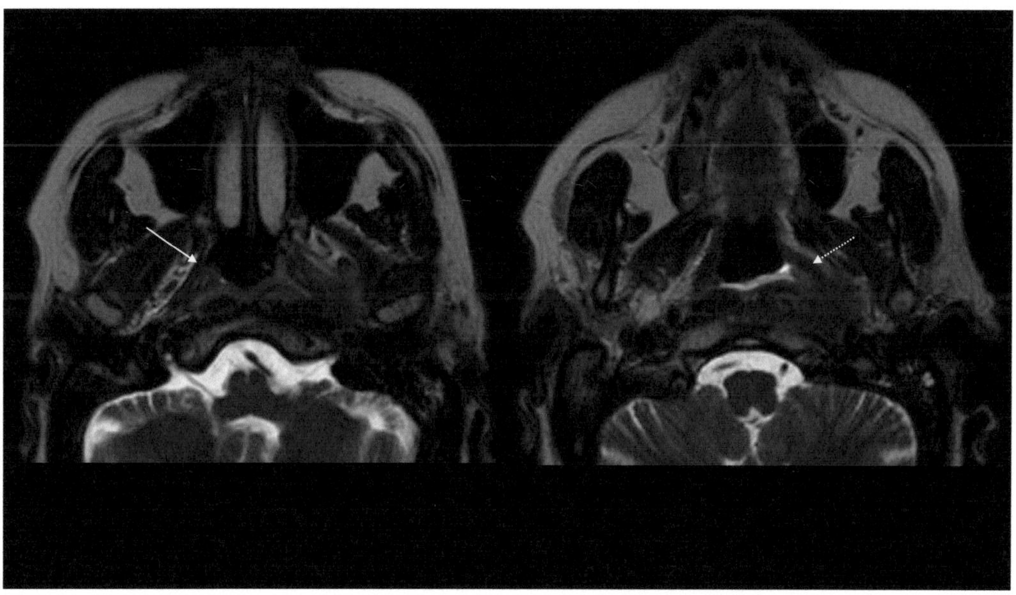

Fig. 8. Axial T2 weighted images shows a carcinoma that has infiltrated lateral to the tensor and levator veli palatini. Solid arrow shows normal tensor veli palatini on the right. Dashed arrow shows the abnormal left levator muscle which is being displaced and the presence of tumor lateral to it.

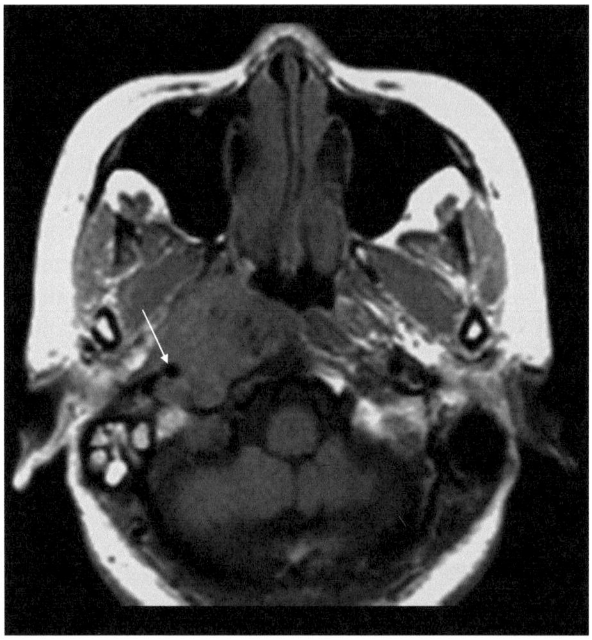

Fig. 9. Axial T1 image shows a large right sided NPC that has extended to encase the right internal carotid artery (arrow).

7.3 T3 NPC

Stage T3 disease is characterized by involvement of the paranasal sinuses and/or the central skull-base structures. Skull base invasion is seen in up to 60% of NPC patients at diagnosis (King *et al.*, 1999; Roh *et al.*, 2004), with the most common sites of involvement being the clivus, pterygoid bones, body of the sphenoid bone, and apices of the petrous temporal bones (King & Bhatia, 2010). In addition, the number of sites involved within the skull base may have prognostic significance (Lu *et al.*, 2004). Assessment of the skull base should focus on five key regions: clivus, right pterygoid base, left pterygoid base, right petrous apex, and left petrous apex (King & Bhatia, 2010). On axial T1-weighted MR sequences, bony skull base disease is detected as a loss of the hyperintense signal, which is characteristic of normal fatty yellow bone marrow. It is replaced with an intermediate signal indicative of either bony reaction or actual invasion. NPC commonly invades posteriorly into the clivus (**Figure 10).** Although normal clival marrow may appear heterogeneous on T1-weighted images, it should still appear more intense than the pons (Goh & Lim, 2009). In addition, up to 25% of patients have tumour spread superiorly into the floor of the sphenoid sinus, often extending up into the sphenoid sinus cavity (Chong & Fan, 1993; Goh & Lim, 2009) (**Figure 11).** The body of the sphenoid is more difficult to assess and may be best studied on coronal images (King & Bhatia, 2010). The sphenoid wings and upper cervical spine should also be assessed. CT scans may also have a role in detecting the presence of cortical erosion and bony sclerosis, which reflects reactive changes due to tumour invasion. It is important, however, to note that sclerosis is a non-specific sign that may arise from adjacent sinus disease, particularly in the sinus margins and the pterygoids.

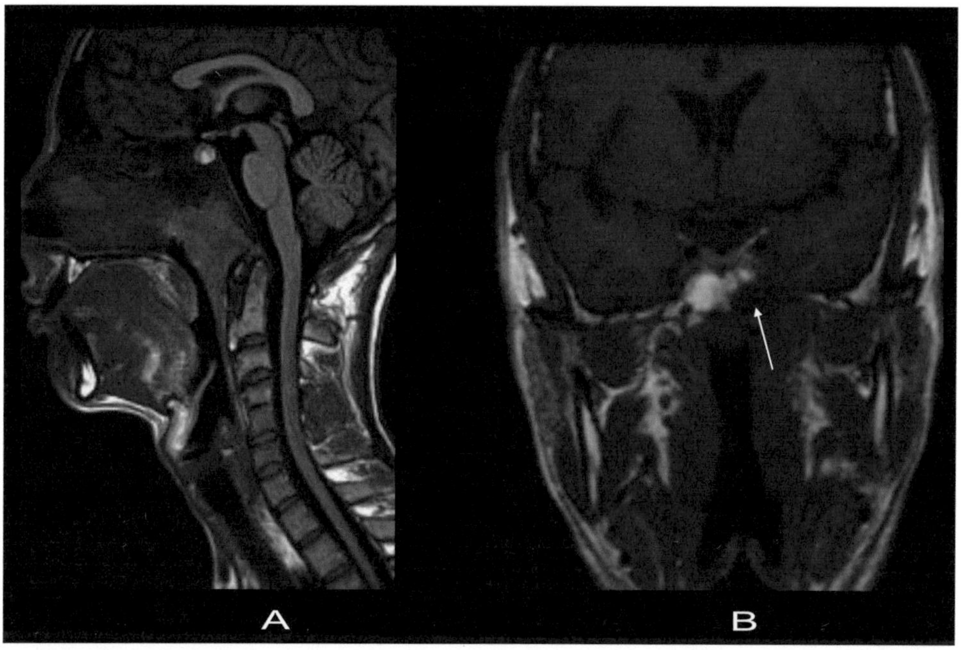

Fig. 10. 10A is a sagittal T1 image that shows NPC invasion into the clivus. There is a loss of the inferior cortical margin of the clivus. The clivus is also of uniform lower signal that reflects sclerotic change. 10B is as coronal T1 image in another patient that shows NPC infiltration into the left aspect of the clivus (arrow).

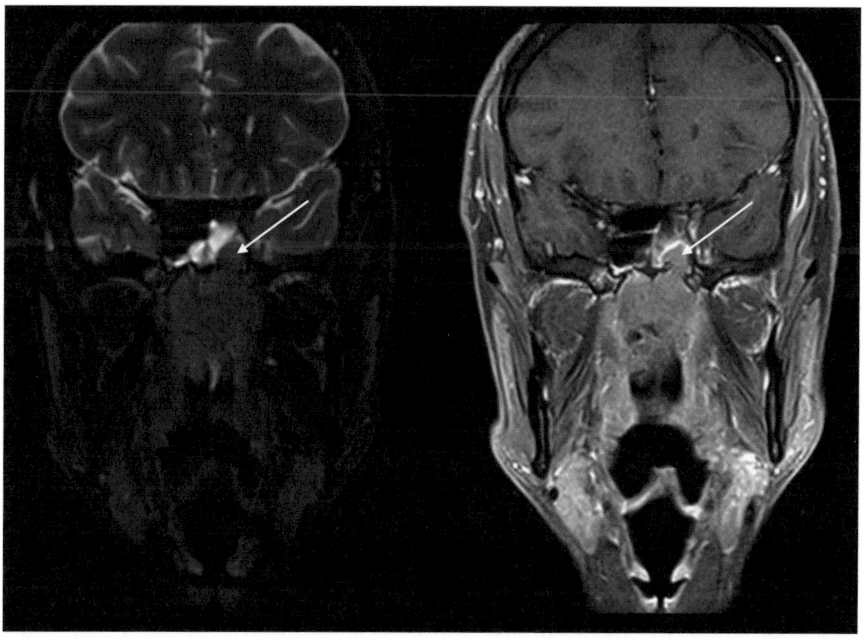

Fig. 11. Coronal T2 (left) and post gadolinium enhanced T1 (right) weighted images show superior extension of NPC through the floor of the sphenoid sinus (arrows).

Next, the skull base foramina and fissures - which include the foramen rotundum (V2 nerve), the vidian canal (vidian nerve), the foramen ovale (V3 nerve), and foramen lacerum - should be examined. Nerve involvement signifies stage T4 disease (see section below). The foramen ovale and lacerum are common routes of tumour extension into the intracranial cavity (King & Bhatia, 2010). While the skull base foramina present an unobstructed route for tumor spread, direct invasion of the bone bordering these foramina is also a common finding. The skull base foramina are best assessed on coronal images. Less common findings include inferior spread of tumor to involve the hypoglossal nerve canal (XII nerve) and jugular foramen (IX-XI nerves) (King & Bhatia, 2010).

It is important to differentiate tumour spread into the paranasal sinuses - which include the ethmoid sinuses, sphenoid sinuses, and maxillary sinuses - from benign mucosal inflammatory changes, which are common in patients with NPC. On MRI, mucosal thickening can be distinguished from NPC by a greater uniform T2-weighted signal and a marked degree of contrast enhancement. With tumor invasion into the ethmoid sinuses, which usually occurs via direct spread from the sphenoid sinus or nasal cavity, there is a reduced chance of shielding the optic nerve from the radiation dose in RT. Involvement of the sphenoid sinus, which is separated from the nasopharynx by only a thin plate of bone, is a common finding (**Figure 11**). In contrast, anteroinferior tumour invasion into the maxillary sinuses is a rare event, except in late disease where there is usually extensive invasion throughout the nasal cavity, other paranasal sinuses, skull base, and brain (King *et al.*, 1999). Sinus involvement is seen on imaging as a loss of contiguity of the sinus walls.

7.4 T4 NPC

T4 disease is denoted by intracranial extension and/or involvement of the cranial nerves, hypopharynx, orbit, or masticator space. Unchecked, NPC can extend superiorly into the cavernous sinus and dura **(Figure 12)**, while direct invasion of the brain is rare at diagnosis (King & Bhatia, 2010). There are multiple routes into the cavernous sinus, including extension from tumour surrounding the horizontal portion of the internal carotid artery or cranial nerve V3, as well as extension from the orbital fissures or the skull base in the region of the foramen ovale or sphenoid sinus (King & Bhatia, 2010). Within the cavernous sinus, cranial nerves III, IV, V1, V2, and VI are vulnerable to tumour invasion. Their involvement is manifested clinically through an abnormal neurological examination, as well as by signs and symptoms of various cranial nerve palsies, including extraocular muscle dysfunction, facial pain, paresthesia and numbness. True perineural spread, however, is uncommon in the pre-treatment setting (King & Bhatia, 2010). Prognostically, cranial nerve involvement has been shown to be associated with a higher rate of distant metastases and decreased survival (Yu *et al.*, 2010). Radiologically, post-contrast T1-weighted MR sequences with fat saturation are used to assess for cranial nerve involvement, especially for V2 along foramen rotundum (**Figure 13**) and V3 in the foramen ovale **(Figure 14).** Contrast-enhanced MRI shows perineural disease extension and cavernous sinus involvement as asymmetric nodular thickening and abnormal enhancement. Skip lesions may also be noted. A late sequelae is expansion of the bony canals in which these nerves travel.

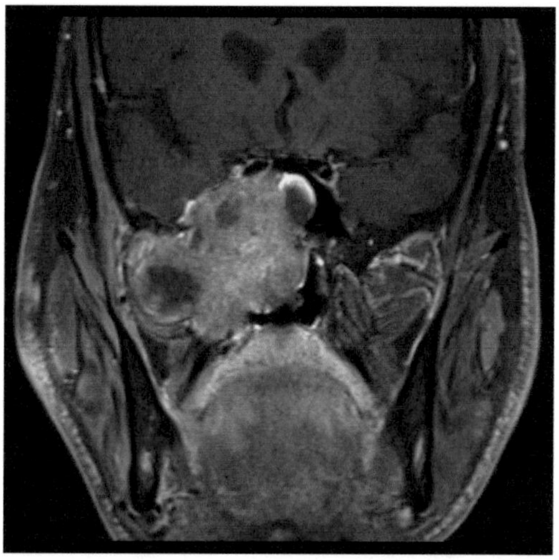

Fig. 12. Coronal postcontrast study shows a large NPC that has extended laterally into the right masticator space as well as superiorly to invade the cavernous sinus, sphenoid sinus and cause mass effect upon the right temporal lobe.

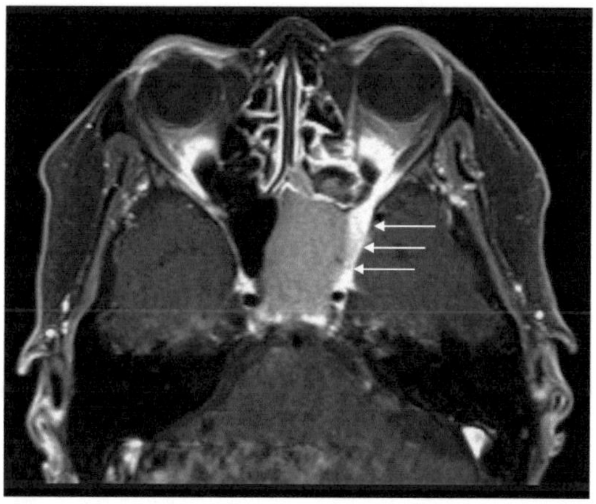

Fig. 13. Axial image shows asymmetric thickening and enhancement along the left V2 nerve (arrows).

Orbital invasion, usually arising from the pterygopalatine fossa via the inferior orbital fissure or directly from the cavernous sinus, denotes the most extensive form of disease (King & Bhatia, 2010) **(Figure 15).** From the PPS, pterygoid base, or pterygomaxillary fissure, NPC can extend laterally to involve masticator space, which includes the medial and lateral pterygoid muscles, temporalis muscle, infratemporal fat, as well as the mandibular division (V3) of the trigeminal nerve **(Figure 14).** Disease involving the masticator space can give rise to trismus and weakness in mastication. In addition, the V3 nerve is vulnerable to tumour infiltration within the masticator space. Both antegrade and retrograde perineural spread along V3 is possible. From the masticator space, NPC can also extend superiorly through the floor of the middle cranial fossa and foramen ovale to gain access to the intracranial cavity and the cavernous sinus.

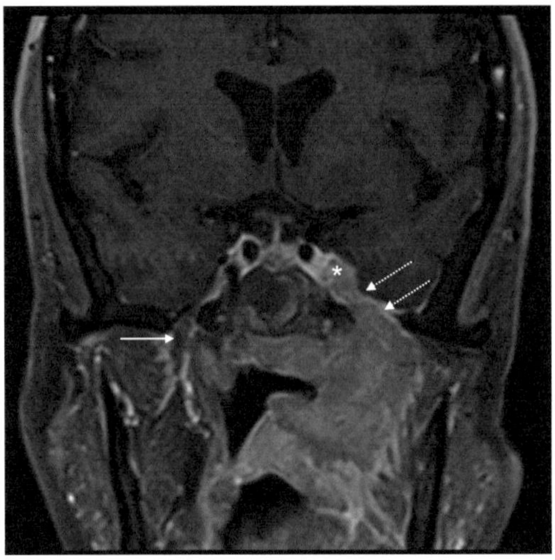

Fig. 14. Coronal image shows NPC that has extended laterally into the left masticator space and subsequent perineural tumor tracking superiorly (dashed arrows) along V3 into the left cavernous sinus (*). Solid arrow shows the normal contralateral V3 nerve.

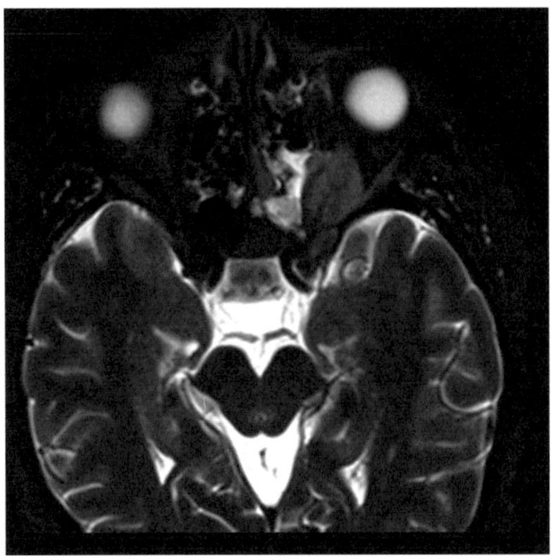

Fig. 15. Axial T2 weighted scan shows intermediate signal tumor that has extended through the superior orbital fissure into the left orbit.

The hypopharynx, which is the most inferior site included in the TMN staging classification, is very rarely involved at diagnosis due to the tendency of NPC to extend superiorly rather than inferiorly (King & Bhatia, 2010).

7.5 Nodal stage

The NPC N classification system differs from other head and neck mucosal malignancies (see Box 1). Up to 60–90% of NPC patients will have nodal metastases at presentation (Glastonbury, 2007; Goh & Lim, 2009), suggesting that only 10-40% of cases present without positive nodal disease (N0). Positive neck nodal disease in NPC is associated with an increased risk of local recurrence and distant metastases (Goh & Lim, 2009). Unlike other head and neck squamous cell carcinomas, nodal disease in NPC is more frequently bilateral.

NPC generally follows a very orderly pathway of nodal spread, beginning with the (lateral) retropharyngeal lymph nodes (RPN) (**Figure 16**) - located medial to the carotid artery - before involving nodal groups along the internal jugular chain (level II to IV), spinal accessory chain (Va and Vb), as well as supraclavicular nodes (Glastonbury, 2007; King *et al.*, 2004). Level IIa or b nodes, located posterior to the jugular vein in the upper neck, are the most common site for non-retropharyngeal node involvement (Mao *et al.*, 2008) (**Figure 17).**

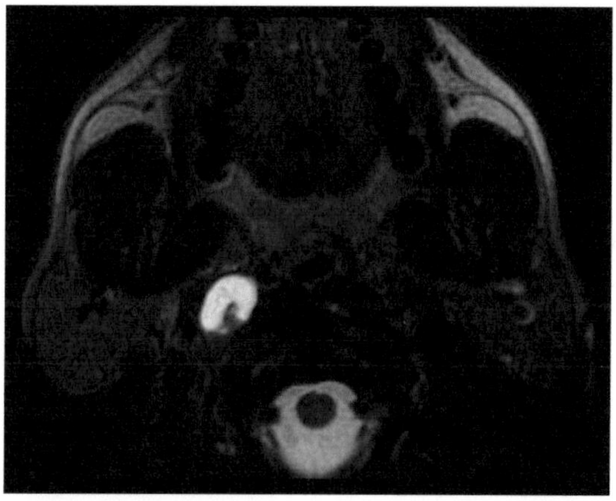

Fig. 16. Cystic right retropharyngeal lymph node.

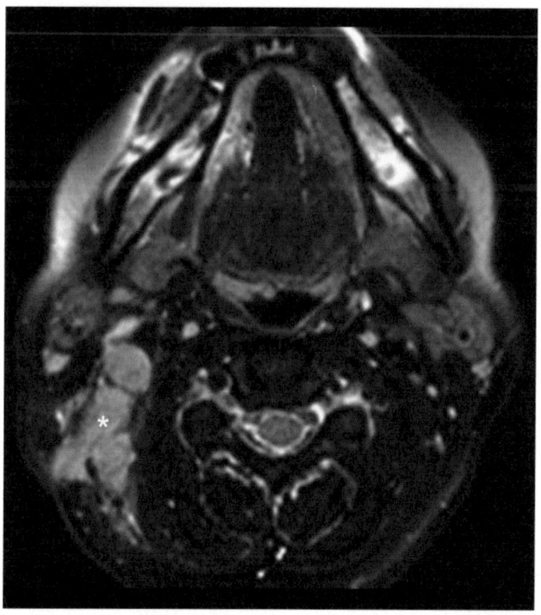

Fig. 17. Right sided level II adenopathy (*).

Nodal disease in the submandibular and parotid/periparotid regions is a rare occurrence (Chong & Fan, 2000; King & Bhatia, 2010), but should be evaluated for radiotherapy planning purposes. Although the RPN are generally considered the first echelon of metastatic spread, studies have shown that this is not true in all cases (Liu *et al.*, 2006; Mao *et al.*, 2008; Ng *et al.*, 2004; Wang *et al.*, 2009). While King *et al.* found that the RPN were bypassed in only 6% of cases to preferentially affect the level II distribution, Ng *et al.* found that 17 of 89 cases of NPC bypassed the RPN (King *et al.*, 2000; Ng *et al.*, 2004). In addition, Ng *et al.* also reported skip metastases in the lower neck lymph nodes and the supraclavicular fossa in 7.9% of cases, and distant metastases to thoracic and abdominal nodes in 3-5% of cases. After radiotherapy, level I nodes may also become involved (Ahuja *et al.*, 1999).

In the current N classification system, N1 disease consists of the presence of unilateral metastasis in cervical lymph node(s) that are 6 cm or less in their greatest dimension, and/or unilateral or bilateral RPN metastasis that are 6 cm or less in their greatest dimension. Nodes greater than 3 cm in size are generally considered "nodal masses" and are indicative of confluent nodes. N2 disease is defined by bilateral metastasis in the cervical lymph node(s) that are again 6 cm or less in greatest dimension. Unlike other carcinomas in the neck, N2 is not further divided into substages. In both N1 and N2 stages, disease is restricted to above the supraclavicular fossa. Once supraclavicular fossa nodal involvement is noted, the disease is upstaged to N3b. Supraclavicular nodes include all lymph nodes seen on the same axial cross-sectional slice as a portion of the clavicle, and include Level IV and Vb nodes. Stage N3a disease is defined by matted nodes greater than 6 cm in their greatest dimension, although this is a rare finding (King & Bhatia, 2010) (**Figure 18**).

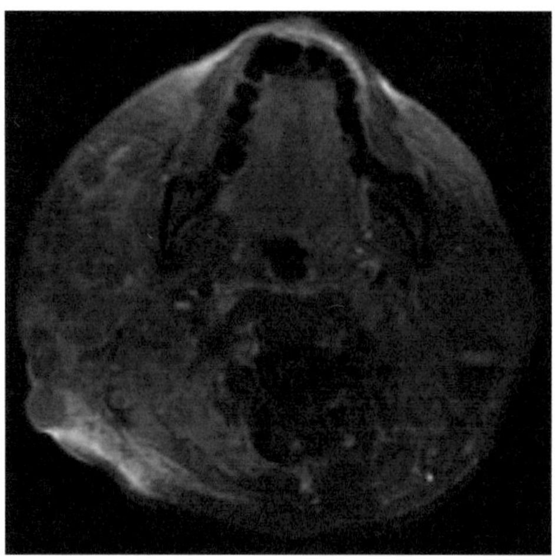

Fig. 18. Massive conglomerate right sided neck adenopathy measuring over 6cm in dimension -N3a disease.

While distinguishing between the primary tumour mass and adjacent RPN is best assessed with MRI, cervical lymph nodes can be evaluated accurately with both MRI and CT (King *et al.*, 2004). T2-weighted imaging with fat saturation shows nodes as bright structures in the posterior cervical fat **(Figure 17).** The higher resolution of CT facilitates the visualization of neck adenopathy, as well as nodal necrosis and extracapsular extension. The latter manifests as a loss or irregularity of the nodal margins, and/or streakiness of the adjacent fat (Yu *et al.*, 2010). Patients with nodes showing necrosis and extranodal spread have a very poor prognosis with a 50% decreased 5-year survival rate (Som *et al.*, 1987).

There are several features on imaging that are suggestive of metastatic nodal disease, including a large size (although there is no accepted size criterion, generally >1.5 cm for levels I and II, >1 cm for levels for levels IV-VII, and >5 mm for RPN using the shortest transaxial diameter is considered suspicious) (Goh & Lim, 2009; King & Bhatia, 2010), a group of 3 or more nodes borderline in size, rounded nodes with loss of the fatty hilum, and necrosis (King & Bhatia, 2010). If identified, necrosis is considered 100% specific. However, due to resolution restrictions, necrosis can only be reliability identified in tumour foci greater than 3 mm, of which approximately one-third reportedly have nodal necrosis (Goh & Lim, 2009; Som & Brandwein, 2003; Yousem *et al.*, 1992). Necrosis or cystic change is hypointense on T1-weighted images with rim enhancement with contrast, and hyperintense on T2-weighted images (**Figure 16**). In CT images, necrosis is seen as a focal area of hypoattenuation with or without rim enhancement (**Figure 19**).

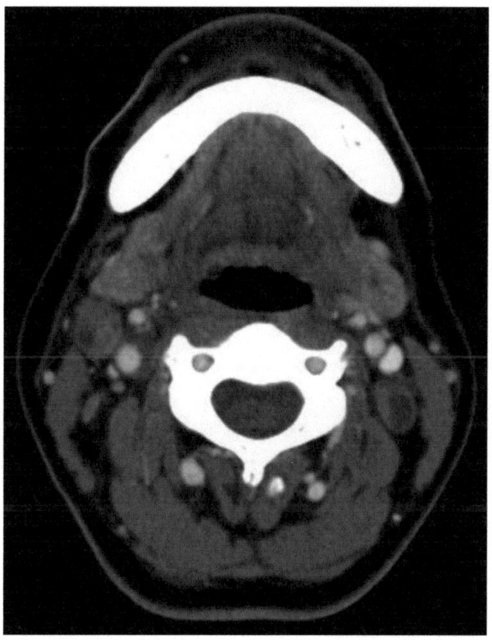

Fig. 19. Bilateral level II adenopathy. Focal areas of lower attenuation on CT is compatible with the presence of necrotic change.

7.6 Distant metastasis (M)

The M stage of NPC is similar to that of other malignancies, whereby M0 signifies the absence of distant metastasis and M1 refers to the presence of such disease. NPC has the highest incidence of distant metastasis among head and neck cancers, with a rate as high as 11% at diagnosis (Kumar *et al.*, 2004; Teo *et al.*, 1996). The likelihood of metastasis increases with increasing T and N stage.

The most commonly affected regions are the bone, lung and liver (Chiesa & De Paoli, 2001) (**Figure 20**). Thus, bones and lung apices should be evaluated for tumour involvement in head and neck MRI studies, especially in patients with risk factors such as metastatic cervical nodes which extend to the supraclavicular fossa (stage N3b).

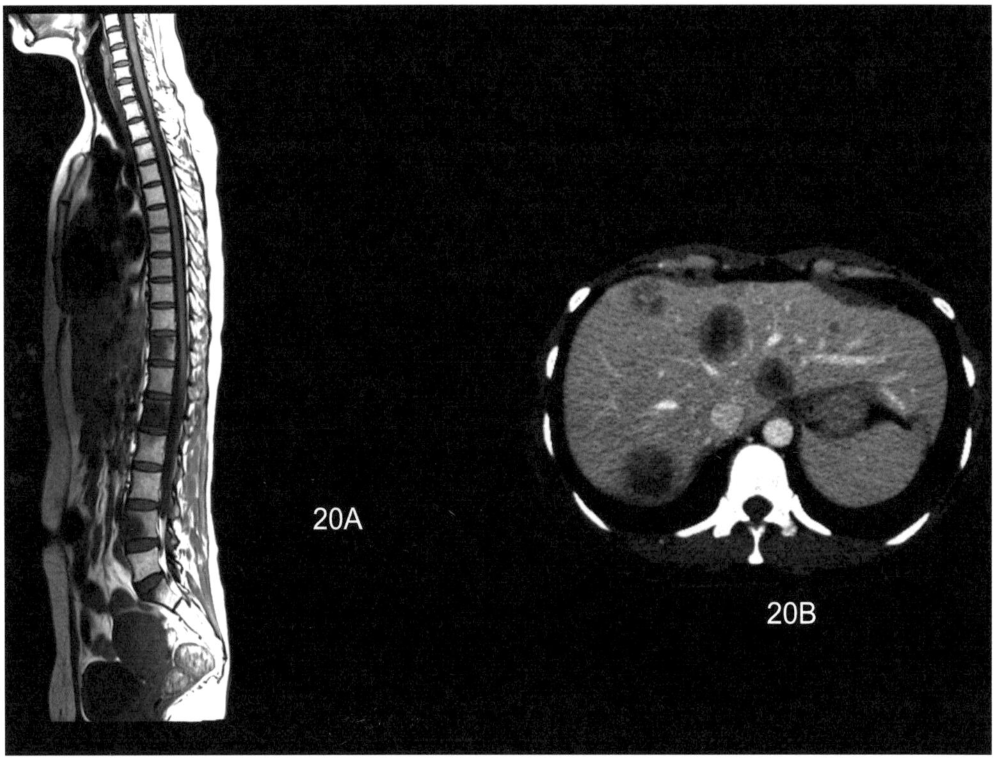

Fig. 20. A and B 20A is a sagittal T1 weighted exam of the spine showing multiple areas of abnormal intermediate signal within vertebral bodies in the lower thoracic and lumbar spine -bony metastases. 20B is a contrast CT of the abdomen that shows the presence of multiple liver metastases.

The presence of M1 disease is associated with shorter survival rates (Teo *et al.*, 1996) and significantly alters patient management, as such patients are generally considered to be incurable. Median survival is under four months and approximately 90% of patients with distant metastases pass away within a year (Goh & Lim, 2009; Khor *et al.*, 1978). The goal of treatment in such instances will be palliation with therapy being applied for locoregional symptom control.

The exact method for the evaluation of distant metastasis will vary from institution to institution. Imaging options include bone scintigraphy, chest x-ray, CT of the thorax, abdomen and pelvis, and PET/CT. Studies have shown fluorodeoxyglucose PET/CT imaging to have a higher sensitivity and specificity in detecting distant metastases (Chen *et al.*, 2006; Chua *et al.*, 2009; Comoretto *et al.*, 2008; King *et al.*, 2008; Lin *et al.*, 2008; Liu *et al.*, 2007; Ng *et al.*, 2009; Wang *et al.*, 2007; Yu *et al.*, 2010).

8. Tumour volume

Tumour volume has also been reported to have significant prognostic relevance outside of the TNM classification system (Wei & Sham, 2005). There is an estimated 1% increase risk of local control failure with every 1 cm^3 increase in tumour volume. The increased risk is attributed to factors such as increase number of tumour clonogens, tumor hypoxia and relative radioresistance, etc (Bentzen *et al.*, 1991; Johnston *et al.*, 1995; Lartigau *et al.*, 1993; Sze *et al.*, 2004). However, issues with standardized methods of volume measurement, the intra- and interobserver reliability due to operator-dependent tracing, as well as the technical challenges associated with implementing this in the clinical setting - including the time it takes to perform this tedious task - have prevented it from being routinely used in daily practice.

9. Summary

Nasopharyngeal carcinoma is a relatively rare neoplasm with a characteristic geographic and ethnic distribution. It most commonly arises in the lateral pharyngeal recess, and has a tendency to invade widely and metastasize. Cervical lymphadenopathy is very common at presentation and is a common presenting complaint.

Diagnosis of NPC can be made on endoscopically-guided biopsy, but effective treatment of NPC requires an accurate mapping of tumor volume and extent with imaging. Imaging allows for evaluation of tumour extent, including submucosal, osseous, and intracranial tumour spread which cannot be assessed clinically or endoscopically. Staging of NPC is based on the new 2010 AJCC guidelines. MRI is the best tool for assessing tumour extent under the current staging system, while high-resolution CT has value for assessing cortical bone erosion and PET/CT is emerging as the most accurate modality for assessing distant metastases and recurrence.

A thorough understanding of the anatomy of the nasopharynx and surrounding structures, as well as the natural history of the disease and patterns of spread, allows for accurate tumour mapping and treatment planning.

10. References

Ahuja AT, Leung SF, Teo P, Ying M, King W, Metreweli C (1999). Submental metastasis from nasopharyngeal carcinoma. *Clin Radiol*. 54:25-8.

Bentzen SM, Johansen LV, Overgaard J, Thames HD (1991). Clinical radiobiology of squamous cell carcinoma of the oropharynx. *Int J Radiat Oncol Bio Phys*. 206:1197-1206.

Brennan B (2006). Nasopharyngeal carcinoma. *Orphanet Journal or Rare Diseases. 1:23.*

Burt RD, Vaughan TL, McKnight B (1992). Descriptive epidemiology and survival analysis of nasopharyngeal carcinoma in the United States. *Int J Cancer*. 52:549 - 56.

Caglar M, Ceylan E, Ozyar E (2003). Frequency of skeletal metastases in nasopharyngeal carcinoma after initiation of therapy: should bone scans be used for follow-up? *Nucl Med Commun*. 24(12):1231

Chang ET & Adami HO (2006). The Enigmatic Epidemiology of Nasopharyngeal Carcinoma. *Cancer Epidemiol Biomarkers Prev.* 15:1765-1777.

Chang JT, Lin CY, Chen TM *et al.* (2005). Nasopharyngeal carcinoma with cranial nerve palsy: the importance of MRI for radiotherapy. *Int. J. Radiat. Oncol. Biol. Phys.* 63(5), 1354–1360.

Chen YK, Su CT, Ding HJ *et al.* (2006). Clinical usefulness of fused PET/CT compared with PET alone or CT alone in nasopharyngeal carcinoma patients. *Anticancer Res.* 26(2B), 1471–1477.

Cheng SH, Tsai SY, Yen KL, Jian JJ, Feng AC, Chan KY, Hong CF, Chu NM, Lin YC, Lin CY, Tan TD, Hsieh CY, Chong V, Huang AT (2005). Prognostic significance of parapharyngeal space venous plexus and marrow involvement: potential landmarks of dissemination for stage I-III nasopharyngeal carcinoma. *Int J Radiat Oncol Biol Phys.* 61: 456-465.

Chiesa F, De Paoli F (2001). Distant metastases from nasopharyngeal cancer. *ORL J Otorhinolaryngol Relat Spec.* 63(4):214.

Chin SC, Fatterpekar G, Chen CY, Som PM. (2003). MR imaging of diverse manifestations of nasopharyngeal carcinomas. *Am. J. Roentgenol.* 180(6), 1715–1722.

Chong VFH (2006). Neoplasms of the nasopharynx. In: *Head and Neck Cancer Imaging*. Baert AL, Sartor K (Eds). Springer, Berlin, Germany, 143–162.

Chong VFH, Fan YF (2000). Facial lymphadenopathy in nasopharyngeal carcinoma. *Clin Radiol.* 55:363-7.

Chong VFH, Fan YF (1993). MRI and CT assessment of paranasal sinus involvement in nasopharyngeal carcinoma. *Clin Radiol.* 48:345.

Chong VF, Fan YF, Khoo JB (1996). Nasopharyngeal carcinoma with intracranial spread: CT and MR characteristics. *J. Comput. Assist. Tomogr.* 20(4), 563–569.

Chua ML, Ong SC, Wee JT *et al.* (2009). Comparison of 4 modalities for distant metastasis staging in endemic nasopharyngeal carcinoma. *Head Neck* 31(3), 346–354.

Chua DT, Sham JS, Kwong DL, Choy DT, Au GK, Wu PM (1996). Prognostic value of paranasopharyngeal extension of nasopharyngeal carcinoma. A significant factor in local control and distant metastasis. *Cancer.* 78(2), 202–210.

Chung NN, Ting LL, Hsu WC, Lui LT, Wang PM (2004). Impact of magnetic resonance imaging versus CT on nasopharyngeal carcinoma: primary tumor target delineation for radiotherapy. *Head Neck.* 26(3), 241–246.

Comoretto M, Balestreri L, Borsatti E, Cimitan M, Franchin G, Lise M (2008). Detection and restaging of residual and/or recurrent nasopharyngeal carcinoma after chemotherapy and radiation therapy: comparison of MR imaging and FDG PET/CT. *Radiology.* 249(1), 203–211.

Dillon WP, Mills CM, Kjos B, et al (1984) Magnetic Resonance imaging of the nasopharynx. *Radiology.* 152:731-738.

Dubrulle F, Souillard R, Hermans R (2007). Extension patterns of nasopharyngeal carcinoma. *Eur Radiol.* 17:2622-2630

Glastonbury CM (2007). Nasopharyngeal Carcinoma The Role of Magnetic Resonance Imaging in Diagnosis, Staging, Treatment, and Follow-up. *Top Magn Reson Imaging.* 18:225-235.

Goh J & Lim K (2009). Imaging of Nasopharyngeal Carcinoma. *Ann Acad Med Singapore.* 38:809-816.

Henderson BE, Louie E, SooHoo Jing J, Buell P, Gardner MB. Risk factors associated with nasopharyngeal carcinoma. *N. Engl. J. Med.* 295(20), 1101–1106 (1976).

Ho HC, Lee MS, Hsiao SH *et al* (2008). Prognostic influence of parapharyngeal extension in nasopharyngeal carcinoma. *Acta Otolaryngol.* 128(7), 790–798.

Ho JHC (1978). An epidemiologic and clinical study of nasopharyngeal carcinoma. *Int J Radiat Oncol Bio Phys.* 4:183-205.

Johnston CR, Thames HD, Huang DT (1995). The tumour volume and clonogens number relationship: tumor control predictions based upon tumor volume estimates derived from computer tomography. *Int J Radiat Oncol Biol Phys.* 332:281-337.

Khor TH, Tan BC, Chua EJ, Chia KB (1978). Distant metastases in nasopharyngeal carcinoma. *Clin Radiol.* 29:27-30.

King AD, Ahuja AT, Leung SF *et al* (2000). Neck node metastases from nasopharyngeal carcinoma: MR imaging of patterns of disease. *Head Neck.* 22(3), 275–281.

King AD, Bhatia KSS (2010). Magnetic resonance imaging staging of nasopharyngeal carcinoma in the head and neck. *World J Radiol.* 2(5):159-165.

King AD, Lam WW, Leung SF, Chan YL, Teo P, Metreweli C (1999). MRI of local disease in nasopharyngeal carcinoma: tumour extent vs tumour stage. *Br. J. Radiol.* 72(860), 734–741.

King AD, Ma BB, Yau YY, Zee B, Leung SF, Wong JKT, Kam MKM, Ahuja T, & Chan ATC (2008). The impact of ^{18}FDG PET/CT on assessment of nasopharyngeal carcinoma at diagnosis. *The British Journal of Radiology.* 81:291-298.

King AD, Teo P, Lam WW, Leung SF, Metreweli C (2000). Paranasopharyngeal space involvement in nasopharyngeal cancer: detection by CT and MRI. *Clin. Oncol. (R. Coll. Radiol.)* 12(6), 397–402.

King AD, Vlantis AC, Tsang RK *et al.* (2006). Magnetic resonance imaging for the detection of nasopharyngeal carcinoma. *Am. J. Neuroradiol.* 27(6), 1288–1291.

King AD, Tse GM, Ahuja AT *et al* (2004). Necrosis in metastatic neck nodes: diagnostic accuracy of CT, MR imaging, and US. *Radiology.* 230(3), 720–726.

Kumar MB, Lu JJ, Loh KS *et al.* (2004). Tailoring distant metastatic imaging for patients with clinically localized undifferentiated nasopharyngeal carcinoma. *Int. J. Radiat. Oncol. Biol. Phys.* 58(3), 688–693.

Lartigau E, Le Ridant AM, Lambin P, Weeger P, Martin L, Sigal R, Lusinchi A, Luboinski B,Eschwege F, Guichard M. (1993). Oxygenation of head and neck tumors. *Cancer.* 717:2319-2325.

Lau KY, Kan WK, Sze WM *e t al* (2004). Magnetic resonance for T-staging of nasopharyngeal carcinoma - the most informative pair of sequences. *Jpn J. Clin. Oncol.* 34(4), 171–175.

Lee AW, Au JS, Teo PM *et al.* (Eds) (2004). *Clin. Oncol. (R. Coll. Radiol.)* 16(4), 269–276.

Lee AW, Poon YF, Foo W, Law SC, Cheung FK, Chan DK, Tung SY, Thaw M, Ho JH (1992). Retrospective analysis of 5037 patients with nasopharyngeal carcinoma treated during 1976-1985: overall survival and patterns of failure. *Int J Radiat Oncol Biol Phys*. 23(2):261.

Liang SB, Sun Y, Liu LZ *et al.* (2009). Extension of local disease in nasopharyngeal carcinoma detected by magnetic resonance imaging: improvement of clinical target volume delineation. *Int. J. Radiat. Oncol. Biol. Phys.* 75(3), 742–750.

Liao XB, Mao YP, Liu LZ, Tang LL, Sun Y, Wang Y, Lin AH, Cui CY, Li L, Ma J (2008). How does magnetic resonance imaging influence staging according to AJCC staging system for nasopharyngeal carcinoma compared with computed tomography? *Int J Radiat Oncol Biol Phys*. 72(5):1368-1377.

Lin XP, Zhao C, Chen MY, Fan W, Zhang X, Zhi SF, Liang PY (2008). Role of 18F-FDG PET/CT in diagnosis and staging of nasopharyngeal carcinoma. *Ai Zheng*. 27(9):974-978.

Liu FY, Lin CY, Chang JT *et al* (2007). ^{18}F-FDG PET can replace conventional work-up in primary M staging of nonkeratinizing nasopharyngeal carcinoma. *J. Nucl. Med.* 48(10), 1614–1619.

Liu MZ, Tang LL, Zong JF *et al.* (2008). Evaluation of sixth edition of AJCC staging system for nasopharyngeal carcinoma and proposed improvement. *Int. J. Radiat. Oncol. Biol. Phys.* 70(4), 1115–1123.

Liu T, Xu W, Yan WL, Ye M, Bai YR, Huang G (2007). FDG-PET, CT, MRI for diagnosis of local residual or recurrent nasopharyngeal carcinoma, which one is best? A systematic review. *Radiotherapy and Oncology*. 85:327-335.

Liu LZ, Zhang GY, Xie CM, Liu XW, Cui CY, Li L (2006). Magnetic resonance imaging of retropharyngeal lymph node metastasis in nasopharyngeal carcinoma: patterns of spread. *Int J Radiat Oncol Biol Phys*. 66: 721-730.

Lu JC, Wei Q, Zhang YQ, Li F (2004). Influence of MRI abnormality in skull base bone on prognosis of nasopharyngeal carcinoma. *Cancer Radiother.* 8: 230-233.

Mao YP, Liang SB, Liu LZ, Chen Y, Sun Y, Tang LL, Tian L, Lin AH, Liu MZ, Li L, Ma J (2008). The N staging system in nasopharyngeal carcinoma with radiation therapy oncology group guidelines for lymph node levels based on magnetic resonance imaging. *Clin Cancer Res.* 14: 7497-7503

Mao YP, Xie FY, Liu LZ *et al (2009)*. Re-evaluation of 6th edition of AJCC staging system for nasopharyngeal carcinoma and proposed improvement based on magnetic resonance imaging. *Int. J. Radiat. Oncol. Biol. Phys.* 73(5), 1326–1334.

Ng S, Chan S, Yen T, Chang JT, Ko S, Wang H, Lin C, Chang K, Lin Y (2010). Comprehensive imaging of residual/recurrent nasopharyngeal carcinoma using whole-body MRI at 3 T compared with FDG-PET-CT. *Eur Radiol*. 20:2229-2240.

Ng S, Chan S, Yen T, Chang JT, Liao C, Ko S, Liu F, Chin S, Fan K, Hsu C (2009). Staging of untreated nasopharyngeal carcinoma with PET/CT: comparison with conventional imaging work-up. *Eur J Nucl Med Mol Imaging*. 36:12-22.

Ng SH, Chang JT, Chan SC, Ko SF, Wang HM, Liao CT, Chang YC, Yen TC (2004). Nodal metastases of nasopharyngeal carcinoma: patterns of disease on MRI and FDG PET. *Eur J Nucl Med Mol Imaging*. 31: 1073-1080.

Ng SH, Chang TC, Ko SF *et al.* (1997). Nasopharyngeal carcinoma: MRI and CT assessment. *Neuroradiology*. 39(10), 741–746.

Olmi P, Fallai C, Colagrande S, Giannardi G (1995). Staging and follow-up of nasopharyngeal carcinoma: magnetic resonance imaging versus computerized tomography. *Int. J. Radiat. Oncol. Biol. Phys.* 32(3), 795–800.

Parkin DM, Bray F, Ferlay J, Pisani P (2005). Global cancer statistics. *CA Cancer J Clin.* 55:74–108.

Parkin DM, Whelan SL, Ferlay J, Teppo L, Thomas DB, editors (2002). Cancer incidence in five continents, vol. VIII. IARC scientific publications No. 155. Lyon: IARC.

Ren EC & Chan SH (1996). Human leucocyte antigens and nasopharyngeal carcinoma. *Clin. Sci. (Lond.)* 91(3), 256–258.

Roh JL, Sung MW, Kim KH, Choi BY, Oh SH, Rhee CS, Ha JW (2004). Nasopharyngeal carcinoma with skull base invasion: a necessity of staging subdivision. *Am J Otolaryngol.* 25(1):26-32.

Sakata K, Hareyama M, Tamakawa M, Oouchi A, Sido M, Nagakura H, Akiba H, Koito K, Himi T, & Asakura K (1999). Prognostic factors of nasopharynx tumors investigated by MR imaging and the value of MR imaging in the newly published TNM staging. *Int J Radiat Oncol Biol Phys.* 43(2):273.

Som PM (1987). Lymph nodes of the neck. *Radiology.* 165:593-600.

Som PM, Brandwein MS. Lymph nodes. In: Som PM, Curtin HD,editors (2003). Head and Neck Imaging. 4th ed. Vol 2. Mosby Inc. 1910-1911.

Som PM, Curtin HD, Mancuso AA (1999). An imaging-based classification for the cervical nodes designed as an adjunct to recent clinically based nodal classifications. *Arch Otolaryngol Head Neck Surg.* 125:388–396.

Su Y, Zhao C, Xie CM, Lu LX, Sun Y, Han F, Wu HB, Cui NJ, Zeng ZY, Lu TX (2006). Evaluation of CT, MRI and PET/CT in detecting retropharyngeal lymph node metastasis in nasopharyngeal carcinoma. *Ai Zheng.* 25(5):521-525.

Sze WM, Lee AW, Yau TK, Yeung RM, Lau KY, Leung SK, Hung AW, Lee MC, Chappell R, Chan K. (2004) Primary tumor volume of nasopharyngeal carcinoma prognostic significance for local control. *Int J Radiat Oncol Biol Phys.* 59:21-27.

Teo PM, Kwan WH, Lee WY, Leung SF, Johnson PJ (1996). Prognosticators determining survival subsequent to distant metastasis from nasopharyngeal carcinoma. *Cancer.* 77(12), 2423–2431.

Teo P, Lee WY, Yu P (1996). The prognostic significance of parapharyngeal tumour involvement in nasopharyngeal carcinoma. *Radiother. Oncol.* 39(3), 209–221.

Wang XS, Hu CS, Ying HM, Zhou ZR, Ding JH, Feng Y (2009). Patterns of retropharyngeal node metastasis in nasopharyngeal carcinoma. *Int J Radiat Oncol Biol Phys.*73(1):194-201.

Wang GH, Lau EW, Shakher R, Binns DS, Hogg A, Drummond E, Hicks RJ (2007). Clinical application of (18)F-FDG PET/CT to staging and treatment effectiveness monitoring of nasopharyngeal carcinoma. *Ai Zheng.*26(6):638-42.

Wei WI & Sham JST (2005). Nasopharyngeal carcinoma. *Lancet.* 365:2041-2054.

Yoshizaki T, Ito M, Murono S, Wakisaka N, Kondo S, & Endo K (2011). Current understanding and management of nasopharyngeal carcinoma. *Auris Nasus Larynx.* Article in press.

Yousem DM, Som PM, Hackney DB, Schwaibold F, Hendrix RA (1992). Central nodal necrosis and extracapsular spread in cervical lymph nodes: MR imaging versus CT. *Radiology*. 182:753-759.

Yu E, O'Sullivan B, Kim J, Siu L, Bartlett E (2010). Magnetic resonance imaging of nasopharyngeal carcinoma. *Expert Rev. Anticancer Ther.* 10(3): 365-375.

Yu MC, Mo CC, Chong WX *et al.* Preserved foods and nasopharyngeal carcinoma: a case–control study in Guangxi, China. *Cancer Res.* 48, 1954–1959 (1988).

Zhang GY, Hu WH, Liu LZ, Wu HB, Gao YH, Li L, Pan Y, Wang QS (2006). Comparison between PET/CT and MRI in diagnosing lymph node metastasis and N staging of nasopharyngeal carcinoma. Zhonghua Zhong Liu Za Zhi. 28(5):381-4.

7

MRI-Detected Cranial Nerve Involvement in Nasopharyngeal Carcinoma

Li Li, Wenxin Yuan, Lizhi Liu and Chunyan Cui
Cancer Center, Sun Yat-Sen University
China

1. Introduction

The incidence of cranial nerve (CN) palsy is not uncommon in patients with untreated nasopharyngeal cancer (NPC). In the 7th edition of the American Joint Committee on Cancer (AJCC) Staging Manual, the AJCC recommended that CN involvement be assessed by neurological evaluation rather than by cross-sectional imaging (computed tomography [CT] and magnetic resonance imaging [MRI]), because CN involvement is considered a poor prognostic indicator in NPC patients, those with CN involvement are staged as T4.

However, evaluation of CN palsy by clinical symptoms and physical examination has limitations. First, the accuracy of the neurological examination depends on the expertise of the examiner and the subjective report of the patient. Second, because CN involvement may be asymptomatic, it is difficult to diagnose CN palsy at an early stage by clinical neurological evaluation. In addition, neurological evaluation is not an optimal diagnostic method for assessing lesion localization and extension, which are critical factors in planning treatment, particularly in delineation of target volume.

With the excellent soft tissue contrast resolution and multiplanar imaging capability of MRI, direct visualization of smaller nerves and nerve branches is possible, making MRI a valuable tool in detecting and defining the extent of CN involvement in NPC. The difference and relationship between MRI findings of CN involvement and the symptoms and signs of CN dysfunction have not been fully addressed.

The goal of this study was to detect the difference and relationship between MRI findings suggestive of CN involvement and the symptoms and signs of CN dysfunction, and to evaluate the prognostic value of MRI-detected CN involvement in a large sample of consecutive patients. These information may contribute to understanding the patterns of spread and biological nature of NPC, and may also prove references in tumor staging and treatment planning.

2. Patients and methods

Patients: From January 2003 to December 2004, 924 consecutive patients with newly diagnosed untreated NPC were included in our study. There were 685 male patients and 239 female patients, with a male-female ratio of 2.9:1, and the median age was 45 years (range, 11-78 years). All patients had a pretreatment evaluation that consisted of a complete history, physical and neurologic examination, hematology and biochemistry profiles, MRI scan of the neck and nasopharynx, chest radiography, and abdominal sonography. Medical records and imaging studies were reviewed retrospectively, and all patients were staged according to criteria in the 6th edition of the AJCC Cancer Staging Manua.

Imaging Protocol: MR scanning was performed with a 1.5-Tesla system (Signa CV/i, General Electric Healthcare) and a head and neck combined coil. The area from the suprasellar cistern to the inferior margin of the sternal end of the clavicle was examined. T1-weighted fast spin-echo images in the axial, coronal, and sagittal planes (repetition time of 500–600 milliseconds, echo time of 10–20 milliseconds, 5-mm slice thickness with 1-mm interslice gap for the axial plane, 6-mm slice thickness with 1-mm interslice gap for coronal and sagittal planes, and a 512*512 matrix) and T2-weighted fast spinecho MR images in the axial plane (repetition time of 4000–6000 milliseconds, echo time of 95–110 milliseconds, 5-mm slice thickness with 1-mm interslice gap, and a 512*512 matrix) were obtained before injection of contrast agent. After intravenous gadolinium diethylenetriamine pentaacetic acid (Gd-DTPA; Magnevist, Schering, Berlin) injection at a dose of 0.1 mmol/kg of body weight, spin-echo T1-weighted axial and sagittal sequences, and spin-echo T1- weighted fat-suppressed coronal sequences were performed sequentially, with parameters similar to those used before Gd-DTPA injection.

2.1 Image assessment and diagnostic criteria

Medical records and imaging studies were retrospectively analyzed. Cranial nerve palsy was diagnosed separately by two radiation oncologists who were unaware of the clinical findings, and clinical nerve palsy was diagnosed by others on the basis of clinical symptoms and a physical examination before treatment. Any disagreements were resolved by consensus. Two radiologists specializing in head and neck cancers, who were unaware of the clinical findings, evaluated the MRI images separately. Any disagreements were resolved by consensus. Soft tissue tumor was observed as intermediate signal intensity on pre-Gd-DTPA T1- and T2-weighted images and an enhancing mass on post-Gd-DTPA T1-weighted images, replacing the normal anatomy of the structure. MRI-detected CN involvement had to meet one of the following criteria: 1) enhancement of soft tissue tumor along the course of the ipsilateral related nerve and replacing the normal structures of the CN on gadolinium-enhanced T1-weighted images [Fig.1]; or 2) perineural spread, defined as an enlargement or abnormal enhancement of the nerve, obliteration of the neural fat pads adjacent to the neurovascular foramina, and neuroforaminal enlargement [Fig.1] [1-3]. Because CNs in the parapharyngeal space could not be identified as isolated structures on MRI, parapharyngeal space invasion could not be regarded as evidence of CN involvement in our study.

MRI-detected CN involvement at the following sites were assessed: extracranial segment of the maxillary nerve (V3), pterygopalatine fossa, foramen rotundum, foramen ovale, jugular foramen, hypoglossal canal, inferior orbital fissure, orbital apex, superior orbital fissure, cavernous sinus segment of CNs III-VI, trigeminal ganglion, and CNs in the cistern. By AJCC criteria, parapharyngeal and skull base invasion were classified as T2 and T3, respectively, and intracranial, infratemporal, hypopharynx, or orbital disease was classified as T4 [4]. Thus, all MRI findings that were suggestive of CN involvement were classified into 2 categories: 1) extracranial or basicranial or 2) intracranial or orbital.

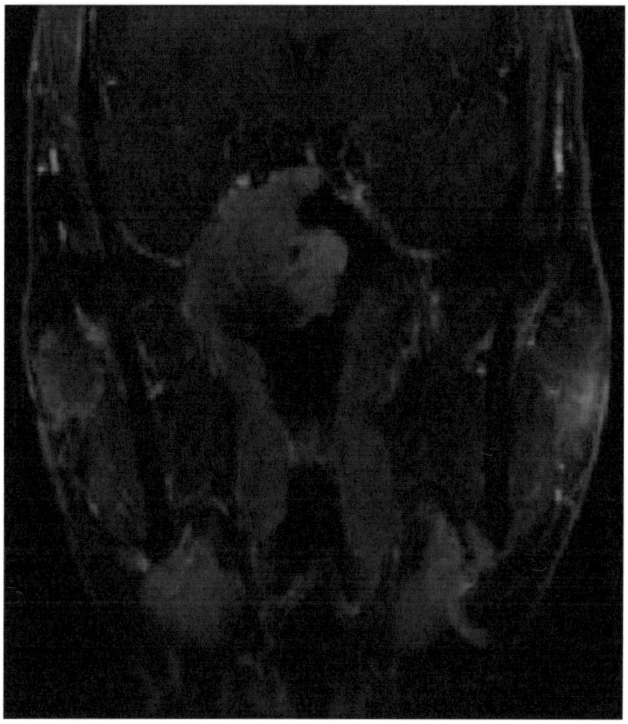

Fig. 1. A palsied cranial nerve V3. The enhanced coronal T1-weighted coronal fat suppression image at the level of the foramen ovale shows the enhancing tumor extending intracranially via the enlarged right foramen ovale along V3 and into the trigeminal cistern.

2.2 Treatment

All patients were treated by definitive-intent radiation therapy. Our policy was to cover the nasopharynx and the retropharyngeal lymph nodes within the primary target in every radical attempt, and to treat patients with gross lymphadenopathy with whole-neck irradiation. Most patients (773 of 924 or 83.7%) were treated with conventional techniques, 12.7% (118 of 924) with intensity-modulated radiation therapy (IMRT), and 3.6% (33 of 924) with 3-dimensional conformal radiation therapy (3-DCRT). Details regarding the radiation therapy techniques at the Cancer Center of Sun Yat-sen University have been reported previously [5-7].

Most patients (517 of 629 or 82.2%) with stage III or stage IV disease (classified as T3-T4 or N2-N3) received neoadjuvant (137 of 629 or 21.8%), concomitant (374 of 629 or 59.5%), or adjuvant chemotherapy (6 of 629 or 1.0%), in conjunction with a platinum-based therapeutic clinical trial. When possible, salvage treatments (including afterloading, surgery, and chemotherapy) were provided in the event of documented relapse or when the disease persisted despite therapy.

2.3 Statistical analysis

Patients were followed up at least every 3 months during the first 2 years; thereafter, patients were followed up every 5 months until death. The median follow-up period for the whole group was 40 months (range, 2-56 months). All events were measured from the date of commencement of the treatment. The following endpoints (time to the first defining event) were assessed: overall survival (OS); local relapse-free survival (LRFS); and distant metastasis-free survival (DMFS). Local recurrence was established by fiberoptic endoscopy and biopsy and/or MRI. Distant metastases were diagnosed based on clinical symptoms, physical examination, and imaging methods including chest radiograph, bone scan, CT, and abdominal sonography.

Statistical analyses were performed using the Statistical Package for the Social Sciences (SPSS Inc., Chicago, IL) 12.0 software. The actuarial rates were calculated by the Kaplan-Meier method [8], and the differences were compared by using the log-rank test. Multivariate analyses with the Cox proportional hazards model were used to test independent significance by backward elimination of insignificant explanatory variables [9]. Host factors (age and sex) were included as the covariates in all tests. The chi-square test was used to analyze the relationship between MRI findings and CN palsies. The criterion for statistical significance was set at a = 0.05. The P values were based on 2-sided tests.

3. Results

3.1 Clinical CN palsies and MRI-detected CN Involvement

Of 924 patients with NPC, 82 (8.9%) patients initially presented with CN palsy. A total of 134 CNs were found to be paralyzed, and 31 patients were detected with multiple CN palsies. In these 82 patients with CN palsy, 79 patients had one or more MRI findings demonstrating CN involvement, and CN V was the most common nerve to be involved. Of all patients, 46 (5.0%) had clinical evidence of trigeminal nerve palsy at presentation, 92 (28%) divisions of palsied trigeminal nerves were clinically identified. Of these 46 patients, 43 (93.5%) had unilateral paresthesia and 3 (6.5%) had bilateral paresthesia. In 5 of these patients with palsied nerves, MRI findings did not correspond to clinical findings. For example, a patient was detected with palsied CN V3, but MRI demonstrated only evidence of CN involvement of CN V2.

A total of 333 (36%) patients demonstrated MRI-detected CN involvement and of the 514 patients with local advanced (T3-4) disease, 332 patients demonstrated MRI-detected CN involvement. The incidence of MRI-detected CN involvement in T3 patients was lower than that in T4 patients (43.8% vs 97.5%, $P = 0.000$). Only 1 patient with T2 disease demonstrated MRI-detected CN involvement. Clinical signs and symptoms of ipsilaterally affected CNs were absent in 259 (77.8%) of patients with MRI-detected CN involvement. The correlation between MRI-detected CN involvement and ipsilateral CN palsy is shown in Table 1.

3.2 Imaging basis of CN palsies

Of the 134 paralyzed CNs, 98 (73.1%) demonstrated ipsilateral intracranial or orbital MRI-detected CN involvement; 21 (15.7%) demonstrated basicranial MRI-detected CN involvement. No MRI evidence of CN involvement was observed in the remaining 15

(11.2%) paralyzed CNs; among these 15 CNs, carotid sheath (n=13) or retropharyngeal lymph node (n = 1) invasion could be identified along the course of the CNs paralyzed on the ipsilateral side; no tumor could be detected along the course of the remaining paralyzed CNs on the MRI images. Of the 92 divisions of palsied trigeminal nerves, 91 trigeminal nerve palsies (98.9%) showed MRI evidence of 1 or more trigeminal nerve involvements. However, no evidence could be found for the remaining 1 palsied V1 case on MR images.

MRI-detecded CN involvement	Sites number*	Palsied CNs, Sites number
Basicranial or extracranial		
Extracranial part of V3	264	V3, 28
Ovale foramen	223	V3, 28
Pterygopalatine fossa	177	V2, 30
Rotundum foramen	86	V2, 19
Jugular foramen	48	IX, 1; X, 2；XI, 0
Hypoglossal foramen	108	XII, 11
Intracranial or orbital		
Superior orbital fissure	6	III,1; IV,2; V1, 2; VI, 1
Orbital apex	11	II, 5
Inferior orbital fissure	36	V2, 14
Cavernous segment of III	41	III,10
Cavernous segment of IV	75	IV, 11
Cavernous segment of V1	130	V1, 20
Cavernous segment of V2	144	V2, 31
Cavernous segment of VI	125	VI, 30
Trigeminal ganglion	86	V, 24
Cisternal part of V CN	9	V, 5
Cisternal part of IX-XI	4	IX-XI, 0
Cisternal part of XII	9	XII, 2

*: Sites number means the number of MRI-detected CN involvement

Table 1. The Correlation between MRI-detected CN Involvement and the Ipsilateral Related CN Palsy.

3.3 Prognosis of MRI-detected CN Involvement in T3-4 disease

In 514 T3-4 patients, significant differences were observed in 3-year OS (75.7% vs 89.2%, $P = 0.001$) and DMFS (77.1% vs 87.8%, $P = 0.002$) rates, with better rates observed in the 182 patients who did not demonstrate MRI-detected CN involvement. No significant difference was observed in 3-year LRFS (86.8% vs 91.8%, $P = 0.067$) rates between the patients with and without MRI-detected CN involvement in T3-4 patients.

Because most (97.5%) T4 patients had MRI-detected CN involvement, the prognoses between the T3 patients with and without MRI-detected CN involvement were also compared. All patients with local advanced disease (T3 and T4) in this series were classified into 3 groups: Group 1, T3 disease without MRI-detected CN involvement; Group 2, T3 disease with MRI-detected CN involvement; and Group 3, T4 disease. Significant differences were observed in OS and DMFS rates between Groups 1 and 2 ($P = 0.009$ and $P = 0.011$, respectively), but no significant differences were observed between Groups 2 and 3 (*P* = 0.322 and *P* = 0.809, respectively). No significant differences were observed in the LRFS rates between Groups 1 and 2 (*P* = 0.750), and no significant difference was observed between Groups 2 and 3 (*P* = 0.079).

Multivariate analysis was performed to adjust for various prognostic factors in T3 and T4 disease. Parameters were included in the Cox proportional hazards model by backward elimination of insignificant explanatory variables: age (50<=years vs >50 years), sex, skull base extension, paranasal sinus extension, intracranial extension, infratemporal extension, orbital extension hypopharynx extension, MRI-detected CN involvement, CN palsy, N classification, radiotherapy technique, and chemotherapy. Both clinical CN palsy and MRI-detected CN involvement were significant predictive factors for the DMFS and OS rates in local advanced disease (Table 2).

Endpoint	Variable	B	Exp(B)	95% CI for Exp(B)	*P*
OS	age	-0.287	0.750	0.550-1.024	0.070
	MRI-detected CN involvement	0.866	2.377	1.620-3.489	0.000
	CN palsy	-0.662	0.516	0.300-0.886	0.016
	intracranial extension	0.511	1.667	1.104-2.516	0.015
	N classification	0.487	1.627	1.396-1.898	0.000
DMFS	MRI-detected CN involvement	0.627	1.871	1.268-2.762	0.002
	CN palsy	-0.506	0.603	0.330-1.102	0.100
	paranasal sinuses extension	0.509	1.665	1.087-2.547	0.019
	N classification	0.576	1.778	1.510-2.094	0.000
LRFS	age	-0.379	0.685	0.457-1.026	0.066
	gender	-0.855	0.425	0.232-0.779	0.006
	intracranial extension	0.787	2.197	1.424-3.389	0.000

OS, overall survival; LRFS, local relapse-free survival; DMFS, metastasis-free survival.

Table 2. Summary of Multivariate Analyses of Prognostic Factors in T3-4 Disease.

3.4 Difference in the prognostic implications between clinical CN palsy and MRI-detected CN involvement

In 336 patients with clinical and/or MRI-detected CN involvement, no significant difference was observed in the 3-year DMFS (74.6% vs 84.6%, *P* = 0.094) or LRFS (86.7% vs 87.9%, *P* = 0.899) rates between patients with and without clinically detected CN palsies. A marginally significant difference was observed in the 3-year OS (74.2% vs 80.1%, *P* = 0.067) rate; however, after adjusting for N classification, there was no significant difference (*P* = 0.102).

3.5 Prognosis of lesion localization in patients with MRI-detected CN involvement

Of the 333 patients with MRI-detected CN involvement, no significant differences were observed with regard to the 3-year OS (78.3% vs 72.9%, *P* = 0.120), LRFS (89.7% vs 84.1%, *P* = 0.154) or DMFS (79.6% vs 74.8%, *P* = 0.466) rates between patients with and without intracranial or orbital MRI-detected CN involvement.

4. Discussion

4.1 Difference between clinical CN palsy and MRI-detected CN involvement

Clinical findings were not consistent with the MRI findings of CN involvement in some cases. Nerves are resistant to tumor, and perineural tumor spread is an insidious and often asymptomatic process. The incidence of MRI-detected CN involvement is high in NPC; patients are often asymptomatic [10]. According to our observation, the incidence of MRI-detected CN involvement was much higher than that of clinical presentation of CN palsy in NPC patients.

With improvement in imaging techniques, direct visualization of smaller nerves and proximal nerve branches have become possible. MRI allows contrast between the nerve fibers and the surrounding cerebrospinal fluid, perineural vascular plexus, and fat pads. Involvement of cranial nerves may be direct or perineural; proposed MRI criteria of cranial nerve involvement in our study include both possibilities. MRI, including the contrast-enhanced fat suppression technique, is particularly helpful in detection of direct and perineural invasion of the nerve in patients with NPC, so we often identified cranial nerve involvement on gadoliniumenhanced T1-weighted images. Perineural spread, in which pathologic conditions spread along the connective tissues of the perineurium, is often associated with malignant disease of the head and neck. The imaging hallmark of this process has been discussed in detail in a previous articles [1-3].

Without contrast between the nerve and the surrounding structures, CNs in the parapharyngeal space could not be identified on MRI; therefore, parapharyngeal space invasion was not defined as evidence of CN involvement in our study. A small number of symptomatic patients with only carotid sheath or retropharyngeal lymph node invasion along the course of ipsilaterally paralyzed CNs were regarded as MRI negative but clinically positive in our series.

Because NPC is a nonsurgical disease, the limitation of our study is that there was no pathologic correlation of CN involvement with MRI findings. Another limitation is the slice thickness of 5 mm used in our study, which may limit the sensitivity of detecting cranial nerve involvement. Ideally, slice thickness should be 3 to 4 mm in future studies; this may lead to earlier identification of CN involvement.

4.2 Prognosis of clinical CN palsy in MRI-detected CN involvement

We observed that most CN palsies had 1 or more MRI findings of intracranial or orbital CN involvement; this may be a reason for the adverse prognostic significance of CN palsies, and patients with CN palsies are determined to be at stage T4 [4].

Several investigators have reported that the perineural tumor spread in patients with non-nasopharyngeal carcinoma of the head and neck is associated with an increased incidence of recurrence [11-14]. However, in our series, MRI-detected CN involvement was not associated with the 3-year LRFS rate in NPC patients with local advanced disease. The primary treatment modality for NPC was radiation therapy, whereas that of other carcinomas of the head and neck was surgery. Lawrence and Cottel reported that postoperative radiotherapy of squamous cell carcinoma with perineural invasion resulted in a much improved survival probability when compared with that observed after conventional surgical excision [13]. Radiation therapy (relatively large treatment volume) provided better LRFS to patients with perineural spread. Early results of improved treatment strategies for nasopharyngeal carcinoma, including the boost technique of 2-dimensional radiation therapy, use of IMRT, and combinationof chemotherapy with radiotherapy, has shown considerable improvement in LRFS [15-16]. Improved treatment might result in no significant difference with regard to the 3-year LRFS rate in patients with T3-4 disease with or without MRI findings of CN involvement.

The LRFS in patients with intracranial or orbital CN involvement was so poor that there was little difference in the 3-year LRFS rate between T3 patients with MRI-detected CN involvement and T4 patients. This poor survival rate may be a result of difficulties encountered in designing a therapeutic strategy for these patients and limitations on the dose escalation for intracranial or orbital disease. Several studies have demonstrated that perineural tumor spread in other head and neck cancers may result in a higher incidence of distant metastases [17-18]. We found that MRI-detected CN involvement was associated with a greater propensity for distant metastasis and resulted in unfavorable outcome in OS. Batsakis reported that carcinoma proliferated along the nerves within the lymphatics of the epineurium and the perineural sheaths [19]. We presume that tumor proliferation within the lymphatics may increase the risk of distant metastasis. On the basis of our data, the pattern of treatment failure in the NPC patients with CN involvement is caused by distant metastases. This implies that tumors with perineural involvement are more aggressive and spread from the primary tumor site to distant organs. Understanding the perineural invasion at the molecular level is an important step toward identification of the prognostic markers and therapeutic targets for NPC treatment.

Both clinical CN palsy and MRI-detected CN involvement were significant and independent predictive factors for the DMFS and OS rates in local advanced disease. In patients with clinical CN palsy or MRI-detected CN involvement, there is no real difference in the OS and DMFS between symptomatic and asymptomatic patients. This implies that MRI-detected involvement of CN itself has a poor prognosis in high-risk NPC irrespective of the clinical symptoms caused by such an involvement. In current *AJCC Cancer Staging Manual*, that CN involvement be assessed by neurological evaluation is recommended, rather than by cross-sectional imaging. Therefore, MRI-detected CN involvement should be involved in the future staging system.

4.3 Clinical value of MRI-detected CN involvement in treatment

Almost all the patients with MRI-detected CN involvement were classified as T3-4. Concurrent chemoradiotherapy has emerged as the treatment of choice for locoregionally advanced (T3-4) NPC. Therefore, all patients with MRI-detected CN involvement should receive concurrent chemoradiotherapy. According to our data, these patients had a high distant metastasis rate; therefore, more intensive chemotherapy regimes should be considered.

Chang et al demonstrated that MRI was associated with improved tumor control of patients with NPC and CN palsy [20]. Because MRI can be used to clearly detect the location and extent of CN invasion, MRI should be considered as a basic imaging modality in the delineation of the target volume, ensuring full coverage of the gross target target volume and high-risk clinical target volume. A higher radiation dose improved tumor control and survival in NPC. We suggest that an adequate dose should be determined for these patients with MRI-detected CN involvement.

4.4 Limitations of our study

Prognosis may depend not only on the extent of disease on MRI but also on the effectiveness of treatment. Variability of treatment may be one of the limitations of our study. In our series, most patients with stage III and IV disease received chemotherapy, but some did not receive chemotherapy (patients with advanced age, heart disease, diabetes, and patients in the control group in a clinical trial). Although 3-DCRT/IMRT techniques were reported to provide excellent locoregional control for NPC, distant metastases are still the main cause of treatment failure [21]. In our series, only a small percentage of patients were treated with IMRT/3-DCRT because of resource limitations; however, when included as a covariate, radiation technique was not an independent prognostic factor for either distant failure or death in multivariate analyses.

5. Summary

The incidence of MRI-detected CN involvement in NPC is high and is often observed in asymptomatic patients, and the incidence of MRI-demonstrable trigeminal nerve involvement is much higher than other nevers. Disease with MRI-detected CN involvement has a poor prognosis, independent of lesion localization and symptoms in local advanced disease.

6. References

[1] Williams LS, Mancuso AA, Mendenhall WM. Perineuralspread of cutaneous squamous and basal cell carcinoma: CT and MR detection and its impact on patient management and prognosis. Int J Radiat Oncol Biol Phys. 2001;49:1061-1069.
[2] Gebarski SS, Telian SA, Niparko JK. Enhancement along the normal facial nerve in the facial canal: MR imaging and anatomic correlation. Radiology. 1992;183:391-394.
[3] Curtin HD, Wolfe P, Snyderman N. The facial nerve between the stylomastoid foramen and the parotid: computed tomographic imaging. Radiology. 1983;149:165-169.
[4] Lin JC, Jan JS. Locally advanced nasopharyngeal cancer: long-term outcomes of radiation therapy. Radiology. 1999;211:513-518.
[5] Jun Ma, Lizhi Liu, Linglong Tang, et al. Retropharyngeal lymphadenopathy in nasopharyngeal carcinoma: prognostic value and staging categories. Clin Cancer Res. 2007;13: 1445-1452.
[6] Zhao C, Han F, Lu LX, et al. Intensity modulated radiotherapy for local-regional advanced nasopharyngeal carcinoma. Ai Zheng. 2004;23:1532-1537.
[7] Wei L, Xiaowu D, Taixiang L. Dosimetric evaluation for 3 dimensional radiotherapy plans for patients with early nasopharyngeal carcinoma. Ai Zheng. 2004;23:605-608.
[8] Kaplan EL, Meier P. Nonparametric estimation from incomplete observations. J Am Stat Assoc. 1958;53:457-481.
[9] Cox DR. Regression models and life tables. J R Stat Soc B. 1972;34:187-220.

[10] Neel HB. Nasopharyngeal carcinoma: clinical presentation, diagnosis, treatment and prognosis. Otolaryngol Clin North Am. 1985;18:479-490.
[11] Feasel AM, Brown TJ, Bogle MA, Tschen JA, Nelson BR. Perineural invasion of cutaneous malignancies. Dermatol Surg. 2001;27:531-542.
[12] Fagan JJ, Collins B, Barnes L, D'Amico F, Myers EN, Johnson JT. Perineural invasion in squamous cell carcinoma of the head and neck. Arch Otolaryngol Head Neck Surg. 1998;124:637-640.
[13] Lawrence N, Cottel WI. Squamous cell carcinoma of skin with perineural invasion. J Am Acad Dermatol. 1994;31:30- 33.
[14] McCord MW, Mendenhall WM, Parsons JT, Flowers FP. Skin cancer of the head and neck with incidental microscopic perineural invasion. Int J Radiat Oncol Biol Phys. 1999;43:591-595.
[15] Xie GF, Cao KJ, Li Y, Huang PY. Impact of dose boost in skull base on recurrence of stage T4 nasopharyngeal carcinoma. Ai Zheng. 2005;24:1246-1248.
[16] Ma J, Mai HQ, Hong MH, et al. Results of a prospective randomized trial comparing neoadjuvant chemotherapy plus radiotherapy with radiotherapy alone in patients with locoregionally advanced nasopharyngeal carcinoma. J Clin Oncol. 2001;19:1350-1357.
[17] Ballantyne AJ, McCarten AB, Ibanez ML. The extension of cancer of the head and neck through peripheral nerves. Am J Surg. 1963;106:651-667.
[18] Byers RM, O'Brien J, Waxler J. The therapeutic and prognostic implications of nerve invasion in cancer of the lower lip. Int J Radiat Oncol Biol Phys. 1978;4:215-217.
[19] Batsakis JG. Nerves and neurotropic carcinomas. Ann Otol Rhinol Laryngol. 1985;94:426-427.
[20] Chang JT, Lin CY, Chen TM, et al. Nasopharyngeal carcinoma with cranial nerve palsy: the importance of MRI for radiotherapy. Int J Radiat Oncol Biol Phys. 2005;63:1354-1360.
[21] Kam MK, Teo PM, Chau RM, et al. Treatment of nasopharyngeal carcinoma with intensity modulated radiotherapy: the Hong Kong experience. Int J Radiat Oncol Biol Phys. 2004;60:1440-1450.

8

Endocrine Complications Following Radiotherapy and Chemotherapy for Nasopharyngeal Carcinoma

Ken Darzy
East & North Hertfordshire NHS Trust
United Kingdom

1. Introduction

Long-term endocrine disorders are the most frequent complications in survivors of adult and paediatric nasopharyngeal carcinoma (NPC). The hypothalamic-pituitary (h-p) axis lies within the field of radiation therapy for NPC. Consequently, neuro-endocrine abnormalities due to radiation-induced damage of the h-p occur in the majority of patients followed long term. Similarly, radiation injury to the thyroid gland can result in primary thyroid dysfunction, particularly hypothyroidism as well as benign and malignant thyroid nodule. Chemotherapy-induced gonadal damage is another frequently seen complication in patients treated with chemotherapy.

Most of the endocrine complications are irreversible and progressive in nature. They may be of sufficient severity to have adverse impact on growth and pubertal development (in children), body image, sexual function, fertility, muscular and skeletal health and ultimately quality of life. It is mandatory that survivors of NPC undergo regular clinical, radiological and/or hormonal surveillance to ensure early diagnosis of these complications and appropriate and timely introduction of hormone replacement therapy and other therapeutic interventions.

2. Radiation-induced hypothalamic-pituitary dysfunction

2.1 Pathophysiology

Radiation damage is a potent cause of hypothalamic-pituitary (h-p) axis dysfunction. Deficiency of one or more of the anterior pituitary hormones may occur following radiotherapy for tumours of the head and neck when the h-p axis falls within the field of radiation. The pathophysiology of radiation-induced damage remains poorly understood. Neuronal cell death and degeneration due to the direct effects of radiation appear to play a major role (Hochberg et al., 1983); however, vascular damage has also been proposed (Chieng et al., 1991).

The onset and severity of radiation-induced hypopituitarism is primarily determined by the total radiation dose, the fraction size and the time allowed between fractions for tissue repair (duration of the radiation schedule) (Thames & Hendry, 1987; Littley et al., 1989a). Radiation schedules utilising the same total dose administered over a shorter duration (larger fraction size) inflict more damage to the h-p axis. To minimise the damage to healthy neuronal tissues (including h-p axis), most radiation schedules have not used more than 2 Gy per fraction and no more than 5 fractions per week. Increasing the fraction size above 2 Gy per fraction (for the same total dose) can induce relatively more injury to the late responding (neuronal) than the early responding (tumour) tissues (Withers, 1994).

Intensive external fractionated radiotherapy in doses exceeding 60 Gy remains the primary treatment for NPC. The radiotherapy field normally covers the nasopharynx and both sides of the neck. The h-p axis is routinely included in the irradiated volume. Consequently, the rate and intensity of neuro-endocrine disturbances complicating treatment of NPC far exceed that seen following less intense therapeutic radiation schedules (18-45 Gy) used for the treatment of brain tumours or haematological malignancies. With modern technological advances in computed tomography and magnetic resonance imaging, it has become possible to use conformal radiotherapy to deliver a higher radiation dose to the main bulk of the tumour while sparing the important nearby structure to reduce long-term complications (Wei, 2001). In addition, shielding the pituitary gland during radiotherapy has been shown to reduce disturbances in pituitary function without compromising tumour control (Sham et al., 1994).

The nature of the neuro-endocrine disturbance following h-p axis irradiation is also determined by the differential radiosensitivity of hypothalamic-pituitary function. This has been shown in animal models (Hochberg et al., 1983; Robinson et al., 2001) and reflected in clinical observations in irradiated patients. Epidemiological studies reveal that the growth hormone (GH) axis is the most radiosensitive followed by the gonadotrophin (FSH & LH), adrenocorticotrophic hormone (ACTH) and thyroid stimulating hormone (TSH) axes (Clayton & Shalet, 1991; Constine et al., 1993; Duffner et al., 1985; Lam et al., 1991; Littley et al., 1989a) (Figures 1& 2).

Low radiation doses of less than 40 Gy mostly affects the most vulnerable GH axis in isolation resulting in variable degrees of GH deficiency (Clayton & Shalet, 1991; Constine et al., 1993; Duffner et al., 1985; Littley et al., 1989a). Deficiencies of other anterior pituitary hormones start to occur when the total radiation dose delivered to the h-p axis exceeds 40 Gy, but much less frequently than GH deficiency. Panhypopituitarism is mostly seen following intensive irradiation with doses exceeding 60 Gy, typically used for the treatment of nasopharyngeal carcinoma and skull base tumours (Chen et al., 1989; Lam et al., 1991; Pai et al., 2001; Samaan et al., 1987, 1982). In contrast, posterior pituitary dysfunction with diabetes insipidus has not been reported even after the most intensive irradiation schedules (Pai et al., 2001).

With less intensive radiation schedules utilising doses of less than 40 Gy, it would appear that age at irradiation influences differential impact on various h-p axes susceptibility to radiation damage. The somatotrophic (GH) axis is more vulnerable to radiation damage in children than adults, while the ACTH axis seems to be more vulnerable to damage in adults than children. These conclusions are based on the relative frequencies of various anterior pituitary hormones deficiencies reported with various radiation schedules, with a dose range of 18-50 Gy, administered to children and adults for non-pituitary brain tumours and leukaemia. For example, isolated GH deficiency is frequently seen in children who received radiation doses of less than 24 Gy (Ogilvy-Stuart et al., 1992) but none in the adults (Littley et al., 1991). In a study of 56 patients irradiated for non-pituitary brain tumours in adulthood, Agha et al (Agha et al., 2005) reported variable degrees of hypopituitarism in 41% of patients. In this study (Agha et al., 2005), GH deficiency (32%) was less frequent that that reported in irradiated children (Clayton & Shalet, 1991; Livesey et al., 1990; Samaan et al., 1987), but ACTH (21%), TSH (9%) and gonadotropin (27%) deficiencies were relatively more common than or similar to that reported in cancer survivors irradiated during childhood (Constine et al., 1993; Livesey et al., 1990; Samaan et al., 1987). The differential influence of age is less clearly defined with intensive irradiation, but it appears to follow the same pattern. Samaan et al (Samaan et al., 1987) in their study of 166 patients aged 6-80 years, who had received high dose irradiation for NPC, showed that children younger than 15 years of age had a higher incidence of GH deficiency soon after radiotherapy than older patients; however, the older age group showed more adrenocortical and luteinizing hormone deficiency.

Irrespective of the intensity of radiation schedule, radiation-induced h-p dysfunction is also time dependent. Both increased incidence and severity of hormonal deficits are seen with longer post-irradiation follow-up intervals (Achermann et al., 2000; Clayton & Shalet, 1991; Lam et al., 1991; Littley et al., 1989b; Samaan et al., 1987; Schmiegelow et al., 2000) (Fig 1 &2). Secondary pituitary atrophy consequent upon lack of hypothalamic releasing/trophic factors accounts for the progressive nature of the hormonal deficits, in addition, to the delayed direct effects of radiotherapy on the axis. There is a belief that radiation may cause delayed brain tissue damage and dysfunction through chronic inflammation and/or enhanced release of proinflammatory cytokines (Chiang et al., 1997; Kyrkanides et al., 1999). The delayed direct radiation damage to the pituitary gland is supported by the gradual decline in the elevated prolactin levels seen in some patients after prolonged periods of follow up post radiotherapy (Littley et al., 1989a).

The predominant site of radiation damage, pituitary vs. hypothalamic, has attracted some controversy. Contrary to what had been believed that the hypothalamus is more radiosensitive than the pituitary and that hypothalamic damage predominates following less intensive radiation schedules (<50 Gy), recent studies by the author et al (Darzy et al., 2005, 2006, 2007, 2009) have strongly suggested the opposite with robust evidence that direct radiation-induced damage to the pituitary still occurs even with low radiation doses and that the pituitary may be the predominant site of radiation damage. However, with higher range of conventional irradiation, i.e. doses in excess of 60 Gy, there is robust clinical evidence to suggest that intensive radiotherapy inflicts dual damage to both the pituitary as well as the hypothalamus resulting in early multiple anterior pituitary hormone deficiencies (Chen et al., 1989; Lam et al., 1991; Pai et al., 2001; Samaan et al., 1982). In addition to direct hypothalamic damage, neuropharmacological studies have suggested that radiation-induced hypothalamic dysfunction may be secondary to radiation damage of the suprahypothalamic neurotransmitter pathways (Jorgensen et al., 1993; Ogilvy-Stuart et al., 1994). Radiation-induced changes at cellular and molecular levels most certainly play a role in the dysfunction of the irradiated h-p axis.

Pituitary damage is demonstrated by impaired GH, LH/FSH, and TSH responses to direct stimulation with exogenous GHRH, LHRH or TRH, respectively. Hypothalamic damage, on

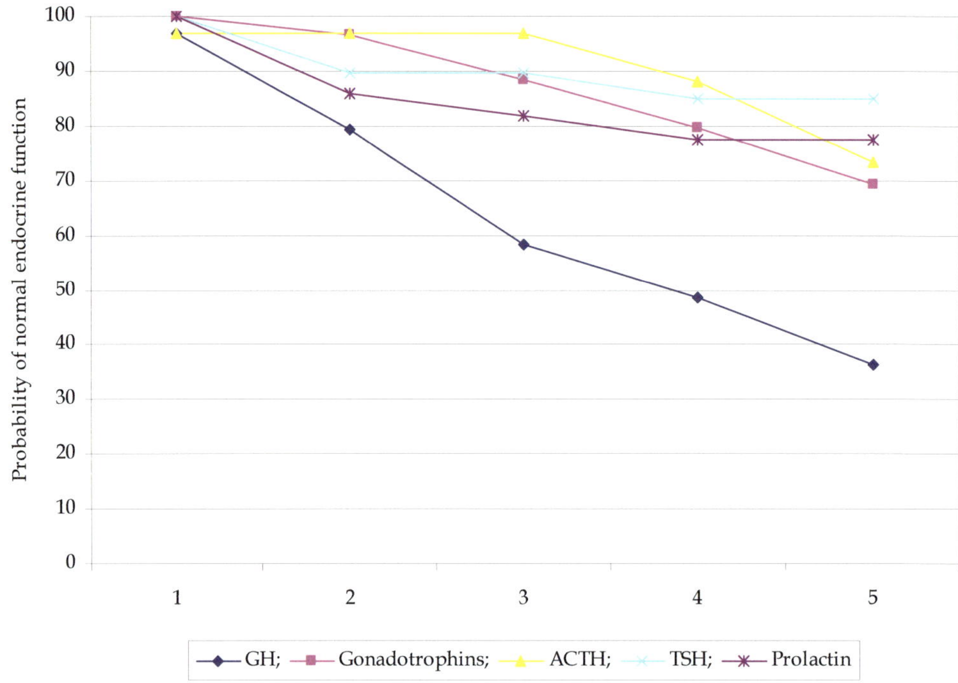

Fig. 1. Cumulative probability of normal endocrine function following radiotherapy for nosopharyngeal carcinoma. Adapted from Lam et al 1991, with permission.

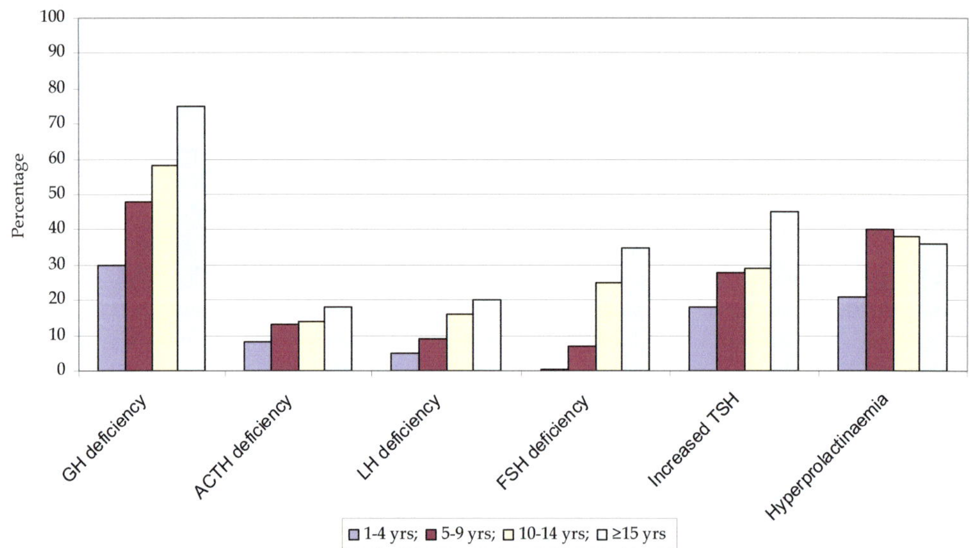

Fig. 2. Percentages of 166 patients with abnormal hormonal levels according to years after radiotherapy for NPC. Adapted from Samaan et al 1987 - Table II, with permission.

the other hand, is characterized by hypothalamic pattern of responses (delayed responses) to LHRH and TRH tests. A robust sign for hypothalamic damage is the occurrence of hyperprolactinaemia due to a reduction in hypothalamic release of the inhibitory neurotransmitter, dopamine. These abnormalities in hypothalamic functions have been clearly described in those intensively irradiated for nasopharyngeal carcinoma (Chen et al., 1989; Lam et al., 1991; Samaan et al., 1987) and skull base tumours (Pai et al., 2001) but much less frequently in those treated for other brain tumours or leukaemia with less intensive radiation schedules (Constine et al., 1993; Rose et al., 1999).

2.2 Growth Hormone (GH) deficiency

2.2.1 Epidemiology and pathophysiology

GH deficiency is the earliest manifestation of neuro-endocrine injury following cranial irradiation. With intensive irradiation used for NPC, the cumulative frequency of GH deficiency is well above 60% after 5 years (Lam et al., 1991). Higher incidence of severe GH deficiency is seen with longer follow up periods reaching well above 80% (Samaan et al., 1987). Given the higher radiosensitivity of the GH axis, GH deficiency is almost always present if deficiencies of one or more of the other anterior pituitary hormones are confirmed. Studies of stimulated GH secretion in children treated for brain tumours indicate that almost all children treated with doses in excess of 35 Gy will have blunted GH secretion within 2-5 years of treatment (Clayton & Shalet, 1991). With the more intensive radiation used for NPC, all children treated for this condition will undoubtedly manifest features of severe GH deficiency soon after irradiation.

Apart from the higher radiosensitivity of the GH axis in children, the higher frequency of severe GH deficiency in children may be explained by the much higher threshold of peak GH response to stimulation used to diagnose GH deficiency in this age group. Children who have been categorised as having severe GH deficiency may in fact be categorised as having normal GH status when retested in adult life. This apparent discrepancy is not related to recovery of the GH axis, but can be attributed to the use of more strict thresholds for the diagnosis of GH deficiency in adults (Shalet et al., 1998).

GH is secreted in a pulsatile manner with a diurnal variation. The latter is characterised by nocturnal increase in GH secretion. This complex pattern of secretion is under hypothalamic control. Recent pathophysiological studies by the author et al of stimulated and spontaneous GH secretion in a cohort of adult cancer survivors irradiated for brain tumours with doses of less than 50 Gy, suggested that hypothalamic regulation of GH secretion in patients with severe GH deficiency is maintained with preserved pulsatility and diurnal variation (Darzy et al., 2005, 2006). The reduction in GH levels appears to be related to a predominant quantitative damage to the pituitary somatotrophs leading to reduced GH pulse amplitude but not frequency. Another study by the author et al (Darzy et al., 2007) has suggested the presence of a compensatory increase in hypothalamic GHRH release to maintain a normal spontaneous GH secretion in patients with reduced pituitary somatotrophs reserve indicated by reduced peak GH responses to direct stimulation with the most potent GHRH and Arginine stimulation test. There has also been a suggestion for the presence of 'compensated GH deficiency' in some patients who would otherwise have been diagnosed with GH deficiency due to impaired peak GH responses to insulin-induced hypoglycaemia (Darzy et al., 2009). It is unknown if the dynamics of GH secretion in patients with GH deficiency following intensive irradiation for NPC, with high probability of hypothalamic damage, are similar to what has been described by the author in patients with history of less intensive irradiation.

2.2.2 Diagnosis

Given the pulsatile nature of GH secretion, a single estimation of GH level is meaningless for the biochemical confirmation of a suspected GH deficiency. Physiological tests of GH secretion, such 24-hour or nocturnal GH profiling are rarely used in routine clinical practice. In current clinical practice, the diagnosis of GH deficiency relies on demonstrating a subnormal peak GH response to pharmacological tests that provoke GH release due to direct stimulation of the pituitary somatotrophs or indirectly through stimulation of the hypothalamus. Various dynamic tests are used in clinical practice; the choice is largely influenced by the experience of the endocrine centre and to some extent by patient's requirement. The insulin tolerance test (ITT) remains the gold standard, especially in the irradiated patients (Lissett et al., 2001), unless contraindicated due to epilepsy or heart disease. Other tests that are commonly used in clinical practice include Glucagon stimulation test, Arginine stimulation test (AST), L-Dopa test, GHRH test and the GHRH+AST.

The cut-off peak GH threshold used to define GH status following various stimuli is arbitrarily defined (Hoffman et al., 1994; Shalet et al., 1998). In children, the peak GH response to the ITT or equipotent tests (Glucagon, AST, L-Dopa or GHRH) below which a child is considered to be suffering from GH deficiency has been gradually increased and currently most GH therapy would be considered, in the appropriate clinical context, if that child failed to achieve a peak GH response above 20mU/L (7μg/L) (Shalet et al., 1998). In adults, however, severe GH deficiency for which GH replacement therapy may be considered is defined as a peak response to ITT or equipotent tests of less than 9mU/L (3μg/L) (Growth Hormone Research Society, 1998) and less than 9μg/L for the GHRH+AST (Aimaretti et al., 1998).

Additional support for diagnosing GH deficiency may be obtained from measuring GH-dependent markers including insulin-like growth factor-I (IGF-I) and IGF binding protein-3 (IGFBP-3). It is to be noted, however, that age and gender-corrected IGF-I and/or IGFBP-3 levels are frequently normal in patients with documented radiation-induced GH deficiency defined by physiological and/or pharmacological tests (Achermann et al., 1998; Cicognani et al., 1999; Tillmann et al., 1998). Thus, it had been thought that neither of these markers can be used as a reliable index of the development of radiation-induced GH deficiency. In general, a reduction in age- and gender-corrected IGF-I levels by 2 standard deviation (SD) is supportive of a diagnosis of GH deficiency providing other causes that reduce IGF-I production have been excluded, such as malnutrition, hypothyroidism, renal failure, liver disease, or diabetes mellitus (Shalet et al., 1998). In patients with panhypoptuitarism, the diagnosis of GH deficiency is almost certain especially if IGF-I levels are significantly reduced and biochemical confirmation can almost always be achieved accurately with a single test.

In addition to biochemical tests, auxological measurements of the irradiated child at regular intervals may provide invaluable information about the GH status. Growth in children is a sensitive marker of GH status. Thus, in the absence of other aetiologies for growth retardation, the presence of significant growth deviation over a one year period, that is, growth velocity below the 25th centile or a drop in height of ≥ 1 standard deviation (SD) is highly suggestive of clinically significant GH deficiency, particularly in the appropriate clinical context, i.e. previous irradiation.

2.2.3 Clinical impact and treatment

GH deficiency is an important cause for impaired linear growth in irradiated children cured from cancer. Ample evidence from studies in brain tumour survivors suggests that GH therapy in those patients prevent further height loss and maintain their initial height centile to adulthood (Clayton et al., 1988; Sulmont et al., 1990) while those who do not receive treatment show further deterioration in their height centiles with a tendency for extreme short stature (Brauner et al., 1989; Clarson & Del Maestro, 1999). In addition, those patients may also need GH replacement therapy in the transition to adulthood to maximize bone density and prevent osteoporosis, which is a frequent finding in the irradiated cancer survivors (Brennan et al., 2005; Murray et al., 1999; Shalet & Rosenfeld, 1998).

In adults, GH deficiency may be associated with symptoms and signs of the well described adult GH deficiency syndrome (Table 1), in particular impaired quality of life (QoL) (de Boer et al., 1995).

GH replacement therapy in the irradiated adult cancer survivors may improve QoL, as in those with GH deficiency due to pituitary tumours (Murray et al., 2002). Thus, it is important that a robust diagnosis of radiation-induced GH deficiency is made so that appropriate GH replacement therapy can be introduced at the right time. Despite the numerous and proven benefits of GH replacement therapy in adults (Table 2), this is currently only recommended to primarily improve QoL. It is given on a trial basis with

1- Increased fat mass (especially truncal) and increased waist/hip ratio
2- Reduced lean body mass (reduced muscle bulk and strength)
3- Osteopenia and Osteoporosis
4- Adverse lipid profile (increased LDL and reduced HDL)
5- Glucose intolerance and insulin resistance
6- Impaired fibrinolysis and nitric oxide generation
7- Altered cardiac function and structure
8- Reduced exercise capacity and muscle strength
9- Reduced quality of life (QoL)
A- Reduced vitality
B- Reduced energy
C- Depressed mood
D-Increased anxiety
E- Increased social isolation
F- Impaired emotional and self-control

Table 1. Features of the adult growth hormone deficiency syndrome.

gradual dose titration to achieve an IGF-I level in the upper quartile of the normal range (Bengtsson et al., 2000). The treatment is administered as a daily subcutaneous injection. Treatment is withdrawn if there is no improvement in QoL after 9 months of treatment. GH therapy for severe osteoporosis, but not QoL issuers, remains controversial.

2.2.4 Timing of testing

Testing for GH deficiency should be initiated at the time when GH therapy is considered safe. It is generally agreed that GH therapy should be avoided in the first 2-3 years after completion of cancer treatment, when the chance of cancer recurrence is greatest. GH therapy offered within this time period may be associated with a number of tumour recurrences and deaths that many families and doctors would associate with GH therapy despite a lack of proof of a causal relationship between GH therapy and tumour recurrence (Shalet et al., 1997; Sklar, 2004; Wilton, 1994).

Given the very high chance of developing severe GH deficiency 2-3 years after intensive radiotherapy in children, offering GH therapy without recourse to GH tests or evidence of impaired growth is an acceptable approach in certain centres. Alternatively, others would consider GH therapy when GH deficiency is established biochemically irrespective of growth rate. These approaches assume, given the epidemiological evidence, that it is highly likely that growth will soon decline in those patients or that an "apparently" normal growth rate is perhaps subnormal. A more selective approach, however, is still adopted by some endocrinologists who would insist on biochemical evidence of GH deficiency and a subnormal growth rate before initiating GH treatment. If GH status appears to be normal and the growth rate is appropriate for pubertal status, then growth is observed closely and the GH stimulation tests are repeated annually.

Testing in adults is only indicated if GH replacement therapy is to be considered in those who manifest symptoms and signs suggestive of severe GH deficiency (de Boeret al., 1995) (Table 1). A normal test 15 years after radiotherapy usually eliminates the need for further annual testing, as further decline in GH secretion is unlikely to occur after that time from radiotherapy.

Radiation-induced GH deficiency is irreversible. However, retesting in adulthood of those who were diagnosed with GH deficiency in childhood is mandatory before adult GH therapy is initiated or continued to address quality of life (QoL) issues. This is because the diagnostic threshold to treat GH deficiency is much lower in adults compared with children.

1- Improved psychological well-being and quality of life
2- Normalisation of body composition (reduced fat mass and increased lean body mass)
3- Increased bone mineral content
4- Increased ECF volume and renal function
5- Improved cardiac function
6- Improved exercise capacity
7- May reduce mortality in hypopituitary patients

Table 2. Benefits of growth hormone replacement therapy in adults.

2.3 Gonadotrophin deficiency

The gonadotrophin axis is the second most vulnerable to radiation damage. Gonadotrophin deficiency is frequently seen after intensive h-p axis irradiation (Chen et al., 1989; Constine et al., 1993; Lam et al., 1991; Rappaport et al., 1982; Samaan et al., 1987).

Gonadotrophin deficiency varies from subtle (subclinical) abnormalities in secretion detected only by GnRH testing to severe impairment associated with diminished circulating sex hormone levels. Although abnormalities in LH/FSH secretion can be demonstrated on dynamic testing, sometimes as early as one month following high dose irradiation (Chen et al., 1989), clinically-significant gonadotrophin deficiency is usually a late complication with a cumulative incidence in excess of 20% after long term follow up whether radiation was administered in childhood or adult life (Agha et al., 2005; Constine et al., 1993; Lam et al., 1991; Rappaport et al., 1982; Samaan et al., 1987). For example, Lam et al (Lam et al., 1991) reported a cumulative incidence of 30.7% 5 years after radiation treatment of NPC, while Samaan et al (Samaan et al., 1987) reported LH and FSH deficiency in 20% and 35% of NCP patients 1-4 years and more than 15 years after radiotherapy, respectively.

The diagnosis of gonadotrophin deficiency is confirmed by normal or low normal basal LH/FSH with diminished circulating sex hormone concentrations. In children, gonadotrophin deficiency may retard pubertal development and linear growth, especially in the context of GH deficiency, which almost always occurs following radiation doses that causes gonadotrophin deficiency. Those children will typically have a delayed bone age as assessed by a wrist radiograph. Treatment with sex steroids is needed to induce and support development of secondary sex characteristics as well as linear growth. It is extremely important that GH deficiency is recognised and treated for some time before introducing sex steroids to maximise the chances of attaining normal height.

In adults, secondary hypogonadism is associated with sexual dysfunction and reduced fertility. In the long term sex steroid deficiency may have adverse impact on metabolic, cardiovascular, muscular, and skeletal health and quality of life (QoL). Patients should be tested at regular intervals and whenever the diagnosis is suspected clinically. Women may present with oligomenorrhoea, amenorrhoea, sweating, and/or hot flushes. Men may complain from reduced libido, erectile dysfunction, reduced shaving frequency, fatigue and tiredness, mood changes and weight increase with central adiposity. Treatment with sex steroid replacement therapy improves QoL and prevent decline in physical and mental health. Gonadotrophin therapy is needed to restore fertility, unless gonadal damage from chemotherapy coexists.

GnRH testing may help to differentiate between hypothalamic and pituitary cause for gonadotrophin deficiency. A delayed peak gonadotrophin response and/or a delayed decline indicate hypothalamic damage; a blunted response indicates pituitary damage or secondary pituitary atrophy; a mixed pattern of responses indicates possible damage at both sites. Repeated intermittent infusion of GnRH may restore pituitary responsiveness and therefore differentiate between primary and secondary pituitary atrophy (Yoshimoto et al., 1975) and with prolonged treatment there is the potential for restoring gonadal function and fertility (Hall et al., 1994).

2.4 ACTH deficiency

The hypothalamic-pituitary-adrenal axis appears to be the most radioresistant in patients irradiated for non-pituitary disorders. Clinically apparent ACTH deficiency occurs in only about 3% of patients receiving a total radiation dose to the h-p axis of 40-50 Gy (Constine et al., 1993; Livesey et al., 1990). In contrast, the frequency of ACTH deficiency in patients treated with intensive irradiation for NPC is significantly higher. Samman et al (Samaan et al., 1987) reported a frequency of 4% in the first 4 years after irradiation and a cumulative frequency of 20% after 15 years, while Lam et al (Lam et al., 1991) reported a cumulative frequency of 30.7% after 5 years. Differences in radiation schedules and diagnostic criteria may explain the higher frequency in the latter study (Lam et al., 1991). In most reported cases, however, ACTH deficiency was partial and only a few patients needed regular hydrocortisone replacement because of symptoms of hypocortisolism (Lam et al., 1991; Samaan et al., 1987; Samaan et al., 1982).

From a clinical perspective, significant as opposed to subtle abnormalities in ACTH secretion, are unlikely to be missed by the ITT, which remains the "gold standard". If the ITT is contraindicated, alternative tests like Glucagon and Synacthen may be considered. Measurements of 9 am cortisol may be adequate; a level in excess of 300 nmol/l almost always excludes significant ACTH deficiency. However, during periods of acute stress or acute illness, a level in excess of 500 nmol/l is required to confirm normality of the ACTH-adrenal axis. Patients with lower levels or those who are symptomatic should be considered for a stimulation test. As ACTH deficiency is a slowly evolving abnormality, it is very unusual to have a normal synacthen test in the context of a clinically significant ACTH deficiency that normally results in secondary adrenal atrophy.

It is to be noted that increased oestrogen levels due to HRT, use of contraceptive pill (OCP) or pregnancy may raise cortisol binding globulin (CBG) resulting in spurious elevation of circulating total cortisol levels by as much as 3 folds or more. Under these circumstances, an apparently normal random cortisol level may occur in the presence of a significant cortisol deficiency. Any assessment of cortisol levels should only be done after withdrawing any oestrogen containing medications for at least 4 weeks. If the patient was on the oral contraceptive pill (OCP) appropriate advice about mechanical contraception should be provided. If the patient is not willing to stop oestrogen replacement therapy or if pregnant, a stimulation test may be needed. The normality of the ACTH-adrenal axis is then determined by a normal cortisol increment rather than by the normality of the absolute basal or stimulated cortisol levels.

Adrenal dysfunction with reduction in spontaneous and/or stimulated cortisol secretion is an important diagnosis to make. Missing a diagnosis of this nature may put patients at risk of acute adrenal crisis during periods of acute stress. Although regular hydrocortisone replacement therapy may not be necessary in asymptomatic patients with partial ACTH deficiency, oral or intravenous hydrocortisone replacement therapy may become necessary during situations that can lead to acute adrenal crisis due to failure of the ACTH-adrenal axis to meet the increased demands for cortisol. Such patients should be properly informed about the emergency use of hydrocortisone during severe stress, acute illness, surgery, and trauma. Patients should also be advised to have a steroid medi-alert bracelet for emergency situations.

Patients with clinically significant ACTH deficiency may experience symptoms of adrenal insufficiency including poor appetite, nausea, vomiting, tiredness, easy fatigability, muscle weakness, and breathlessness on exertion. Weight loss may not occur due to coexisting GH deficiency and/or hypothyroidism, which cause central obesity. Regular replacement therapy is strongly recommended in those patients.

2.5 TSH deficiency

Like the ACTH axis, the hypothalamic-pituitary-thyroid axis appears to be the least vulnerable to radiation damage and the latter is highly dose-dependent (Constine et al., 1993; Lam et al., 1991; Littley et al., 1989a). With radiation doses of less than 50 Gy, the frequency of TSH deficiency remains as low as 3-6%, such as that found in survivors of non-pituitary brain tumours (Livesey et al., 1990; Oberfield et al., 1992). Patients irradiated during adulthood for non-pituitary brain tumours were reported to have 9% rate of secondary hypothyroidism (Agha et al., 2005). A higher incidence of overt secondary hypothyroidism is noted in patients with pituitary tumours (Littley et al., 1989a), but more frequently following intensive irradiation schedules utilizing doses in excess of 50 Gy, typically used for head and neck tumours including NPC (Chen et al., 1989; Constine et al., 1993; Lam et al., 1991; Pai et al., 2001; Samaan et al., 1987). For example Lam et al (Lam et al., 1991) reported a cumulative incidence of secondary hypothyroidism of 14.9% after 5 years of follow up. The exact incidence of TSH deficiency may be under-estimated in NPC patients due to the high frequency of co-existing primary thyroid dysfunction causing TSH elevation.

Annual testing of thyroid function is indicated in patients irradiated for NPC who are particularly at much greater risk of primary hypothyroidism due to radiation-induced damage of the thyroid gland. The diagnosis of frank central hypothyroidism is straightforward - subnormal T4 level with normal or low basal TSH concentration. Given the wide range of normal free T4 levels, a significant decline in free T4 levels over time with normal or low normal TSH levels may signify a diagnosis of evolving central hypothyroidism or a mixed (primary and secondary) hypothyroidism even before free T4 levels drop below the lower normal limit. This should be highly suspected in the presence of gonadotrophin and/or ACTH deficiency or if there is history of thyroidal irradiation and it may warrant a therapeutic trial with thyroxin in the presence of a supportive clinical picture.

Thyroxine replacement therapy may precipitate symptomatic acute adrenal insufficiency in an otherwise asymptomatic individual with unrecognised ACTH deficiency. It is mandatory that reduced cortisol production be ruled out with certainty before starting thyroxine therapy. If cortisol deficiency coexists, it should be treated first before intruding thyroxine therapy. It is also important to continue to assess the ACTH-adrenal axis at regular intervals after commencing thyroxine replacement therapy.

With the difficulty in diagnosing evolving central hypothyroidism by a single test, it has been claimed that the presence of a hypothalamic TSH response to a TRH test and/or diminished nocturnal TSH surge despite a normal free T4 level may imply a diagnosis of so-called "hidden" central hypothyroidism in a substantial proportion of irradiated children (Rose et al., 1999). In a recent study by the author et al (Darzy & Shalet, 2005), however, it was demonstrated that, like in some normal individuals, the loss of nocturnal TSH surge seen in about 20% of euthyroid adult cancer survivors did not reflect a genuine loss of diurnal rhythm, but simply occurred as a result of a physiological shift in the timing of the peak TSH (acrophase) and/or the nadir TSH levels potentially leading to an erroneous diagnosis of "hidden" central hypothyroidism. Therefore, serial thyroid testing to demonstrate a decline in T4 levels provides the only means for diagnosing "hidden" central hypothyroidism.

2.6 Hyperprolactinaemia

Radiation-induced hyperprolactinaemia is mostly seen following intensive irradiation due to hypothalamic damage leading to a reduction in the inhibitory neurotransmitter dopamine. It has been described in both sexes and all age groups but is most frequently encountered in the adult female with radiation doses in excess of 40 Gy. In these patients, a mild to modest elevation in prolactin level is noticed in 20-50% (Agha et al., 2005; Constine et al., 1993; Lam et al., 1991; Littley et al., 1989a; Samaan et al., 1987) compared with less than 5% in children (Rappaportet al., 1982) and after low radiation doses (Littley et al., 1991). A much higher incidence is seen following intensive irradiation; Chen et al (Chen et al., 1989) reported hyperpractinaemia in 21% and 36% in the first 4 years and after 15 years of radiotherapy in NCP, respectively.

Radiation-induced hyperprolactinaemia is not clinically significant in the vast majority of patients. Occasionally, it may be of sufficient severity to impair gonadotrophin secretion and cause pubertal delay or arrest in children, decreased libido and impotence in adult males and galactorrhoea and/or ovarian dysfunction in women (Samaan et al., 1982). A gradual decline in the elevated prolactin level may occur with time and can normalize in some patients. This may reflect time-dependent slowly evolving direct radiation-induced damage to the pituitary lactotroph (Littley et al., 1989b).

Radiation-induced hyperprolactinaemia responds very well to treatment with dopamine agonists. Galactorrhoea resolves soon after normalising prolactin levels. However, treatment with dopamine agonists will only restore gonadal function and fertility if there is no co-existing gonadotrophin deficiency or primary chemotherapy-induced gonadal damage.

3. Radiation-induced primary thyroid dysfunction

Primary hypothyroidism is the most common clinical consequence of radiotherapy to the cervical area. It is well described in patients treated for Hodgkin's disease with a cumulative incidence of 44% after 25 years of radiotherapy (Hancock et al., 1991). The intensity of the damage, and hence, the degree of thyroid dysfunction is both dose- and time-dependent (Sklar et al., 2000). Primary hypothyroidism has been reported with fractionated radiotherapy with doses exceeding 25 Gy (Shalet et al., 1977). The probability of developing primary thyroid failure is significantly increased beyond 45 Gy (Bhandare et al., 2007). Chemotherapy has not been shown to influence the development of thyroid dysfunction following standard radiation therapy for head and neck cancers (Miller & Agrawal, 2009).

The pathophysiological mechanisms underlying radiation-induced thyroid dysfunction remain controversial. Various mechanisms have been proposed including radiation-induced autoimmune thyroiditis, direct radiation-induced damage to the follicular epithelium, direct microvascular and macrovasular damage resulting in thyroid tissue hypoxemia and nutrient-poor environment leading to reduced synthetic and secretory capacity, and radiation-induced fibrosis that may prevent compensatory hypertrophy of the gland (Miller & Agrawal, 2009). The development of thyroid antibodies after radiotherapy may predict a higher chance of thyroid dysfunction in the long-term.

Subtle thyroid dysfunction occurs soon after radiotherapy for NPC; Chen et al (Chen et al., 1989) have demonstrated increased peak TSH responses to TRH stimulation a month after radiotherapy and more so after 15-18 months of radiotherapy. More severe degrees of thyroid dysfunction with increased TSH and reduced free T4 tend to occur in the long term. However, hypothyroidism may occasionally develop as early as 6 weeks after completion of high dose radiotherapy to the neck.

A cumulative incidence of increased TSH of 18% and 45% was reported in 166 patients treated for NPC in the first 4 years and after 15 years of follow up, respectively (Samaan et al., 1987). In a prospective study of 408 patients who had received radiation therapy for NPC; the estimated incidences for clinical hypothyroidism were 5.3%, 9.0%, and 19.1% and for sub-clinical hypothyroidism were 9.7%, 15.7%, and 20.5% at 3, 5 and 10 years after radiotherapy, respectively (Wu et al., 2010). This study has also showed that clinical hypothyroidism occurred more frequently in younger patients, female sex and following conformal radiotherapy. Some reports have also suggested a higher incidence of radiation-induced hypothyroidism in the younger age group treated for Hodgkin's disease (Shalet et al., 1977) or for NPC (Zubizarreta et al., 2000), while other reports did not (Daoud et al., 2003; Kupeli et al., 2006). These rates of radiation-induced hypothyroidism are significantly higher than the reported rates of 0.3-1.3% in the general population (Wu et al., 2010). Much higher rated of hypothyroidism are seen in other head and neck tumours that involved thyroid surgery in addition to radiotherapy (Wu et al., 2010).

The diagnosis of primary hypothyroidism is straight forward. Frank (clinical) hypothyroidism is associated with increased TSH and subnormal free T4. Sub-clinical cases are characterised by increased TSH but apparently normal free T4. The presence of radiation-induced hypothalamic-pituitary damage with TSH deficiency may compound the biochemical picture and interpretation of the thyroid functions tests. Significant reduction in free T4 levels, albeit in the normal range, may be seen in the presence of normal or slightly elevated TSH levels. Under these circumstances a trend showing a progressive decline in free T4 levels despite a stable/mild increase in TSH levels following radiotherapy supports the diagnosis of central hypothyroidism or a combined primary and secondary hypothyroidism that may warrant a trial of thyroxine replacement therapy.

It is recommended that all patients have a thyroid function test at baseline and every 6-12 months after radiotherapy. Symptoms and signs of hypothyroidism should be explored during any consultation. The symptoms of overt hypothyroidism include weight gain or difficulty loosing weight, intolerance to cold, dry skin, hair loss, constipation, menorrhagia or intermenstrual spotting, decrease physical activity, lethargy, easy fatigability, muscle cramps, and slow mentation. The signs include periorbital oedema, loss of eyebrows, cool and dry skin, a prolonged relaxation phase of deep tendon reflexes, and pleural or pericardial effusions. If the biochemical diagnosis is uncertain, a trial of thyroxine replacement therapy in those with "sub-clinical" hypothyroidism with "normal" free T4 levels is worth considering with a proper assessment of the response.

In contrast to hypothyroidism, the frequency of hyperthyroidism due to Garves' disease is slightly increased post-irradiation (Jereczek-Fossa et al., 2004).

4. Radiation-induced thyroid nodules and tumours

The development of thyroid nodules and benign and malignant neoplasms is well described in patients who received neck irradiation for Hodgkin's lymphoma (Oeffinger et al., 2003) or as part of cranio-spinal irradiation for brain tumours (Shalet et al., 1977). There is no literature on this complication following treatment of NPC.

A significantly increased risk is seen in children irradiated before the age of 10 years. Other risk factors include female sex, longer duration of follow up and increased radiation dose above 2 Gy with no reduction in risk with high radiation doses reaching 60 Gy. Most of these thyroid nodules are benign in nature and may regress (Jereczek-Fossa et al., 2004). The risk of nodules being malignant is significantly higher if irradiation was administered before age 16 years and the tumourigenic effects of radiation in this age group can last up to 40 years post treatment (Schneider et al., 1993).

The frequency of diagnosed thyroid nodules after irradiation depends on the diagnostic method used. Clinical examination is usually not robust enough to detect small nodules less than 2cm in size. High-resolution thyroid ultrasound has increased the detection frequency (Mihailescu et al., 2005). Thyroid ultrasonography also helps to identify suspicious nodules that need a diagnostic fine needle aspiration (FNA). Routine surveillance ultrasonography of the thyroid remains a controversial issue, as it may increase anxiety and unnecessary diagnostic interventions. However, patients at high risk of radiation-induced thyroid cancer should undergo regular surveillance ultrasonography. FNA should be performed for suspicious nodules by virtue of size, rapidity of growth and/or ultrasonographic appearance. A diagnostic partial thyroidectomy may also be needed if the FNA was inconclusive.

5. Chemoptherapy-induced gonadal damage

The gonads are extremely sensitive to chemotherapy. Gonadotoxicity with resulting gonadal failure is a significant complication, which is seen more frequently than before due to increased use of chemotherapy in NPC, in particular Cisplatinum, which is highly gonadotoxic.

5.1 Chemoptherapy-induced ovarian damage

Chemotherapy-induced ovarian damage depends on the type and the total dose of the drugs used. The chemosensitivity of the ovary is age-dependent with progressively smaller doses being required to produce ovarian failure with increasing age (Rivkees & Crawford, 1988). Chemotherapeutic agents known to be gonadotoxic include alkylating agents, in particular Cyclophosphamide, Vinca-alkaloids, Antimetabolites, Platinum agents (Cisplatinum) and others such as Procarbazine.

Cisplatinum is the most commonly used agent in the treatment of NPC. The pathophysiological mechanisms underlying chemotherapy-induced ovarian damage are not fully understood. They are thought to be related to the cytotoxic effects of the drugs on ovarian follicles leading to impairment of follicular maturation and/or depletion of primordial follicles.

Chemotherapy-induced ovarian damage is unlikely to occur in the pre-pubertal patients. However, it is quite frequent in women with a frequency reaching 50% in those who received Alkylating agents. Acute ovarian failure may occur shortly after completion of chemotherapy. Recovery of acute ovarian failure is variable and can occur after many months or even years of amenorrhoea. Patients who retain their ovarian function after completion of chemotherapy and those who recover from acute ovarian failure are still at risk of early or premature ovarian failure later in life (Howell & Shalet, 1998).

Depending on severity, chemotherapy-induced ovarian damage can lead to delayed, arrested or absent pubertal development (in children), oligomenorrhoea, amenorrhoea, infertility, or sub-fertility. Oestrogen deficiency symptoms such as hot flushes, sweating, sexual dysfunction, and psychosomatic complaints are common especially with acute ovarian failure. These symptoms can have very negative impact on quality of life and physical well-being. In the long-term early ovarian failure may lead to accelerated decline in bone density and osteoporosis, increased cholesterol levels and possible increased risk of cardiovascular disease. Adequate oestrogen replacement therapy is recommended to relieve symptoms and preserve bone density, especially in younger people providing there are no contra-indications for their use. The decision to use HRT and its duration should be individualised and agreed with the patient taking into account the benefits and the long-term risks of HRT.

Biochemically, ovarian damage is characterised by reduced oestrogen levels and increased gonadotrophin levels and/or impaired ovulation tests. The compensatory increase in FSH/LH levels may be attenuated or completely absent if radiation-induced gonadotrophin deficiency coexists.

Fertility preservation in young women, if resources allow, should be considered and offered to certain patients depending on their age, presence of a partner, desire for fertility, psychosocial issues, and the extent of the disease and prognosis. Methods to preserve fertility in women include freezing (embryo crypreservation, oocyte cryopreservation, and ovarian tissue cryopreservation) and ovarian suppression with GnRH analogues or antagonists. Unfortunately, fertility preservation techniques are not widely available and each method has its own advantages and disadvantages with no guaranteed outcome (Howell & Shalet, 2002).

5.2 Chemotherapy-induced testicular damage

Temporary or permanent chemotherapy-induced testicular damage occurs at all ages of life (Howell & Shalet, 2001, 2005). Unlike in females, children seem to be more susceptible to the damaging effects of cytotoxic agents. Although all chemotherapeutic drugs may have some effects on fertility, some are known to be more gonadotoxic than others. Alkylating agents are the most gonadotoxic; others include Cisplatinum, Cytarabine, Dacarbazine and Procarbazine. The germinal epithelium in the seminiferous tubules is more chemo-sensitive than Leydig cells. Germinal epithelium damage following chemotherapy can be seen in the presence of normal Leydig cell function. Depending on the type and number of agents administered and the total dose, damage to the germinal epithelium and the supporting Sertoli cells, with consequent oligo-or azoo-spermia, occurs in 20-90% of patients following chemotherapy. Recovery of spermatogenesis is not unusual and can be seen several years after chemotherapy (Howell & Shalet, 2005). In patients treated for testicular cancer, for example, variable degrees of recovery of spermatogenesis are seen in 50-80% after 2 to 5 years following completion of cisplatinum-based chemotherapy (Howell & Shalet, 2005). However, patients who have fully preserved or recovered spermatogenesis still have reduced sperm count compared with healthy men. Damage to the germinal epithelium causes gradual atrophy of the testes with reduced volume, reduced inhibin B and increased FSH secretion.

Although less vulnerable to the cytotoxic effects of chemotherapy than the germinal epithelium, Leydig cell dysfunction following chemotherapy is well described. It is often fully compensated with normal testosterone levels and significantly increased LH levels (Howell & Shalet, 2001). The effects of chemotherapy on the production of testosterone from Leydig cells are only seen at much higher doses. The doses required to cause Leydig cell failure will invariably have resulted in damage to the germinal epithelium. However, subtle degrees of Leydig cell dysfunction may be seen in the presence of normal spermatogenesis (Howell & Shalet, 2001). Co-existing radiation-induced gonadotrophin deficiency may impair the extent of compensation and result in combined primary and secondary hypogonadism.

The impact of mild/subclinical Leydig cell insufficiency is unclear (Howell et al., 1999). However, the manifestations of severe degrees of Leydig cell dysfunction depend upon the age of the patient. Loss of Leydig cell function before the onset of, or during puberty will be associated with failure to enter puberty spontaneously or arrest of pubertal development. Leydig cell failure following the development of normal secondary sexual characteristics manifests clinically with reduced libido, erectile dysfunction, fatigue and mood changes. In the long-term, Leydig cell failure may adversely affect skeletal, muscular, cardiovascular, and metabolic health as well as cognitive functions (Bhasin et al., 2010). If not contraindicated, testosterone replacement therapy is recommended for symptomatic men with classical androgen deficiency aimed at inducing and maintaining secondary sex characteristics and at improving their sexual function, sense of well-being, and bone mineral density. Clinical monitoring of testosterone therapy at regular intervals to assess response, compliance and adverse effects is important. Assessment of bone density every 1-2 years in osteoporotic men and annual monitoring of the haematocrit and the PSA (in men 40 yr of age or older) are also important particularly in the long-term (Bhasin et al., 2010).

With regard to fertility preservation, cryopreservation of spermatozoa before sterilizing chemotherapy (sperm banking) in the sexually mature male is currently the only established clinical option. In men with spermatogenic arrest, sperm extraction for intracytoplasmic sperm injection (ICSI) is a potentially successful approach. Other fertility preservation techniques such as cryopresvation of testicular tissues, germ cell transplantation, testis tissue xenografting and hormonal manipulation are largely experimental (Howell & Shalet, 2002).

6. Conclusions

Treatment of NPC with radiotherapy is associated with a high risk of radiation-induced hypothalamic-pituitary dysfunction. More than 80% of NPC survivors will have at least one anterior pituitary hormone deficiency and hyperprolactinaemia is frequently seen in women. Irradiation of the thyroid is associated with a significant risk of primary hypothyroidism. In the long-term there is increased risk of thyroid nodules and thyroid cancer, especially in children. These abnormalities in the endocrine functions are progressive and irreversible and can result in significant morbidity and impaired quality of life. In addition, chemotherapy may cause transient or permanent direct gonadal damage and hypogonadism. Regular endocrine surveillance is mandatory to achieve early detection of these abnormalities and timely treatment.

7. References

Achermann, J. C., Brook, C. G. & Hindmarsh, P. C. (2000). The GH response to low-dose bolus growth hormone-releasing hormone (GHRH(1-29)NH2) is attenuated in patients with longstanding post-irradiation GH insufficiency. *European Journal of Endocrinology*, Vol. 142, No. 4, April 2000. pp: 359-64.

Achermann, J. C., Hindmarsh, P. C. & Brook, C. G. (1998). The relationship between the growth hormone and insulin-like growth factor axis in long-term survivors of childhood brain tumours. *Clinical Endocrinology (Oxford)*, Vol. 49, No. 5, November 1998. pp: 639-45.

Agha, A., Sherlock, M., Brennan, S., O'Connor, S. A., O'Sullivan, E., Rogers, B., Faul, C., Rawluk, D., Tormey, W. & Thompson, C. J. (2005). Hypothalamic-pituitary dysfunction after irradiation of nonpituitary brain tumors in adults. *Journal of Clinical Endocrinology & Metabolism*, Vol. 90, No. 12, December 2005. pp: 6355-60.

Aimaretti, G., Corneli, G., Razzore, P., Bellone, S., Baffoni, C., Arvat, E., Camanni, F. & Ghigo, E. (1998). Comparison between insulin-induced hypoglycemia and growth hormone (GH)-releasing hormone + arginine as provocative tests for the diagnosis of GH deficiency in adults. *Journal of Clinical Endocrinology & Metabolism*, Vol. 83, No. 5, May 1998. pp: 1615-8.

Bengtsson, B. A., Johannsson, G., Shalet, S. M., Simpson, H. & Sonken, P. H. (2000). Treatment of growth hormone deficiency in adults. *Journal of Clinical Endocrinology & Metabolism*, Vol. 85, No. 3, March 2000. pp: 933-42.

Bhandare, N., Kennedy, L., Malyapa, R. S., Morris, C. G. & Mendenhall, W. M. (2007). Primary and central hypothyroidism after radiotherapy for head-and-neck tumors. *International Journal of Radiation Oncology. Biology. Physics*, Vol. 68, No. 4, July 2007. pp: 1131-9.

Bhasin, S., Cunningham, G. R., Hayes, F. J., Matsumoto, A. M., Snyder, P. J., Swerdloff, R. S. & Montori, V. M. (2010). Testosterone therapy in men with androgen deficiency syndromes: an Endocrine Society clinical practice guideline. *Journal of Clinical Endocrinology & Metabolism*, Vol. 95, No. 6, June 2010. pp: 2536-59.

Brauner, R., Rappaport, R., Prevot, C., Czernichow, P., Zucker, J. M., Bataini, P., Lemerle, J., Sarrazin, D. & Guyda, H. J. (1989). A prospective study of the development of growth hormone deficiency in children given cranial irradiation, and its relation to statural growth. *Journal of Clinical Endocrinology & Metabolism*, Vol. 68, No. 2, February 1989. pp: 346-51.

Brennan, B. M., Mughal, Z., Roberts, S. A., Ward, K., Shalet, S. M., Eden, T. O., Will, A. M., Stevens, R. F. & Adams, J. E. (2005). Bone mineral density in childhood survivors of acute lymphoblastic leukemia treated without cranial irradiation. *Journal of Clinical Endocrinology & Metabolism*, Vol. 90, No. 2, February 2005. pp: 689-94.

Chen, M. S., Lin, F. J., Huang, M. J., Wang, P. W., Tang, S., Leung, W. M. & Leung, W. (1989). Prospective hormone study of hypothalamic-pituitary function in patients with nasopharyngeal carcinoma after high dose irradiation. *Japanese Journal of Clinical Oncology*, Vol. 19, No. 3, September 1989. pp: 265-70.

Chiang, C. S., Hong, J. H., Stalder, A., Sun, J. R., Withers, H. R. & McBride, W. H. (1997). Delayed molecular responses to brain irradiation. *International Journal of Radiation Biology*, Vol. 72, No. 1, July 1997. pp: 45-53.

Chieng, P. U., Huang, T. S., Chang, C. C., Chong, P. N., Tien, R. D. & Su, C. T. (1991). Reduced hypothalamic blood flow after radiation treatment of nasopharyngeal cancer: SPECT studies in 34 patients. *American Journal of Neuroradiology*, Vol. 12, No. 4, July-August 1991. pp: 661-5.

Cicognani, A., Cacciari, E., Pession, A., Pasini, A., De Iasio, R., Gennari, M., Alvisi, P. & Pirazzoli, P. (1999). Insulin-like growth factor-I (IGF-I) and IGF-binding protein-3 (IGFBP-3) concentrations compared to stimulated growth hormone (GH) in the evaluation of children treated for malignancy. *Journal of Pediatric Endocrinology & Metabolism*, Vol. 12, No. 5, September-October 1999. pp: 629-38.

Clarson, C. L. & Del Maestro, R. F. (1999). Growth failure after treatment of pediatric brain tumors. *Pediatrics*, Vol. 103, No. 3, March 1999. pp: E37.

Clayton, P. E. & Shalet, S. M. (1991). Dose dependency of time of onset of radiation-induced growth hormone deficiency. *Journal of Pediatrics*, Vol. 118, No. 2, February 1991. pp: 226-8.

Clayton, P. E., Shalet, S. M. & Price, D. A. (1988). Growth response to growth hormone therapy following craniospinal irradiation. *European Journal of Pediatrics*, Vol. 147, No. 6, August 1988. pp: 597-601.

Constine, L. S., Woolf, P. D., Cann, D., Mick, G., McCormick, K., Raubertas, R. F. & Rubin, P. (1993). Hypothalamic-pituitary dysfunction after radiation for brain tumors. *New England Journal of Medicine*, Vol. 328, No. 2, January 1993. pp: 87-94.

Daoud, J., Toumi, N., Bouaziz, M., Ghorbel, A., Jlidi, R., Drira, M. M. & Frikha, M. (2003). Nasopharyngeal carcinoma in childhood and adolescence: analysis of a series of 32 patients treated with combined chemotherapy and radiotherapy. *European Journal of Cancer.*, Vol. 39, No. 16, November 2003. pp: 2349-54.

Darzy, K., Pezzoli, S., Thorner, M. & Shalet, S. (2005). The dynamics of GH secretion in adult cancer survivors with severe GH deficiency acquired following brain irradiation in childhood for non-pituitary brain tumors: evidence for preserved pulsatility and diurnal variation with increased secretory disorderliness. *Journal of Clinical Endocrinology & Metabolism*, Vol. 90, No. 5, May 2005. pp: 2794-2803.

Darzy, K. H., Murray, R. D., Gleeson, H. K., Pezzoli, S. S., Thorner, M. O. & Shalet, S. M. (2006). The impact of short-term fasting on the dynamics of 24-hour GH secretion in patients with severe radiation-induced GH deficiency. *Journal of Clinical Endocrinology & Metabolism*, Vol. 91, No. 3, March 2006. pp: 987-94.

Darzy, K. H., Pezzoli, S. S., Thorner, M. O. & Shalet, S. M. (2007). Cranial irradiation and growth hormone neurosecretory dysfunction: a critical appraisal. *Journal of Clinical Endocrinology & Metabolism*, Vol. 92, No. 5, May 2007. pp: 1666-1672.

Darzy, K. H. & Shalet, S. M. (2005). Circadian and stimulated thyrotropin secretion in cranially irradiated adult cancer survivors. *Journal of Clinical Endocrinology & Metabolism*, Vol. 90, No. 12, 2005. pp: 6490-7.

Darzy, K. H., Thorner, M. O. & Shalet, S. M. (2009). Cranially irradiated adult cancer survivors may have normal spontaneous GH secretion in the presence of discordant peak GH responses to stimulation tests (compensated GH deficiency). *Clinical Endocrinology (Oxford)*, Vol. 70, No. 2, February 2009. pp: 287-93.

de Boer, H., Blok, G. J. & Van der Veen, E. A. (1995). Clinical aspects of growth hormone deficiency in adults. *Endocrine Reviewes*, Vol. 16, No. 1, 1995. pp: 63-86.

Duffner, P. K., Cohen, M. E., Voorhess, M. L., MacGillivray, M. H., Brecher, M. L., Panahon, A. & Gilani, B. B. (1985). Long-term effects of cranial irradiation on endocrine function in children with brain tumors. A prospective study. *Cancer*, Vol. 56, No. 9, 1985. pp: 2189-93.

Growth Hormone Research Society. (1998). Consensus guidelines for the diagnosis and treatment of adults with growth hormone deficiency: summary statement of the Growth Hormone Research Society Workshop on Adult Growth Hormone Deficiency. *Journal of Clinical Endocrinology & Metabolism*, Vol. 83, No. 2, February 1998. pp: 379-81.

Hall, J. E., Martin, K. A., Whitney, H. A., Landy, H. & Crowley, W. F., Jr. (1994). Potential for fertility with replacement of hypothalamic gonadotropin-releasing hormone in long term female survivors of cranial tumors. *Journal of Clinical Endocrinology & Metabolism*, Vol. 79, No. 4, October 1994. pp: 1166-72.

Hancock, S. L., Cox, R. S. & McDougall, I. R. (1991). Thyroid diseases after treatment of Hodgkin's disease. *New England Journal of Medicine*, Vol. 325, No. 9, August 1991. pp: 599-605.

Hochberg, Z., Kuten, A., Hertz, P., Tatcher, M., Kedar, A. & Benderly, A. (1983). The effect of single-dose radiation on cell survival and growth hormone secretion by rat anterior pituitary cells. *Radiation Research*, Vol. 94, No. 3, June 1983. pp: 508-12.

Hoffman, D. M., O'Sullivan, A., Baxter, R. C. & Ho, K. K. (1994). Diagnosis of growth-hormone deficiency in adults. *Lancet*, Vol. 343, No. 8905, April 1994. pp: 1064-8.

Howell, S. & Shalet, S. (1998). Gonadal damage from chemotherapy and radiotherapy. *Endocrinology Metabolism Clinics of North America*, Vol. 27, No. 4, December 1998. pp: 927-43.

Howell, S. J., Radford, J. A., Ryder, W. D. & Shalet, S. M. (1999). Testicular function after cytotoxic chemotherapy: evidence of Leydig cell insufficiency. *J Clin Oncol*, Vol. 17, No. 5, May 1999. pp: 1493-8.

Howell, S. J. & Shalet, S. M. (2001). Testicular function following chemotherapy. *Human Reproduction Update*, Vol. 7, No. 4, July-August 2001. pp: 363-9.

Howell, S. J. & Shalet, S. M. (2002). Fertility preservation and management of gonadal failure associated with lymphoma therapy. *Current Oncology Reports*, Vol. 4, No. 5, September 2002. pp: 443-52.

Howell, S. J. & Shalet, S. M. (2005). Spermatogenesis after cancer treatment: damage and recovery. *Journal of the National Cancer Institute Monographs*, Vol. No. 34, 2005. pp: 12-7.

Jereczek-Fossa, B. A., Alterio, D., Jassem, J., Gibelli, B., Tradati, N. & Orecchia, R. (2004). Radiotherapy-induced thyroid disorders. *Cancer Treatment Reviews*, Vol. 30, No. 4, June 2004. pp: 369-84.

Jorgensen, E. V., Schwartz, I. D., Hvizdala, E., Barbosa, J., Phuphanich, S., Shulman, D. I., Root, A. W., Estrada, J., Hu, C. S. & Bercu, B. B. (1993). Neurotransmitter control of growth hormone secretion in children after cranial radiation therapy. *Journal of Pediatrics Endocrinol*, Vol. 6, No. 2, April 1993. pp: 131-42.

Kupeli, S., Varan, A., Ozyar, E., Atahan, I. L., Yalcin, B., Kutluk, T., Akyuz, C. & Buyukpamukcu, M. (2006). Treatment results of 84 patients with nasopharyngeal carcinoma in childhood. *Pediatric Blood Cancer*, Vol. 46, No. 4, April 2006. pp: 454-8.

Kyrkanides, S., Olschowka, J. A., Williams, J. P., Hansen, J. T. & MK, O. B. (1999). TNF alpha and IL-1beta mediate intercellular adhesion molecule-1 induction via microglia-astrocyte interaction in CNS radiation injury. *Journal of Neuroimmunology*, Vol. 95, No. 1-2, March 1999. pp: 95-106.

Lam, K. S., Tse, V. K., Wang, C., Yeung, R. T. & Ho, J. H. (1991). Effects of cranial irradiation on hypothalamic-pituitary function--a 5-year longitudinal study in patients with nasopharyngeal carcinoma. *Quarterly Journal of Medicine*, Vol. 78, No. 286, February 1991. pp: 165-76.

Lissett, C. A., Saleem, S., Rahim, A., Brennan, B. M. & Shalet, S. M. (2001). The impact of irradiation on growth hormone responsiveness to provocative agents is stimulus dependent: results in 161 individuals with radiation damage to the somatotropic axis. *Journal of Clinical Endocrinology & Metabolism*, Vol. 86, No. 2, February 2001. pp: 663-8.

Littley, M. D., Shalet, S. M., Beardwell, C. G., Robinson, E. L. & Sutton, M. L. (1989a). Radiation-induced hypopituitarism is dose-dependent. *Clinical Endocrinology (Oxford)*, Vol. 31, No. 3, September 1989. pp: 363-73.

Littley, M. D., Shalet, S. M., Beardwell, C. G., Ahmed, S. R., Applegate, G. & Sutton, M. L. (1989b). Hypopituitarism following external radiotherapy for pituitary tumours in adults. *Quarterly Journal of Medicine*, Vol. 70, No. 262, February 1989. pp: 145-60.

Littley, M. D., Shalet, S. M., Morgenstern, G. R. & Deakin, D. P. (1991). Endocrine and reproductive dysfunction following fractionated total body irradiation in adults. *Quarterly Journal of Medicine*, Vol. 78, No. 287, March 1991. pp: 265-74.

Livesey, E. A., Hindmarsh, P. C., Brook, C. G., Whitton, A. C., Bloom, H. J., Tobias, J. S., Godlee, J. N. & Britton, J. (1990). Endocrine disorders following treatment of childhood brain tumours. *British Journal of Cancer*, Vol. 61, No. 4, April 1990. pp: 622-5.

Mihailescu, D. V., Collins, B. J., Wilbur, A., Malkin, J. & Schneider, A. B. (2005). Ultrasound-detected thyroid nodules in radiation-exposed patients: changes over time. *Thyroid*, Vol. 15, No. 2, February 2005. pp: 127-33.

Miller, M. C. & Agrawal, A. (2009). Hypothyroidism in postradiation head and neck cancer patients: incidence, complications, and management. *British Journal of Cancer*, Vol. 17, No. 2, April 2009. pp: 111-5.

Murray, R. D., Brennan, B. M., Rahim, A. & Shalet, S. M. (1999). Survivors of childhood cancer: long-term endocrine and metabolic problems dwarf the growth disturbance. *Acta Paediatrica Supplement*, Vol. 88, No. 433, December 1999. pp: 5-12.

Murray, R. D., Darzy, K. H., Gleeson, H. K. & Shalet, S. M. (2002). GH-deficient survivors of childhood cancer: GH replacement during adult life. *Journal of Clinical Endocrinology & Metabolism*, Vol. 87, No. 1, January 2002. pp: 129-35.

Oberfield, S. E., Sklar, C., Allen, J., Walker, R., Mcelwain, M., Papadakis, V. & Maenza, J. (1992). Thyroid and gonadal function and growth of long-term survivors of medulloblastoma / PNET, In *Late effects of treatment for childhood cancer*, D.M. Green and G.J. D'Angio, Editors, pp. (55-62), Wiley-Liss, Inc: New York.

Oeffinger, K. C., Sklar, C. A. & Hudson, M. M. (2003). Thyroid nodules and survivors of Hodgkin's disease. *American Family Physician*, Vol. 68, No. 6, September 2003. pp: 1016-19.

Ogilvy-Stuart, A. L., Clark, D. J., Wallace, W. H., Gibson, B. E., Stevens, R. F., Shalet, S. M. & Donaldson, M. D. (1992). Endocrine deficit after fractionated total body irradiation. *Archives of Disease in Childhood,* Vol. 67, No. 9, September 1992. pp: 1107-10.

Ogilvy-Stuart, A. L., Wallace, W. H. & Shalet, S. M. (1994). Radiation and neuroregulatory control of growth hormone secretion. *Clinical Endocrinology (Oxford),* Vol. 41, No. 2, August 1994. pp: 163-8.

Pai, H. H., Thornton, A., Katznelson, L., Finkelstein, D. M., Adams, J. A., Fullerton, B. C., Loeffler, J. S., Leibsch, N. J., Klibanski, A. & Munzenrider, J. E. (2001). Hypothalamic/pituitary function following high-dose conformal radiotherapy to the base of skull: demonstration of a dose-effect relationship using dose-volume histogram analysis. *Journal of Radiation Oncology. Biology. Physics,* Vol. 49, No. 4, March 2001. pp: 1079-92.

Rappaport, R., Brauner, R., Czernichow, P., Thibaud, E., Renier, D., Zucker, J. M. & Lemerle, J. (1982). Effect of hypothalamic and pituitary irradiation on pubertal development in children with cranial tumors. *Journal of Clinical Endocrinology & Metabolism,* Vol. 54, No. 6, June 1982. pp: 1164-8.

Rivkees, S. A. & Crawford, J. D. (1988). The relationship of gonadal activity and chemotherapy-induced gonadal damage. *Journal of the American Medical Association,* Vol. 259, No. 14, April 1988. pp: 2123-5.

Robinson, I. C., Fairhall, K. M., Hendry, J. H. & Shalet, S. M. (2001). Differential radiosensitivity of hypothalamo-pituitary function in the young adult rat. *Journal of Endocrinology,* Vol. 169, No. 3, June 2001. pp: 519-26.

Rose, S. R., Lustig, R. H., Pitukcheewanont, P., Broome, D. C., Burghen, G. A., Li, H., Hudson, M. M., Kun, L. E. & Heideman, R. L. (1999). Diagnosis of hidden central hypothyroidism in survivors of childhood cancer. *Journal of Clinical Endocrinology & Metabolism,* Vol. 84, No. 12, December 1999. pp: 4472-9.

Samaan, N. A., Schultz, P. N., Yang, K. P., Vassilopoulou-Sellin, R., Maor, M. H., Cangir, A. & Goepfert, H. (1987). Endocrine complications after radiotherapy for tumors of the head and neck. *Journal of Laboratory and Clinical Medicine,* Vol. 109, No. 3, March 1987. pp: 364-72.

Samaan, N. A., Vieto, R., Schultz, P. N., Maor, M., Meoz, R. T., Sampiere, V. A., Cangir, A., Ried, H. L. & Jesse, R. H., Jr. (1982). Hypothalamic, pituitary and thyroid dysfunction after radiotherapy to the head and neck. *International Journal of Radiation Oncology. Biology. Physics,* Vol. 8, No. 11, November 1982. pp: 1857-67.

Schmiegelow, M., Lassen, S., Poulsen, H. S., Feldt-Rasmussen, U., Schmiegelow, K., Hertz, H. & Muller, J. (2000). Growth hormone response to a growth hormone-releasing hormone stimulation test in a population-based study following cranial irradiation of childhood brain tumors. *Hormone Research,* Vol. 54, No. 2, 2000. pp: 53-9.

Schneider, A. B., Ron, E., Lubin, J., Stovall, M. & Gierlowski, T. C. (1993). Dose-response relationships for radiation-induced thyroid cancer and thyroid nodules: evidence for the prolonged effects of radiation on the thyroid. *Journal of Clinical Endocrinology & Metabolism,* Vol. 77, No. 2, August 1993. pp: 362-9.

Shalet, S. M., Brennan, B. M. & Reddingius, R. E. (1997). Growth hormone therapy and malignancy. *Hormone Research,* Vol. 48, Suppl 4, 1997. pp: 29-32.

Shalet, S. M. & Rosenfeld, R. G. (1998). Growth hormone replacement therapy during transition of patients with childhood-onset growth hormone deficiency into adulthood: what are the issues? *Growth Hormone & IGF Research,* Vol. 8, Suppl B, April 1998. pp: 177-84.

Shalet, S. M., Rosenstock, J. D., Beardwell, C. G., Pearson, D. & Jones, P. H. (1977). Thyroid dysfunction following external irradiation to the neck for Hodgkin's disease in childhood. *Clinical Radiology*, Vol. 28, No. 5, 1977. pp: 511-5.

Shalet, S. M., Toogood, A. A., Rahim, A. & Brennan, B. M. D. (1998). The diagnosis of growth hormone deficiency in children and adults. *Endocrine Reviews*, Vol. 19, No. 2, 1998. pp: 203-23.

Sham, J., Choy, D., Kwong, P. W., Cheng, A. C., Kwong, D. L., Yau, C. C., Wan, K. Y. & Au, G. K. (1994). Radiotherapy for nasopharyngeal carcinoma: shielding the pituitary may improve therapeutic ratio. *International Journal of Radiation Oncology. Biology. Physics*, Vol. 29, No. 4, July 1994. pp: 699-704.

Sklar, C., Whitton, J., Mertens, A., Stovall, M., Green, D., Marina, N., Greffe, B., Wolden, S. & Robison, L. (2000). Abnormalities of the thyroid in survivors of Hodgkin's disease: data from the Childhood Cancer Survivor Study. *Journal of Clinical Endocrinology & Metabolism*, Vol. 85, No. 9, September 2000. pp: 3227-32.

Sklar, C. A. (2004). Growth hormone treatment: cancer risk. *Hormone Research*, Vol. 62, Suppl 3, 2004. pp: 30-4.

Sulmont, V., Brauner, R., Fontoura, M. & Rappaport, R. (1990). Response to growth hormone treatment and final height after cranial or craniospinal irradiation. *Acta Paediatrica Scandinavica*, Vol. 79, No. 5, May1990. pp: 542-9.

Thames, H. D. & Hendry, J. H. (1987). Response of tissues to fractionated irradiation: effect of repair, In: *Fractionation in Radiotherapy*. pp (53-99) Taylor & Francis: London.

Tillmann, V., Shalet, S. M., Price, D. A., Wales, J. K., Pennells, L., Soden, J., Gill, M. S., Whatmore, A. J. & Clayton, P. E. (1998). Serum insulin-like growth factor-I, IGF binding protein-3 and IGFBP-3 protease activity after cranial irradiation. *Hormone Research*, Vol. 50, No. 2, 1998. pp: 71-7.

Wei, W. I. (2001). Nasopharyngeal cancer: current status of management: a New York Head and Neck Society lecture. *Archives of Otolaryngology-Head & Neck Surgery*, Vol. 127, No. 7, July 2001. pp: 766-9.

Wilton, P. (1994). on behalf of the International Board of the Kabi Pharmacia International Growth Study. Safety of growth hormone (GH) - Value of a large data base. *Clinical Pediatric Endocrinology*, Vol. 3, Suppl 5, 1994. pp: 61-71.

Withers, H. R. (1994). Biology of radiation oncology, In: *Current radiation oncology*, J.S. Tobias and P.R.M. Thomas, Editors, pp. (5-23), Edward Arnold: London.

Wu, Y. H., Wang, H. M., Chen, H. H., Lin, C. Y., Chen, E. Y., Fan, K. H., Huang, S. F., Chen, I. H., Liao, C. T., Cheng, A. J. & Chang, J. T. (2010). Hypothyroidism after radiotherapy for nasopharyngeal cancer patients. *International Journal of Radiation Oncology. Biology. Physics*, Vol. 76, No. 4, March 2010. pp: 1133-9.

Yoshimoto, Y., Moridera, K. & Imura, H. (1975). Restoration of normal pituitary gonadotropin reserve by administration of luteinizing-hormone-releasing hormone in patients with hypogonadotropic hypogonadism. *New England Journal of Medicine*, Vol. 292, No. 5, January 1975. pp: 242-5.

Zubizarreta, P. A., D'Antonio, G., Raslawski, E., Gallo, G., Preciado, M. V., Casak, S. J., Scopinaro, M., Morales, G. & Sackmann-Muriel, F. (2000). Nasopharyngeal carcinoma in childhood and adolescence: a single-institution experience with combined therapy. *Cancer*, Vol. 89, No. 3, August 2000. pp: 690-5.

9

Ear-Related Issues in Patients with Nasopharyngeal Carcinoma

Wong-Kein Christopher Low and Mahalakshmi Rangabashyam
Department of Otolaryngology, Singapore General Hospital
Singapore

1. Introduction

Nasopharyngeal carcinoma (NPC) is the sixth most common cancer in Singapore amongst males. Each year, there are 300-400 new cases diagnosed (Singapore cancer registry 2005-2009). NPC is endemic in Southeast Asia, North Africa, and parts of the Mediterranean basin, with the highest prevalence in Southern China where an average of 80 cases per 100,000 populations is reported each year (Loong et al., 2008).

The nasopharynx is at a point where the ear, nose and upper pharynx converge. NPC is relevant to the Otologist although the nasopharynx is located outside the precincts of the anatomical confines of the ear, since it frequently manifests itself in the form of ear-related symptoms. The ear deserves special attention not only during diagnosis, but also in treatment and follow-up of patients with NPC. NPC is extremely radiosensitive and potentially curable provided the diagnosis is made early. As ear structures are often included in the radiation fields, ear-related complications of radiotherapy are common as well.

Early diagnosis is important as it has better treatment outcomes. Patients with early stages of the disease may present with ear-related complaints. In advanced disease, adjuvant chemotherapy may become necessary. Chemotherapy usually involves using Cisplatin (CDDP), which is potentially ototoxic. It is of concern that only 10% of patients are diagnosed early at stage I (van Hasselt and Woo, 2008). According to Leong et al.(1999), patient factors identified which contributed to delayed diagnosis included deferment in seeking medical help, defaulting follow up visits and refusing investigations. Other factors contributing to further delay in diagnosis were Clinicians not considering a diagnosis of NPC and Clinicians suspecting NPC but misled by the results of investigations. These factors contributed to nearly a fifth of patients with NPC having delayed diagnosis. Many of the factors responsible for the delays appear to be preventable by better patient education and counseling, doctors having sharper clinical acumen and skills in NPC diagnosis and the hospital administration having a system of tracking down high risk patients who default. Therefore, Clinicians should be familiar with the ear-related manifestations of NPC, which may help in its early diagnosis

This review aims to highlight ear-related issues in NPC patients from 2 perspectives: 1) as a manifestation of the disease itself and 2) ear-related complications arising from treatment of

NPC namely, radiotherapy with and without chemotherapy. There is a relative paucity of world literature focusing on the impact of NPC on the Otologist. A major part of this review is from the principal author's previous work spanning 2 decades and review of other relevant literature.

2. Otological manifestations of NPC

Middle ear effusion resulting from NPC is a well-known presenting feature. However, there are other less common otological presentations including otalgia, giddiness, heamotympanum, barotrauma and periauricular mass which one should be mindful of (Low and Goh 1999).

2.1 Middle ear involvement

The link between the middle ear and nasopharynx by the Eustachian tube is one of the important reasons why the middle ear is frequently involved in patients with NPC.

A small tumor in the Fossa of Rosenmüller of the nasopharynx does not necessarily impair the Eustachian tubal function, but involvement of the Fossa by NPC seems necessary for Eustachian tube dysfunction to occur (Su et al., 1993). Tumour may spread outward via the mucosa and submucosa, or along the muscle bundles within the fibro-fatty tissue planes that surround the muscles or along the neuro-vascular planes (Miura et al., 1990).

2.1.1 Middle ear effusion

Middle ear effusion (MEE) is a common otological manifestation of NPC and may be the only presenting symptom of the disease. The resulting conductive hearing loss is usually unilateral and is due to the tumour causing Eustachian tube dysfunction.

Sham et al. (1992) evaluated the relationship between the paranasopharyngeal extension of tumor and the presence of MEE using CT scans (1992). The Eustachian tube traverses the paranasopharyngeal space and the presence of tumor in this region was likely to have an impact on tubal function, either mechanical or functional. The degree of paranasopharyngeal extension of tumor, erosion of petrous temporal bone and the obliteration of pharyngeal recess were found to be significantly related to the development of MEE, but not sex and age. Erosion of the petrous temporal bone was not as strong a risk factor for MEE as paranasopharyngeal involvement. The functional derangement of the cartilaginous part of the Eustachian tube was more important than its bony part in the development of MEE.

Despite numerous studies, uncertainty exists with regards to the exact patho-physiological process culminating in MEE. Although Eustachian tube dysfunction can be caused by inflammation within the lumen and invasion of the tubal orifice, there is mounting evidence pointing towards functional pathology rather than true mechanical obstruction of the tubal lumen (Bluestone 1983; Choa, 1981). More recent studies showed that in patients with NPC-associated MEE; the Eustachian tube was actually patent (Young & Hsieh, 1992). This led to the evolution of various theories to explain the observed functional rather than mechanical obstruction.

2.1.1.1 Muscle infiltration theory

Sadé (1994) argued that MEE in NPC was usually the consequence of faulty middle ear aeration, due to the inability to introduce air through the Eustachian tube. This was because of its muscles being affected and not because of it's opening in the nasopharynx being blocked by a tumor. He observed that in animal studies, MEE could be produced experimentally by damaging the tensor veli palatini muscles in monkeys (Casselbrandt *et al*, 1988 as cited in Sadé 1994). In post-mortem studies, histological examination of the Eustachian tube in patients with NPC revealed that while sometimes the tumour infiltrated the Eustachian tube submucosa and cause obstruction (Cundy *et al.*, 1973 as cited in Sadé 1994); it usually infiltrated the Eustachian tube muscles and did not involve the Eustachian tube opening or its lumen at all (Cundy *et al.*, 1973; Takahara *et al.*, 1986 as cited in Sadé 1994). In various clinical studies, (Honjo, 1988 as cited in Sadé 1994; Sham *et al.*, 1992) demonstrated a direct relationship between the frequency of MEE in NPC and the extent of its infiltration to the parapharyngeal region where the Eustachian tube muscles were probably infiltrated. Myers *et al.*, (1984) also pointed to the presence of MEE in cases of other head or neck tumours such as maxillary sinus carcinoma and its surgery. They showed that in these cases, damage to the Eustachian tube muscles rather than obstruction of the Eustachian opening or lumen led to the effusion.

2.1.1.2 Neurogenic theory

Su et al., (1993) conducted an electromyogenic (EMG) study of the tensor veli palatini (TVP) and levator veli palatini (LVP) muscles in NPC patients. An abnormal TVP wave pattern coincided with a symptomatic ear whereas the non-symptomatic ear had a normal wave pattern. A paralyzed LVP with intact TVP did not result in effusion. NPC invasion generally did not demonstrate a myopathic EMG finding in both muscles. This led to the conclusion that neurogenic paralysis of TVP muscle on the lesion side played an important role in the pathogenesis of functional obstruction of the Eustachian tube leading to MEE. The tough pharyngobasilar fascia not only separated the TVP and LP, but also kept the tensor lateral to it. Anatomically the nerve to TVP was placed in a more vulnerable position and hence, a neurogenic cause of TVP paralysis was more likely (Su et al., 1993; Miura et al 1990).

2.1.1.3 Cartilage erosion theory

Low et al. (1997) found in a MRI study that NPC patients who had associated MEE had a tendency for the Eustachian tube cartilage to be eroded by tumour. Based on these findings and other observations relating to MEE, the authors postulated that the effect of tumour on Eustachian tube cartilage played an important role in the genesis of MEE in NPC.

The authors argued that MEE could not be explained by simple mechanical obstruction of the Eustachian tube alone. The 'hydrops-ex-vacuo' theory of MEE based on the concept that continuous gaseous absorption occurs in a closed biological air pocket until very high negative pressures capable of inducing MEEs develop, had largely been discredited (Grontved ***et al.***, 1990). More recent studies had shown that in an unventilated middle-ear cavity, bidirectional gaseous exchange took place between the middle ear and the circulatory system of the local tissues until an equilibrium was reached, resulting in middle-ear pressures which were only slightly negative or even positive (Hergils and Magnuson, 1990; Sadé and Luntz, 1991). It had been postulated that pressure-regulatory mechanisms in the middle ear, prevent the formation of excessively high negative middle-ear pressure from gaseous absorption through the middle-ear mucosa (Grontved *et al.*, 1990). This had been supported by animal studies where the prevention of middle ear ventilation by ligating the Eustachian tube led to maximum middle-ear pressures of only 116 mm water (Proud *et al.*, 1971). In humans, it had been observed that inadequate middle ear ventilation from organic obstruction by antro-choanal polyps and some other nasopharyngeal tumors seldom led to MEE formation (Sadé, 1994).

However, for many years, the compliance of the Eustachian tube had been thought to be a factor causing MEE in children (Bluestone, 1985). More recently, the MEE's associated with cleft palate and Down's syndrome was believed to be the result of poorly developed Eustachian cartilages with abnormal compliances (Shibahara and Sando, 1989).

It is therefore reasonable to postulate that abnormal compliance of the Eustachian tube could also result from tumor erosion of the cartilaginous part of the tube and this may also play a role in the pathogenesis of NPC-associated MEE. Low et al. (1997) suggested that when tumour has affected the lamina and the hinge portion of the cartilage, it could lead to a change of tubal compliance, resulting in MEE formation.

2.1.2 Ear blockage and negative middle ear pressures

NPC-induced Eustachian tube dysfunction could present as a sensation of ear blockage. Low and Goh (1999) illustrated this with a case study:

A 50-year-old Chinese man presented with the complaint of a sensation of blockage in his left ear lasting for two weeks. He had no preceding upper respiratory tract infection. Examination of the ears was normal. Examination of his nasopharynx with the flexible nasal-endoscope was unremarkable. Epstein-Barr viral serology (as an NPC screen) was positive for both viral capsid and early antigens. Random nasopharyngeal biopsies revealed undifferentiated carcinoma on the left side. Magnetic resonance scan showed a small T 1 submucosal lesion on the left side of the nasopharynx

Ear blockage is the result of negative middle ear pressures (MEPs) without actually developing MEE. Low (1995) carried out a prospective study to investigate MEPs in patients with NPC. Newly diagnosed patients with NPC were studied before and at three to 12 months (mean 7.5 months) after radiotherapy. MEPs were measured by tympanometry. The mean MEP before and after radiotherapy was -55.2 mm water (range -250 to 45 mm water) and -73.1 mm water (range -215 to 35 mm water) respectively. About two-thirds of assessable ears had an increase in negative MEPs after irradiation and the rest had less negative MEPs after irradiation. Those ears that developed post-irradiation middle ear effusions were found to have pre-irradiation negative middle ear pressures of at least -45 mm water. It was concluded that tympanometry before radiotherapy may prove to be useful in identifying ears with a high risk of developing post-irradiation MEE.

2.1.3 Barotrauma

Sub-clinical Eustachian tube dysfunction caused by NPC might present clinically as barotrauma. Low & Goh (1999) illustrated this in a case report of a 40-year-old Chinese female complaining of right earache and blockage after descending from an air-flight. She did not have history of rhinitis prior to nor during the flight. She was diagnosed by her general practitioner to have sustained barotrauma and was treated medically with partial improvement of symptoms. The blockage in her right ear however, deteriorated a month later and was diagnosed by an Otolaryngologist as due to middle-ear effusion. Post-nasal space examination revealed a tumor on the right side, which was histologically proven to be NPC.

2.1.4 Tumor invading the middle ear

NPC may spread and occupy the middle ear space. It has been proposed that the routes of spread of NPC to the middle ear are via the eustachian tube, direct invasion from the parapharyngeal space and spread from the cavernous sinus through the carotid canal and into the middle ear (Low, 2002).

The incidence of middle ear invasion of NPC is probably higher than what has been reported, considering the anatomic communication and close proximity. Diagnosis may not necessarily be straightforward. Low (2002) reported a case where middle ear invasion by nasopharyngeal carcinoma was misdiagnosed as simple post-radiotherapy middle ear effusion for which myringotomy and ventilation tube insertion were performed. In a patient who had been previously irradiated, a recurrent tumour in the ear can be confused with other related conditions such as osteo-radionecrosis (Figure 1).

2.2 Cerebello-pontine angle involvement

In the work-up of a space occupying lesion cerebello-pontine angle (CPA), metastatic NPC is normally not considered. Although it is a rare complication, NPC should be kept in mind in a population where NPC is endemic (Yuh et al., 1993). It was observed in a study that when NPC involved the cerebello-pontine, it occurred in patients with advanced or recurrent disease (Low et al., 2000).

Involvement of the CPA can present a varied clinical picture. NPC manifesting as sensorineural hearing loss is rare (Bergstrom et al., 1977). It can be the result of the tumor affecting the cochlear nerve but it seldom affects the cochlea because of the tough otic capsule (Pringle et al., 1993). Although the resulting hearing loss is usually insidious in nature, it may occasionally present as sudden hearing loss (Low and Goh, 1999; Young, 2001). NPC involving the CPA can also affect the vestibular component of the 8th cranial nerve causing vestibular symptoms. This usually occurs insidiously and results in imbalance rather than true vertigo (Ramsden, 1987). NPC in the CPA can also affect the facial nerve resulting in facial palsy (Low, 2002).

Clinical diagnosis of NPC involvement at the CPA can be difficult. A patient who has received irradiation for NPC in the past may come to the Otologist with sensorineural deafness caused by recurrent NPC in the CPA. The attending physician may miss the diagnosis if he/she simply assumes the deafness to be radiation-induced (Low and Fong, 1998). Similarly, dizziness may be assumed to be the result of metabolic abnormalities and other post irradiation effects (Singh and Slevin 1991). Even facial palsy as the presenting symptom of NPC involvement of the CPA can be misleading because doctors are ever eager to attribute it to Bell's palsy, given that facial palsy as a consequence of NPC is rare (Skinner et al., 1991). The maxim, "All that palsies is not Bell's," is particularly relevant with respect to

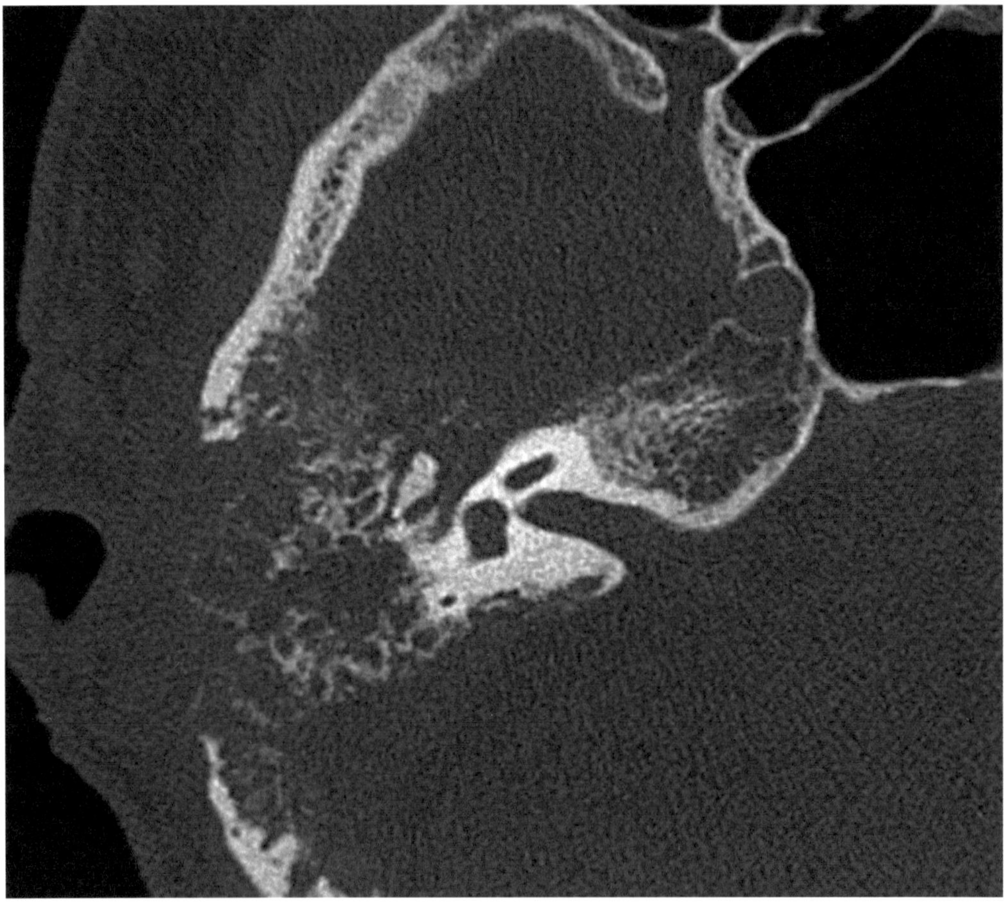

Fig. 1. Axial CT Scan of the right temporal bone ear showing tumor recurrence of the middle ear and mastoid.
This 50 year old Chinese man who had radiotherapy for NPC 2 years ago presented with chronic right ear discharge. Examination of the right ear showed narrowed edematous external ear canal. The eardrum could not be seen from auroscopy. The CT scan showed bony involvement. The list of differential diagnoses included tumour recurrence, osteo-radionecrosis and malignant otitis externa. He underwent surgical exploration and biopsy, which confirmed tumour recurrence. He was treated with palliative chemotherapy.

patients who have previously been treated for advanced NPC. In these patients, recurrent or persistent NPC involving the CPA, temporal bone, or parotid should be excluded (Low 2002). A factor that makes the diagnosis even more elusive is that postnasal space was often free of disease (Gouliamos et al, 1996).

Low et al (2000) reported the following case report, which illustrated the typical features of CPA involvement by NPC. A 53-year-old man was found to have NPC (stage T4N2, UICC 1997) when he experienced left vocal cord palsy (CN 10) and left CN 12 palsy. He was treated with radical radiotherapy. Two years later, he experienced left facial palsy (CN 7), giddiness, and left sensorineural hearing loss (CN 8). The giddiness was described as a sense of imbalance and light-headedness but not vertigo. The postnasal space was clinically free of tumor, and biopsy did not show malignancy. A CT scan showed a deep submucosal recurrent NPC with bony erosion of the left jugular foramen and extending to the left posterior cranial fossa. He was subsequently treated with gamma knife radio-surgery.

There are a few possible mechanisms by which NPC can involve the CPA. Isolated lesions in the CPA that did not have tumor involvement of the skull base can involve the CPA, suggesting spread from the hematogenous route (Gouliamos et al. 1996). Yuh et al. (1993) suggested that metastatic cancers to the CPA could also arise from direct leptomeningeal spread or from dissemination through cerebrospinal fluid. The jugular foramen also offers a route of communication between the region of the para-nasopharynx and the posterior cranial fossa (Low et al 2000). Goh and Lim et al. (2009) suggested it could be as a result of perineural tumor spread.

According to Low et al. (2000), CPA manifestations of NPC can be as a result of inadequacies of standard radiotherapy techniques in the treatment of advanced NPC. The design of radiotherapy fields is based on the principle of maximal dose delivery to tumor-bearing tissues and maximal sparing of normal structures. A normal tissue or organ is considered to be "dose limiting" if its tolerance to radiation is so poor that it affects the maximum dose deliverable to the adjacent tumor-bearing tissues. Such structures around the postnasal space include the contents of the orbits, the optic nerves and chiasm, the hypothalamic-pituitary axis, the inner ear, the spinal cord, the temporal lobes of the brain, and the brainstem. Encephalomyelopathy is a feared complication in NPC treatment. To minimize the dose to the brainstem, standard radiotherapy techniques to the postnasal space mandate a brainstem shield. Thus, even microscopic disease in this area is under-treated. Geographic under treatment of an initially advanced cancer may result in a patient's returning for treatment at a later stage with clinical manifestations of tumor involving the CPA. Low et al (2000) concluded that this might represent progression of persistent tumor than a true relapse.

Treatment of NPC in the CPA is clinically challenging because when the standard radiotherapy techniques for NPC are applied to this region, the brainstem is at great risk. Gross disease extension into the CPA evident on CT scan is probably not radio-curable for this reason. In our center, such patients would be treated with initial chemotherapy in the hope that the tumor would shrink sufficiently to be encompassed by standard radiotherapy fields. Unfortunately, as illustrated by Low et al. (2000), NPC in the CPA may not respond well to chemotherapy.

Where a tumor is localized in the CPA, focal means of delivering radiotherapy in the form of radiosurgery as delivered by the gamma knife or fractionated stereotactic Linac radiotherapy, may be considered. Such focal means of delivering radiotherapy have the advantage of depositing a high dose to a well-defined volume of tumor-bearing tissues, with rapid dose fall off to the surrounding structures. The disadvantage is that there is a 4-cm upper limit in diameter of tumor size beyond which the dose-sparing feature of this modality is rapidly lost. Where the tumor is larger than is feasible for stereotactic radiotherapy, a standard wedge pair technique may be feasible. The caveat, which cannot be overemphasized, is that the larger the tumor volume, the higher the likelihood of incurring critical damage to surrounding structures (Low et. al., 2000)

2.3 Referred otalgia

Referred otalgia is pain felt in the ear but originating from a non-otologic source. Ear pain is a diagnostic dilemma when otoscopy reveals normal external ear and tympanic membrane. As the ear is innervated by sensory contributions of the the 5th, 7th, 9th and 10th cranial nerves as well as spinal nerves C2 and C3, lesions arising from areas supplied by these nerves may result in pain referred to the ear.

Theoretically, NPC can present as referred otalgia by involving the 9th cranial nerve. We concur with the observation by van Hasselt & Gibb (1991) that otalgia is less common than one might expect. We agree with the view that the most common description of pain is not "sharp" but "aching, dull or pressing" (Epstein and Jones, 1993). This is illustrated by a case report by Low & Goh (1999):

A 48 year old man complained of a sensation of fullness in the left peri-auricular region, just antero-inferior to the tragus lasting for a month. Examination by manual palpation failed to reveal any mass in the region. CT scan of the parotid was normal. Nasal-endoscopy however, revealed a discrete mass in the left side of the post-nasal space. Biopsy of this nasopharyngeal mass showed undifferentiated nasopharyngeal carcinoma. His symptom resolved after radiation therapy.

2.4 Tinnitus

It is common for patients to consult the Otologist for the complaint of tinnitus in the absence of other ear symptoms or signs. If unilateral, the Otologist often considers the possibility of an early acoustic neuroma and investigates as such. It is however, highly unlikely that NPC presents as tinnitus as an isolated symptom in the absence of other features relating to the ear, a view shared by van Hasselt & Gibb (1991). If present, it is normally a result of Eustachian tube, middle ear or auditory nerve involvement with the resulting associated aural manifestations as well.

2.5 Peri-auricular mass

Although NPC metastasizing to the parotid is rare with only 14 cases reported in the literature (Wanamaker et al., 1994), this possibility should be considered in high-risk patients presenting with parotid masses. Batsakis and Bautina (1990) cautioned that some cases of 'primary undifferentiated carcinoma of nasopharyngeal type' in the major salivary glands might in fact be metastatic nasopharyngeal carcinoma. Low (2002) reported a case of metastatic NPC to the parotid and presenting with facial palsy as follows.

A 50-year-old man was treated for nasopharyngeal carcinoma overseas. Two years later, he exhibited complete left lower motor neuron facial nerve palsy. Examination revealed a hard mass in the left parotid over the region of the facial trunk in addition to multiple swollen cervical nodes (figure 3). The postnasal space was clinically free of tumor, and the appearance of the ears was unremarkable. Chest x-ray showed multiple metastases. Analysis of a fine-needle aspiration sample of the parotid mass identified an undifferentiated carcinoma consistent with metastatic nasopharyngeal carcinoma. The patient refused further treatment and died 3 months later.

Parotid metastasis is most commonly due to lymphatic spread (Wanamaker et al., 1994). The parotid is made up of a rich network of lymphatic vessels and interconnecting intra-glandular and peri-glandular lymph nodes. NPC can affect the retropharyngeal lymph nodes, which can drain into the parotid nodes. From the parotid nodes, the tumor has access to the lymphatic plexus, parotid parenchyma, facial nerve, and even the parapharyngeal space (Batsakis & Bautina 1990).

3. Otologic complications arising from treatment of NPC

As NPC is highly radiosensitive, radiation treatment stands as the primary modality of management. The aim of treatment is eradication of tumor through targeted delivery of radiation to the tumor bed, at tolerable doses to minimize acute and late complications. It is a challenge to balance cure on one hand, and prevention of complications from treatment on the other. The focus in this section is to highlight the impact of treatment of NPC on ear structures.

3.1 Radiation therapy

Megavoltage external beam radiotherapy is the primary treatment of choice. There are two lateral opposing and one anterior field beams. This is meant to cover the sides of the neck and entire nasopharynx. Radiotherapy is given prophylactically to the neck assuming there is occult disease.

A typical convention technique used by us involves patients treated with six megavolt (6MV) X-rays from linear accelerators. Chemotherapy was not part of the protocol for any patient. The primary volume covered the nasopharynx including the Eustachian tube, adjacent parapharynx to the level of the inferior border of C2, and posterior third to half of the nasal cavity and maxillary antra (Figures 2 and 3). As shown, the brainstem was shielded throughout on the lateral fields and the inner ear would be at the edge of this shield. A total dose of 66 - 70 Gys in 2 Gy daily increments was prescribed. The neck received 60 Gy electively, with palpable nodes boosted to 70 Gy.

3.1.1 Post-irradiation otitis media

3.1.1.1 Middle ear effusion

MEE is a common finding among patients who have been irradiated for NPC patients and is generally attributed to Eustachian tube dysfunction. Post-irradiated ultra-structural findings of the Eustachian tubal mucosa showed ciliary loss, intercellular and intracellular vacuolation and ciliary dysmorphism (Lou et al., 1999). Most of these pathologic findings were observed to be persistent and did not resolve with time suggesting that radiation had caused long-term damage to the Eustachian tube epithelium. The Eustachian tube could grossly manifest in differing ways ranging from patulous Eustachian tube, adhesion, incomplete and complete obstruction (Zhou et al., 2003).

MEE could be present in the early post-radiotherapy period and some persist in the long-term. Low & Fong (1998) studied the factors, which could possibly influence the development of long-term middle ear effusion in patients irradiated for NPC. Thirty-five patients (70 ears) were studied for 2-8 years (mean 5.5 years) post-radiotherapy. The factors studied were (a) sex (b) age (c) tumour size and (d) presence of pre-radiotherapy MEE. Only

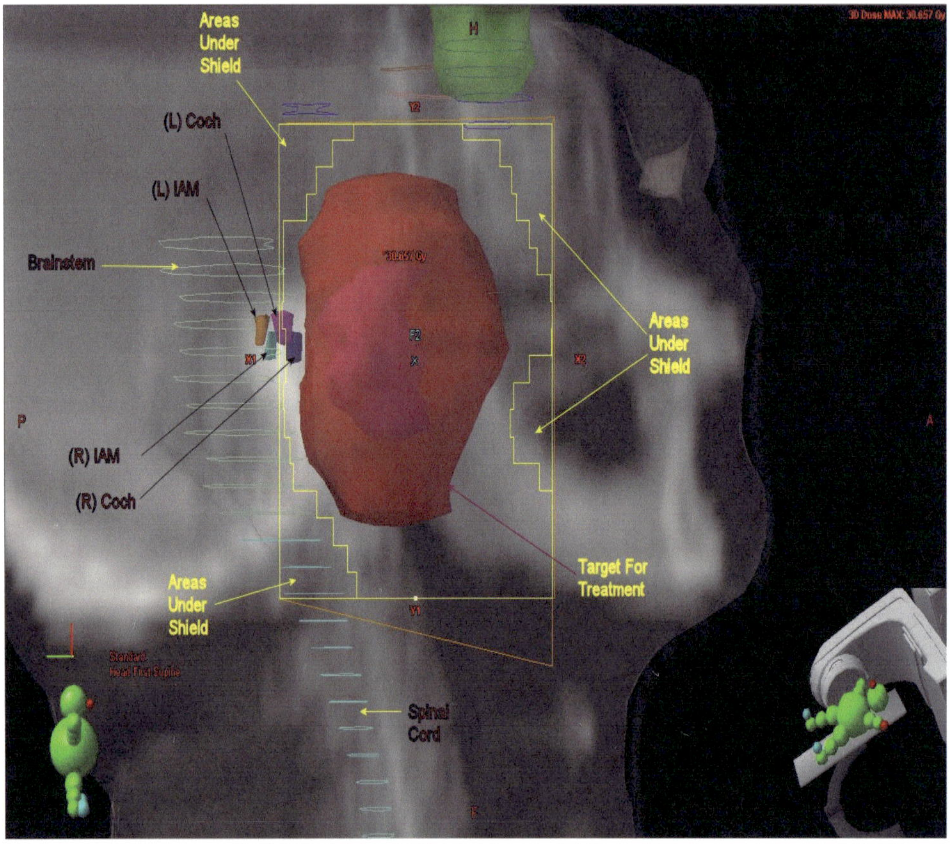

Fig. 2. Beam's Eye View (BEV) of lateral post-nasal space field.
The field (yellow box) is superimposed on a digitally reconstructed radiograph (DRR) by the planning computer. The solid red area represents the target volume where a uniform high dose is deposited. Critical structures are shielded to reduce exposure. These structures include the brain stem and spinal cord, optic chiasma (blue), and the inner ear as much as is feasible.

the presence of pre-radiotherapy MEE was found to be statistically significant (P = 0.004, Fisher's exact test). Stepwise multiple regression analysis showed the presence of pre-radiotherapy MEE was a predictor of post-radiotherapy MEE with an odds ratio of 0.67. Hence, an ear with pre-irradiation MEE was almost seven times more likely to have long-term post-irradiation MEE than an ear without pre-irradiation MEE. It was postulated that irreversible Eustachian tube dysfunction occurred only when the tube that had been damaged by tumour was further damaged by irradiation. It may well be that tumour and irradiation had induced change in the compliance of the Eustachian tube resulting in the development of long-term post-radiotherapy MEE.

As the mechanism of post-radiotherapy MEE is likely to be different from MEE commonly found in children, its principles of management are also different. Unlike in children, the use of ventilation tubes has the tendency to result in chronic infection, which was are often persistent and troublesome. They also tend to be associated with persistent perforations.

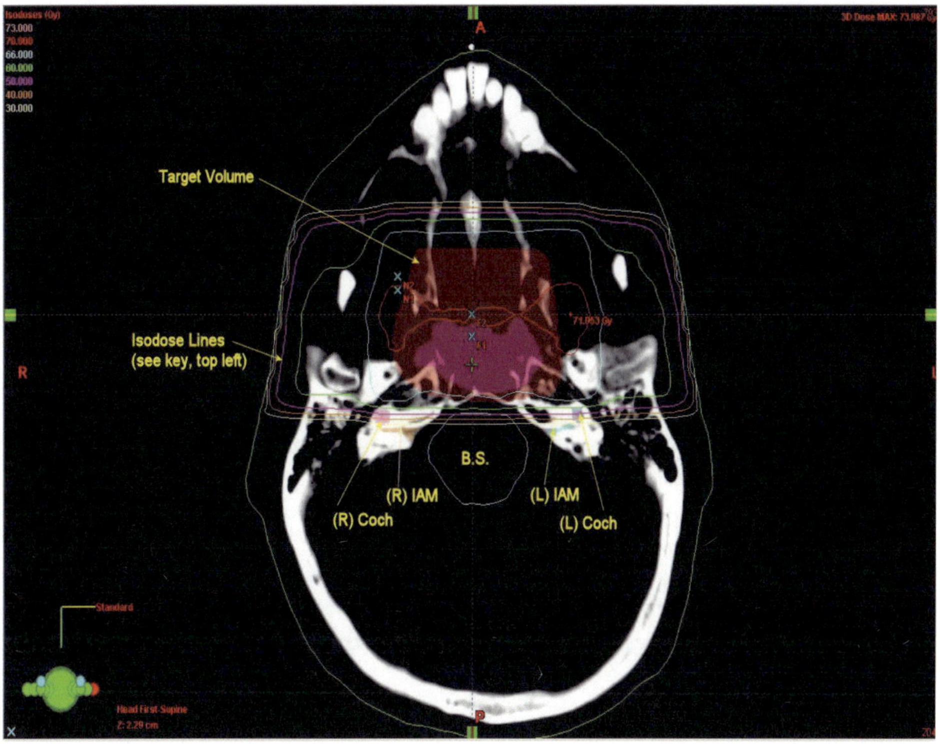

Fig. 3. Axial CT scan of the nasopharynx showing a computer generated isodose plan. This shows the distribution of radiation dose as determined by the specific beam arrangement. The dose to the target volume and various structures of interest can be assessed.

Therefore, hearing loss resulting from post-radiotherapy MEE should preferably be addressed by amplification with hearing aids rather than drainage with ventilation tubes (Skinner & van Hasselt, 1991).

3.1.1.2 Chronic suppurative otitis media

Chronic Suppurative Otitis Media (CSOM) was found in 24.5% of NPC patients who developed otological complications after radiotherapy (Yuen and Wei, 1994). Perforation of the eardrum may occur after ventilation tube insertion for MEE or spontaneously as a result of radiotherapy-induced spontaneous Eustachian tube dysfunction (Wei et al, 1988).

Some Otologists in managing CSOM in post-irradiated NPC patients prefer a conservative approach, presumably because of the belief that impaired healing is more likely in irradiated tissues and radiation-induced Eustachian tube dysfunction may lead to lesser chance of successful repair. Yuen and Wei (1994) however, recommended tympanomastoidectomy for NPC patients with active CSOM who fail to respond to conservative treatment, citing a nearly 70% chance of success after surgery.

3.1.2 Post-irradiation sensorineural hearing loss

Radiotherapy of head and neck cancers including NPC is well known to result in sensorineural hearing loss (SNHL), when the ear structures are included in the radiation fields. The reported post-radiation therapy hearing loss rates based on audiometric evaluation varied between 0% and 54% (Ho et al., 1999; Kwong et al., 1996; Raajmakers et al., 2002). This is attributed to radiation-induced damage to the sensorineural auditory pathways.

It is important to know whether the auditory nerve, the central nervous pathways or both, are damaged by radiotherapy. This is important in the context of treating profound hearing loss in post-irradiated ears using the cochlear implant. The cochlear implant works by stimulating the auditory nerve fibres directly, without the need for functioning cochlear hair cells. Its success therefore, depends largely on a functional auditory nerve and its central nervous pathways.

If the auditory nerve and central nervous structures are indeed spared and that damage occurs primarily in the cochlea, it will then be useful to understand the cellular and molecular processes involved in radiation-induced cochlear hair-cell damage. This is because it has relevance in preventive measures where medications are used to target the cellular and molecular pathways involved.

3.1.2.1 Pathogenesis

It was demonstrated in chinchillas that cochlear nerve fiber degeneration occurred after exposure to high radiation doses. In ears exposed to 40 to 50Gy and 60 to 90Gy of radiation, the incidence rates were 31% and 62% respectively, (Bohne et al., 1985) confirming that radiation induced damage is dose dependent.

To find out if radiation damages retro-cochlear auditory pathways, we prospectively studied newly diagnosed NPC patients treated by radiotherapy alone (Low et al., 2005). Audiograms including evoked response audiometry which could assess the integrity of retro-cochlear auditory pathways, were carried out prior to and after radiotherapy (at 3, 18 and 48 months). There was no statistically significant difference in inter-waves latencies recorded before and after RT ($p > 0.05$, Wilcoxon Signed Ranks Test), suggesting that the retro-cochlear auditory pathways were functionally intact. Analysis of dose-volume histograms confirmed that the cochlea and internal auditory meatus received significant doses of radiation, ranging from 24.1-62.2 and 14.4 - 43.4 Gy respectively.

It is believed that etiologies of SNHL such as ageing and drug toxicity, share similar cell death mechanisms leading to a final common apoptotic pathway (Atar et al., 2005). Radiation-induced apoptosis has been well demonstrated in non-cochlear cell systems and is generally accepted as an important mechanism of radiation-induced cell death in vivo (Shinomiya 2001; Verheij & Bartelink 2000) Therefore, by relating our findings to what is already known, it is not unreasonable to expect radiation-induced apoptosis occurring in cochlear hair-cells in vivo.

It is well accepted that radiation-induced SNHL is progressive in nature. The integrity of normal tissues or organs depends on the maintenance of a certain number of normally functioning mature cells. When the depletion of functioning cells reaches a critical level, a clinically detectable effect becomes apparent (Awwad 1990). In the case of radiation-induced SNHL the cochlea consists of a finite number of post-mitotic non-regenerating hair cells. A patient may experience hearing loss when a critical mass of hair cells is lost and it may take several months or years after radiation exposure before this stage is reached. Radiation-induced SNHL has been described to have either early or late-onset. Early-onset

SNHL occur within hours or days after completion of RT, whereas late-onset radiation-induced SNHL may manifest months or years after exposure. Hence, "late"-onset radiation-induced SNHL may possibly represent the later stages of the progression in hair cell degeneration initiated by direct cellular injury during irradiation. Alternatively, the initial radiation-induced injury could have rendered the cells more susceptible to apoptosis following subsequent exposure to insults such as noise and ototoxic medications (Low et al., 2009).

There has been compelling evidence in animal models, implicating reactive oxygen species (ROS) in the damage associated with non-radiation causes such as cochlear ischemia, noise trauma, presbycusis, meningitis-associated hearing loss and aminoglycoside and cisplatin ototoxicity (Seidman and Vivek, 2004).

In radiation-induced apoptosis in the OC-k3 inner ear cell line, Low et al., (2006a), demonstrated dose-dependant intracellular generation of ROS at 1 hour post-irradiation and was believed to be an important triggering factor in the apoptotic process. ROS could explain the observation that high frequency hearing is preferentially damaged by radiation (Rybak & Whitworth 2005). In an animal study on aminoglycoside ototoxicity, outer hair-cell death in the Organ of Corti was observed to follow a base-to-apex gradient, which was eliminated by the addition of antioxidants (Sha et al., 2001). This was attributed to the outer hair cells in the basal coil (respond to higher frequency sounds) having much lower levels of glutathione than those in the apical region (respond to lower frequency sounds) and therefore, a lower antioxidant capacity (Rybak & Whitworth 2005).

In the OC-k3 inner ear cell line, Low et al., (2006a) found up- regulation of p53 related genes from micro-array studies. Western blotting confirmed up-regulation of p53 at 72 hours and phosphorylation at 3, 24, 48 and 72 hours after irradiation. It is well known that p53 can induce apoptosis.

Nevertheless, a number of different mechanisms leading to cell deaths may also be involved in radiation-induced ototoxicity. These include necrotic cell death, p53-independent mechanisms and caspase-independent programmed cell death. Multiple cellular organelles may trigger several pathways that may act independently or in concert (Leist & Jaattela 2003).

3.2 Prevention

For NPC and other tumours that are treated mainly by radiation, improved radiotherapy techniques such as intensity modulated RT help to reduce unnecessary radiation exposure to the ear. This may be facilitated by early detection when the tumours are still small and situated away from ear structures.

Accurate delineation of the middle and inner ear is a prerequisite to achieve dose constraint to those structures. The size and proximity of the middle and inner ear to the tumor, renders it susceptible to damage. As deviation during contouring can have a profound impact on post treatment sequelae (Wang et al., 2011), Pacholke et al. (2005) established guidelines for contouring the middle ear and the two major components of the inner ear. These guidelines have been of practical help to radiation oncologists.

Improving tumor control rate is the aim, but another important goal is to reduce radiation-induced complications and to improve the quality of life of survivors. The application of 3D conformal radiation therapy (3D-CRT) and intensity-modulated radiation therapy (IMRT) signified a major improvement over conventional 2D radiation therapy. A randomized controlled clinical study showed that at 12 months post-radiation therapy, quality of life scores were significantly higher in the IMRT group than the conventional radiation therapy group for patients with NPC (86.5 versus 58.3; $P < 0.001$) (Pow et al., 2006). The incidence of chronic otitis media and abnormal vestibular evoked myogenic potentials in NPC patients treated by IMRT were significantly lower when compared with those treated by 2DRT, demonstrating the superiority of IMRT in decreasing unwanted otologic complications. However, occurrence of MEE, which was related with advanced T stage, cannot be reduced by IMRT (Hsin et al., 2010).

Clinically effective preventive measures can potentially be applied based on the above proposed ROS-linked p-53 dependent apoptotic model of radiation-induced ototoxicity. It also provides a basis for the use of anti-oxidants and anti-apoptotic factors in its prevention. Antioxidants look promising as effective agents to prevent radiation-induced ototoxicity; they target upstream processes leading to different cell death mechanisms that may co-exist in the population of damaged cells (Low et al., 2009). An anti-oxidant, L-N-Acetylcysteine (L-NAC), was demonstrated in the same cell line to have a protective effect (Low et al., 2008). With its track record of safety in humans and efficacy as an anti-oxidant, L-NAC appears promising as an agent to prevent radiation-induced SNHL in the near future. High doses can potentially be delivered trans-tympanically into the middle ear with minimal systematic side effects, and entry to the inner ear is facilitated by its low molecular weight.

3.3 Treatment

Efforts to regenerate hair cells represent a large and important field of research and appear promising in animal studies. However, integrating transplanted stem cells into damaged epithelium and generating the correct number of cells in the correct parts of the Organ of Corti will be a challenge. Given that much of cochlear function depends on the precise mechanical properties of the Organ of Corti, excess or inappropriately placed cells are likely to cause problems. Moreover, the possible effects of radiation on the supporting and vascular structures of the Organ of Corti, may also complicate regenerative efforts.

For now, the best therapeutic strategy would be effective rehabilitation of SNHL after RT.

3.3.1 Cochlear implantation

In patients with profound SNHL, cochlear implants may be effective if the retro-cochlear auditory pathways remained intact. To substantiate that the retro-cochlear auditory pathways remained intact after RT (Low et al., 2005), a case-control study of cochlear implant recipients who had prior irradiation for NPC was conducted in our clinic (Low et al 2006b). They received their RT 11-28 years prior to cochlear implantation and the post-implant follow-up period ranged from 9 to 46 months. The implanted ear of each patient had favourable pre-operative promontory stimulation results. Post-implant, all patients were satisfied with their hearing outcomes and the improvement in speech discrimination scores was comparable to the controls.

There are specific issues related to cochlear implantation in post-irradiated ears that one should consider:

3.3.1.1 Surgery

Adhesions in middle ear could complicate surgery, including posing difficulties during identification of the round window niche. Post radiation obliteration of the cochlea lumen is possible, which could compromise smooth insertion of electrode array during implantation (Formanek et al., 1998).

In cochlear implantation of patients who had been irradiated for NPC, two aspects ought to be highlighted. Firstly, these patients not infrequently have perforated eardrums and middle ear infections, with the Eustachian tube openings in the nasopharynx completely obliterated. For these patients, conventional techniques of cochlear implantation do not apply and modified techniques such as subtotal petrosectomy, fat obliteration and blind sac closure become necessary. Secondly, NPC has a racial predilection and is common in the Chinese. Racial differences in mastoid morphology exist and such differences had even been used in race identification during forensic and anthropology investigations. Indeed, a study of Chinese temporal bones had revealed differences in the course of the facial nerve in the mastoid and in the origin of the chorda tympani, as compared to those described in Western textbooks (Low, 1999). Knowledge of such racial anatomical variations may reduce the risk of facial nerve injury during mastoid surgery, especially in irradiated ears where the bone is usually more friable than normal.

3.3.1.2 Surveillance imaging

A part of the internal component of the cochlear implant is a small magnet, which is required to secure the external component to the skin of the patient. In an NPC patient who had been treated previously, magnetic resonance imaging is sometimes required to exclude the possibility of tumor recurrence. Should magnetic resonance imaging be indicated in a patient who is already a cochlear implant recipient, there may be a need to remove the magnet from the internal device before the scan.

3.3.1.3 Re-irradiation

In recurrent tumors, further radiotherapy may be indicated. Fortunately, the internal device had been shown to be resistant to damage by radiation (Ralston et al., 1999). However, cumulative radiation doses from further radiotherapy could inflict severe damage to the auditory nerve, which could compromise the post-implant hearing outcome.

3.3.2 Bone-anchored hearing aids

Conventional hearing aids may effectively address conductive hearing loss resulting from MEE. However, they may aggravate otorrhea, and ear moulds traumatize osteoradionecrosis ulcers in the ear canal. An alternative for patients is the bone-anchored hearing aids (BAHA). BAHA has been shown to have successful osseointegration in post-irradiated NPC patients (Soo et al., 2009). Improved subjective hearing clarity, reduced ear discharge rates, and extended BAHA usage times accounted for high patient satisfaction with the BAHA hearing system. Soo et al (2009) therefore, recommended the BAHA hearing system for the treatment of chronic suppurative otitis media-related hearing problems in NPC patients.

3.3.3 Active middle ear implants

Compared to conventional hearing aids, active middle ear implants such as the Vibrant Soundbridge provide more mechanical energy into the inner ear. However, they still rely on viable cochlear hair cells in order to convert mechanical energy into electrical energy for onward transmission through the auditory nerve to the brain. In radiation-induced SNHL, there may be progressive cochlear hair cell loss. Patients with post-radiotherapy SNHL affecting only the higher frequencies may initially be suitable for middle ear implants. However, it's use should be cautioned as the natural progressive nature of radiation-induced SNHL might affect the effectiveness of these devices in the longer term.

3.3.4 Chemo-radiation and their combined ototoxic effects

Combined chemo-radiotherapy is increasingly being used clinically to treat advanced head and neck cancers. In radiotherapy of tumours in the head and neck region, the auditory pathways are often included in the radiation fields and radiation-induced SNHL may result. Cisplatin (CDDP), widely used as an effective anti-neoplastic drug for these cancers, is also well known to cause ototoxicity. Therefore, in combined therapy, the synergistic ototoxic effects of CDDP and radiation could theoretically be catastrophic for the patient and is a clinical issue that deserves more attention.

Skinner et al. (1990) remarked that previous or concurrent use of other ototoxic agents with CDDP, may increase toxicity by more than simple algebric summation. Indeed, there have been a number of reports that described enhanced radiatiation-induced ototoxicity when used with CDDP. In a study by Schnell et al (1989) it was found that children and young adults treated with CDDP suffered an additional 20-30dB SNHL if they had received prior cranial RT. In a study on children and adolescents who had received CDDP for the treatment of solid tumours, Skinner et al. (1990) reported more severe CDDP ototoxicity in patients who had previously received RT encompassing the ear. Similarly, Merchant et at (2004) observed enhanced ototoxicity in a study on children with brain tumours who were treated by pre-RT ototoxic chemotherapy. Miettinen et al (1997) also found that radiotherapy enhanced the ototoxicity of CDDP in the higher speech frequencies. The results of these studies were consistent with those from case reports, which supported the idea that RT should be considered cautiously in children treated with CDDP for intracranial malignancies (Sweetow & Will, 1993; Walker et al, 1989)

We conducted a single blinded randomized trial to investigate the true differences in extent, onset and clinical course of SNHL between newly diagnosed nasopharyngeal carcinoma (NPC) patients treated by RT alone and by combined chemo-RT (Low et al 2006c). Bone conduction thresholds were performed before treatment and at 1 week, 6 months, 1 year and 2 years after completion of RT. Statistical analysis was performed using the Mann-Whitney test. Hearing thresholds averaged over 0.5, 1 and 2kHz were found to be poorer in the chemo-RT group (116 ears) compared to the radiotherapy group (114 ears), at 1 year ($p=0.001$) and 2 years ($p=0.03$) post-treatment. Hearing thresholds at 4kHz were significantly worse for patients in the chemo-RT arm at all the post-treatment time points studied and were more severely affected than those at lower frequencies.

3.4 Osteo-radionecrosis

Osteo-radionecrosis (ORN) is an uncommon complication of radiation treatment. In post-irradiated NPC patients, it may occur in the temporal bone and presents as chronic or recurrent ear discharge. To the unwary Clinician, this can potentially be misdiagnosed as the symptoms of chronic suppurative otitis media and otitis externa, both of which are common in post-irradiated NPC patients.

Radiation may result in hypoxia, hypovascularity and hypocellularity of canal skin. These impair normal collagen synthesis and cell production and lead to tissue breakdown and eventual ORN (Hao et al., 2007). Obliterative vasculitis also causes a direct radiation-induced avascular necrosis of the bone (Schuknecht & Karmody, 1966). This is more likely to occur in the presence of tumor involvement (Lederman, 1965). There is a positive relationship between the size of the radiation dose and the degree of necrosis (Thornley et al., 1979).

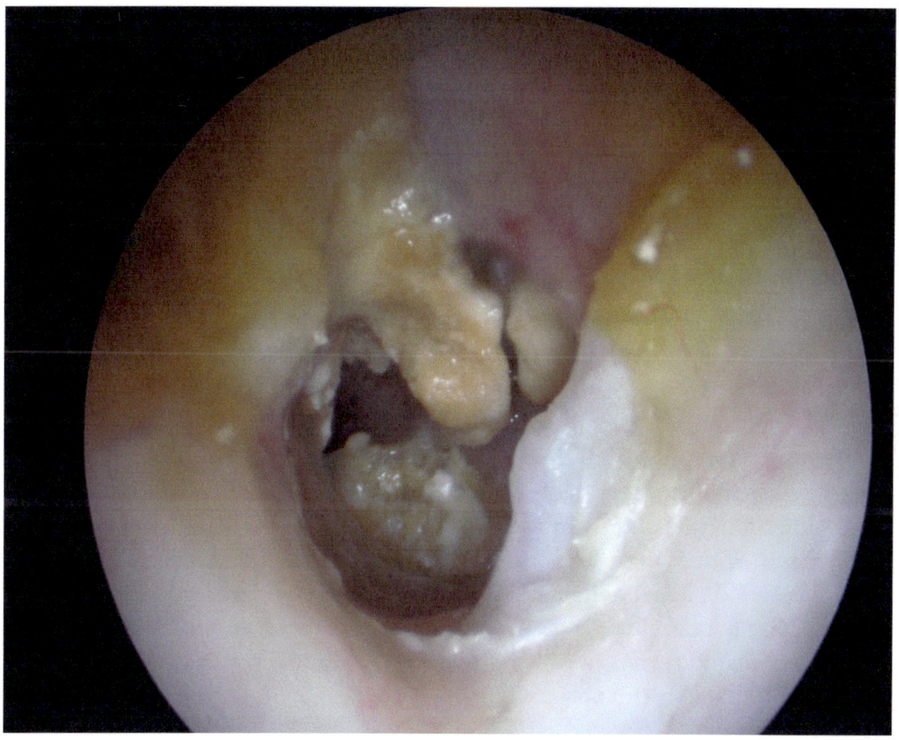

Fig. 4. Endoscopic view of the left external and middle ear showing osteo-radionecrosis. This 60 year old woman had radiotherapy for NPC 15 years ago and had remained disease free since. She presented with chronic left ear discharge 12 years after radiotherapy. Examination showed necrotic in the external ear canal and middle ear. CT scan showed that the bony lesions did not involve the rest of the temporal bone. She was closely followed up with regular aural toilet and topical antibiotics. She was not keen for other treatment options like hyperbaric oxygen and sequestrectomy.

Ramsden et al (1975) classified osteoradionecrosis of the temporal bone as either localized or diffuse. In localized osteoradionecrosis, the disease is generally confined to the external auditory canal, and symptoms manifest according to the site and stage of the disease. In diffuse osteoradionecrosis it extends beyond the temporal bone to the base of the skull and its surrounding structures. The affected patients presented with more severe symptoms of profuse and pulsatile otorrhea and significant pain. The diffuse form is associated with a greater likelihood of complications, including trismus, intracranial infection, facial nerve palsy, labyrinthitis, chronic mastoiditis, CSF leak, and internal carotid artery aneurysm. (John et al., 1993)

The type that is more commonly seen is the localized type where the ORN is heralded by unhealed ulcer, foul discharge, exposed bone and accompanying granuloma. It is typically seen in the lower external canal skin, an area predisposed to downward pressure-induced trauma from wearing hearing aids or iatrogenically traumatized during aural toileting or ear-picking. Sometimes, it involves the middle ear (Figure 4). As suggested by Hao et al, treatment ranges from thorough aural toilet, otic drops, hyperbaric oxygen (Rudge 1993) that reverses the ill effects of radiation induced skin changes, and finally sequestrectomy. Most important though rare, high degree of suspicion and awareness is the key in detection and early management of this condition before serious complication ensues. Lim et al (2005) reported an interesting case of a 44-year-old Chinese man with a history of nasopharyngeal carcinoma that was treated with radiotherapy presented with fluid in the middle ear. A myringotomy was performed and subsequently a diagnosis of cerebrospinal fluid leakage secondary to osteoradionecrosis of the temporal bone was made.

3.5 Radiation-associated tumors

Radiation-associated tumours (RATS) are rare complications of radiotherapy. Goh et al (1999) studied RATs in the temporal bones of patients who were previously irradiated for cancers of the nasopharynx. Of the 7 patients studied, 5 had squamous cell carcinomas, 1 osteogenic sarcoma and 1 chondrosarcoma. This distribution of the type of cancer is interesting as radiation-induced cancers are more associated with sarcoma than with squamous cell carcinoma. A possible reason for this observation may be related to the chronic ear infections that are commonly present in post-irradiated ears. The combined long-term effects of radiation and chronic infections may well predispose the ear to squamous cell carcinoma. In another study of patients with malignant tumors of the external auditory canal and temporal bone, the 1-year cumulative recurrence for the RAT group was 100%, but there was no recurrence in the non-RAT group ($P = 0.001$) suggesting a poorer prognosis in RATS patients (Lim et al 2000)

Delayed diagnosis is not uncommon in this condition. Almost two thirds of the patients in the series reported by Lim et al. (2000) had T3 disease at the time of presentation. One reason could be that otorrhea, the most common presentation, was often mistaken to be due to chronic otitis externa.

Another reason for misdiagnosis is difficulty in getting histological confirmation in the Clinic. Lim et al (2000) gave the example of a patient with an initial diagnosis of pseudoepitheliomatous hyperplasia. This was based on superficial small punch biopsy specimens obtained under local anesthesia. It was only upon larger and deeper specimens obtained under general anesthesia from the mastoid that revealed the true diagnosis.

RATs may be uncommon, but with refinement in radiotherapy techniques and the resultant increase in patient survival, there may be more patients with radiation-associated tumours in the future. It remains imperative for clinicians to be vigilant when patients previously irradiated for NPC present with otological symptoms as the key to the successful management of this condition lies in the early detection and expedient treatment of this difficult disease.

4. Conclusion

Because of the close relation between the nasopharynx and ear structures, NPC frequently has Otological manifestations. Attending Physicians must be mindful of these manifestations as they may aid early diagnosis with consequently better treatment outcomes.

Treatment of NPC with radiotherapy or chemo-radiation also has great impact on the practice of Otology. Improved RT techniques have reduced unnecessary radiation exposure to ear structures, with lesser chances of developing ear complications. Nevertheless, it is inevitable in many instances. With greater emphasis in the use of chemo-RT in advanced head and neck cancers, chemo-radiation-induced SNHL has also assumed greater significance. Although recent technology such as cochlear implants have been highly successful in rehabilitating profound hearing loss, prevention is still the best practice in the management of radiation-induced SNHL. A proposed ROS-dependent apoptotic model of hair-cell damage offers the prospect of prevention at a molecular level in the near future.

5. Acknowledgement

We thank Dr Fong Kam Weng, Senior Consultant of the Therapeutic Radiology Department, Singapore National Cancer Centre, for the illustrations

6. References

Atar O, Avraham KB. Therapeutics of hearing loss: expectations vs reality. Drug Discov Today; 2005 Oct 1;10 (19):1323-30.

Awwad HK. Late reacting tissues: radiation damage to central nervous system. Radiation Oncology: The Netherlands: 1990 Nov; Kluger Academic Publishers.

Batsakis JG, Bautina E. Metastases to major salivary glands. Ann Otol Rhinol Laryngol. 1990 Jun; 99:501-03.

Bergstrom L, Baker, BB, Sando I. Sudden deafness and facial palsy from metastatic bronchogenic carcinoma. J Laryngol Otol. 1977 Sep; 91: 787-89.

Bluestone CD. Current concepts in Eustachian tube function as related to otitis media. Auris-Nasus-Larynx (Tokyo) 1985; 12 (Suppl 1): 1-4.

Bluestone CD.Eustachian tube function: physiology, pathophysiology, and role of allergy in pathogenesis of otitis media. J allergy Clin. Immunol. 1983 Sep; 72:242-51.

Bohne BA, Marks JE, Glasgow GP. Delayed effects of ionizing radiation on the ear. Laryngoscope 1985 Jul; 95:818-28.

Casselbrandt ML, Cantekin EI, Dirkmat Dc, Doyle WJ, Bluestone CD. Experimental paralysis of tensor veli palatini muscle, Acta Otolaryngologica (Stolkholm) 1988 Sep-Oct; 106:178-85

Choa GB, Nasopharyngeal carcinoma. In: Otolaryngology, Vol. 5 ed. G.M. Philadelphia: Harper & Row,1981; 1-35.

Cundy LR, Sando I, Hemingway WG. Middle ear extension of nasopharyngeal carcinoma via eustachian tube. Arch Otolaryngol. 1973 Aug; 98: 131-33.

Epstein JB, Jones CK. Presenting signs and symptoms of nasopharyngeal carcinoma. Oral Surg Oral Med Oral Pathol. 1993 Jan; 75(1):32-36.

Formanek M, Czerny C, Gstoettner W, Kornfehl J. Cochlear implantation as a successful rehabilitation for radiation-induced deafness. Eur Arch Otorhinolaryngol. 1998; 255:175–78.

Goh J, Lim K. Imaging of nasopharyngeal carcinoma. Ann Acad Med Singapore. 2009 Sep; 38(9):809-16.

Goh YH, Chong VF, Low WK. Temporal bone tumours in patients irradiated for nasopharyngeal neoplasm. J Laryngol Otol. 1999 Mar; 113(3):222-28.

Gouliamos AD, Athanassopoulou A, Moulopoulou L, et al. MRI nasopharyngeal carcinoma to the cerebellopontine angle. Neuroradiol. 1996 May; 38:375–77.

Grontved A, Moller A, Jorgenson L. Studies on gas tension in the normal middle ear. Acta Otolaryngologica (Stockholm)1990 Mar; 109:271-77.

Hao SP, Tsang NM, Chang KP, Chen CK, Chao WC. Osteoradionecrosis of external auditory canal in nasopharyngeal carcinoma. Chang Gung Med J. 2007 Mar-Apr; 30(2): 116-21.

Hao SP, Chen HC, Wei FC, Chen CY, Yeh AR, Su JL. Systematic management of osteoradionecrosis in the headand neck. Laryngoscope; 1999 Aug; 109:1324-27.

Hergils L, Magnuson B. Human ear gas composition studied by mass spectrometry. Acta Otolaryngologica (Stockholm) 1990 Jul-Aug; 110:92-99.

Ho, WK, Wei WI, Kwong DL, Sham JS, Tai PT, Yuen AP, Au DK. Long-term sensorineural hearing deficit following radiotherapy in patients suffering from nasopharyngeal carcinoma: a prospective study. Head Neck; 1999 Sep; 21, 547–53.

Honjo, I. Nasopharyngeal Carcinoma on Otitis Media with Effusion in Eustachian Tube and Middle Ear Diseases. Springer-Verlag, Tokyo-Berlin-Heidelberg-New York-London-Paris, 1988; 91-111.

Hsin CH, Chen TH, Young YH, Liu WS. Comparison of otologic complications between intensity-modulated and two-dimensional radiotherapies in nasopharyngeal carcinoma patients. Otolaryngol Head Neck Surg. 2010 Nov;143(5):662-68.

John DG, Porter MJ, van Hasselt CA. Beware bleeding from the ear. J Laryngol Otol 1993 Feb; 107:137-9.

Kwong DLW, Wei WI, Sham JST, Ho WK, Yuen PW, Chua DTT, Au DKK, Wu PM, Choy DTK. Sensorineural hearing loss in patients treated for nasopharyngeal carcinoma: A prospective study of the effect of radiation and cisplatin treatment. Int J Rad Oncol Biol Phys. 1996 Sep; 36: 281-89.

Lederman M. Malignant tumours of the ear. J Laryngol Otol. 1965 Feb: 79: 85-119.

Leist M, Jaattela M. Caspase-independent cell death. In: Grimm S, editor. Genetics of Apoptosis. UK: BIOS Scientific Publishers Ltd,Trowbridge, 2003.

Leong JL, Fong KW, Low WK. Factors contributing to delayed diagnosis in nasopharyngeal carcinoma. J Laryngol Otol. 1999 Jul; 113(7):633-36.

Lim BY, Pang KP, Low WK, Tan HM. CSF otorrhea complicating temporal bone osteoradionecrosis in a patient with nasopharyngeal carcinoma. Ear Nose Throat J. 2005 Jan; 84(1):39-40.

Lim LH, Goh YH, Chan YM, Chong VF, Low WK. Malignancy of the temporal bone and external auditory canal. Otolaryngol and Head Neck Surg. 2000 Jun;122(6):882-86.

Loong HH, Ma BB, Chan AT. Update on the management and therapeutic monitoring of advanced nasopharyngeal cancer. Hematol Oncol Clin North Am. 2008 Dec; 22(6): 1267-78

Lou PJ, Chen WP, Tai CC. Delayed irradiation effects on nasal epithelium in patients with nasopharyngeal carcinoma. An ultrastructural study. Ann Otol Rhinol Laryngol. 1999 May; 108(5):474-80.

Low WK. Facial palsy from metastatic nasopharyngeal carcinoma at various sites: Three reports. Ear, Nose Throat J. Feb. 2002; 81(2):99-101.

Low WK. Surgical anatomy of the facial nerve in Chinese mastoids. ORL J Otorhinolaryngol Relat Spec. 1999 Nov-Dec; 61(6):341-44.

Low WK. Middle ear pressures in patients with nasopharyngeal carcinoma and their clinical significance. Journal of Laryngology and Otology. 1995 May; 109:390-93.

Low WK, Burgess R, Fong KW, Wang DY. Effect of radiotherapy on retro-cochlear pathways. Laryngoscope; 2005 Oct; 115:1823-26.

Low WK, Fong KW, Chong VF. Cerebellopontine angle involvement by nasopharyngeal carcinoma. Am J Otol. 2000 Nov; 21(6):871-76.

Low WK, Fong KW. Long-term hearing status after radiotherapy for nasopharyngeal carcinoma. Aurus Nasus Larynx; 1998 Jan; 25:21–24.

Low WK, Goh YH, Uncommon otological manifestations of nasopharyngeal carcinoma, J Laryngol Otol. 1999 Jun; Vol.113, 558-60.

Low WK, Gopal K, Goh LK, Fong KW. Cochlear implantation in postirradiated ears: outcomes and challenges.Laryngoscope; 2006b Jul; 116(7):1258-62.

Low Wk, Lim TA, Fan YF, Balakrishnan A, Pathogenesis of middle ear effusion in nasopharyngeal carcinoma: a new perspective. J Laryngol Otol. 1997 May; 111(5): 431-34.

Low WK, Sun L, Tan MG, Chua AW, Wang DY. L-N-Acetylcysteine protects against radiation-induced apoptosis in a cochlear cell line. Acta Otolaryngol. 2008 Apr; 128(4):440-45.

Low WK, Tan MG, Chua AW, Sun L, Wang DY. 12th Yahya Cohen Memorial Lecture: The cellular and molecular basis of radiation-induced sensori-neural hearing loss. Ann Acad Med Singapore. 2009 Jan; 38(1):91-94.

Low WK, Tan MG, Sun L, Chua AW, Goh LK, Wang DY. Dose- dependant radiation-induced apoptosis in a cochlear cell-line. Apoptosis 2006a Dec; 11:2127-36.

Low WK, Toh ST, Wee J, Fook-Chong SM, Wang DY. Sensorineural hearing loss after radiotherapy and chemoradiotherapy: a single, blinded, randomized study. J Clin Oncol. 2006c Apr; 20;24(12):1904-09.

Merchant TE, Gould CJ, Xiong X, Robbins N, Zhu J, Pritchard DL, Khan R, Heideman RL, Krasin MJ, Kun LE. Early neuro-otologic effects of three-dimensional irradiation in children with primary brain tumors. Int J Radiat Oncol Biol Phys. 2004 Mar 15; 58(4): 1194-207.

Miettinen S, Laurikainen E, Johansson R, Minn H, Laurell G, Salmi TT. Radiotherapy enhanced ototoxicity of cisplatin in children. Acta Otolaryngol Suppl. 1997; 529:90-94.

Miura T, Hirabuki N, Nishiyama K, Hashimoto T, Kawai R, Yoshida J, Sasaki R, Matsunaga T, Kozuka T. Computed tomographic findings of nasopharyngeal carcinoma with skull base and intracranial involvement. Cancer. 1990 Jan; 65(1): 29-37.

Myers EN, Beery QC, Bluestone CD, Rood SR, Sigler BA. Effect of certain head and neck tumors and their management on the ventilatory function of the eustachian tube. Ann Otol Rhinol Laryngol Suppl. 1984 Nov-Dec; 114:3-16.

Pacholke HD, Amdur RJ, Schmalfuss IM, Louis D, Mendenhall WM. Contouring the middle and inner ear on radiotherapy planning scans. Am J Clin Oncol. 2005 Apr; 28(2): 143-47.

Pow EH, Kwong DL, McMillan AS, Wong MC, Sham JS, Leung LH, Leung WK. Xerostomia and quality of life after intensity-modulated radiotherapy vs. conventional radiotherapy for early-stage nasopharyngeal carcinoma: initial report on a randomized controlled clinical trial. Int J Radiat Oncol Biol Phys. 2006 Nov; 66(4): 981-91.

Pringle MB, Jefferis AF, Barrett GS. Sensorineural hearing loss caused by metastatic prostatic carcinoma: a case report. J Laryngol Otol. 1993 Oct; 107(10):933-4.

Proud GO, Odoi H, Toledo PS. Bullar pressure changes in eustachian tube dysfunction. Ann Otol Rhinol Laryngol. 1971 Dec; 80(6):835-7.

Raaijmakers E, Engelen AM. Is sensorineural hearing loss a possible side effect of nasopharyngeal and parotid irradiation? A systematic review of the literature. Radiother Oncol. 2002 Oct; 65(1): 1-7.

Ralston A, Stevens G, Mahomudally E, Ibrahim I, Leckie E. Cochlear implants: response to therapeutic irradiation. Int. J Radiat Oncol Biol Phys 1999 Apr; 44(1):227–31.

Ramsden RT. Acoustic neuroma. In: Booth JB, Kerr AG. Scotts-Brown otolaryngology: otology, 5th ed. London: Butterworth, 1987; 500–33

Ramsden RT, Bulman CH, Lorigan BP. Osteoradionecrosis of the temporal bone. J Laryngol Otol. 1975 Sep; 89:941-55.

Rudge FW.Osteoradionecrosis of the temporal bone: Treatment with hyperbaric oxygen therapy. Mil Med. 1993 Mar; 158(3):196-8.

Rybak L. P, Whitworth C. A. Ototoxicity:therapeutic opportunities. Drug Discov Today; 2005 Oct; 10(9):1313-21.

Sadé J. The nasopharynx, Eustachian tube and otitis media. J Laryngol Otol. 1994 Feb; 108: 95-100.

Sadé J, Luntz M. Gas diffusions in the middle ear. Acta Otolaryngologica (Stockholm); 1991; 111(2): 354-57.

Schell M, McHaney VA, Green AA, Kun LE, Hayes FA, Horowitz M, Meyer WH. Hearing loss in children and young adults receiving cisplatin with and without prior cranial irradiation. J Clin Oncol. 1989 Jun; 7(6):754-60.

Schuknecht HF, Karmody CS. Radionecrosis of the temporal bone. Laryngoscope; 1966 Aug; 76(8):1416-28.

Seidman MD, Vivek P. Intratympanic treatment of hearing loss with novel and traditional agents. Otolaryngol Clin North Am. 2004 Oct; 37(5): 973-90.

Sha SH, Taylor R, Forge A, Schacht J. Differential vulnerability of basal and apical hair cell is based on intrinsic susceptibility to free radicals. Hear Res. 2001 May; 155(1-2):1-8.

Sham, JSI, Weis I, Lau SK, Yau CC, Choy D. Serous otitis media and paranasopharyngeal extension of nasopharyngeal carcinoma. Head and Neck. 1992 Jan-Feb; 14(1): 19-23.

Shibahara Y, Sando I. Congenital anomalies of the Eustachian tube in Down Syndrome. Histopathologic case report. Ann Otol Rhinol Laryngol. 1989Jul; 98: 543-7.

Shinomiya N. New concepts in radiation-induced apoptosis: 'premitotic apoptosis' and 'postmitotic apoptosis'. J Cell Mol Med. 2001 Jul-Sep; 5(3):240-53.

Singapore Cancer Registry Interim Report 2001-2005

Singh IP, Slevin NJ. Late audio-vestibular consequences of radical radiotherapy to the parotid. Clin Oncol. 1991 Jul; 3 (4):217–19.

Skinner DW, van Hasselt CA. A study of the complications of grommet insertion for secretory otitis media in the presence of nasopharyngeal carcinoma. Clin Otolaryngol Allied Sci. 1991 Oct; 16(5):480-82

Skinner DW, van Hasselt CA, Tsao SY. Nasopharyngeal carcinoma: modes of presentation. Ann Otol Rhinol Laryngol. 1991 Jul; 100(7): 544–51

Skinner R, Pearson ADJ, Amineddine HA, Mathias DB, Craft AW. Ototoxicity of cisplatinum in children and adolescent. Br J Cancer. 1990 Jun; 61(6):927-31.

Soo G, Tong MC, Tsang WS, Wong TK, To KF, Leung SF, van Hasselt CA. The BAHA hearing system for hearing-impaired post-irradiated nasopharyngeal cancer patients: a new indication. Otol Neurotol. 2009 Jun; 30(4):496-501.

Su CY, Hsu SP, Lui CC. Computed tomography, magnetic resonance imaging and electromyographic studies of tensor veli palatini muscles in patients with nasopharyngeal carcinoma. Laryngoscope; 1993 Jun; 103(6): 673-78.

Sweetow RW, Will TI . Progression of hearing loss following the completion of chemotherapy and radiation therapy: case report. J Am Acad Audiol. 1993 Nov; 4:360-63.

Takahara T, Sando I, Bluestone CD, Myers EM. Lymphoma invading the anterior Eustachian tube. Temporal bone histopathology of functional tubal obstruction. Ann Otol Rhinol Laryngol. 1986 Jan-Feb; 95: 101-105.

Thornley GD, Gullane PJ, Ruby RR, Heeneman H. Osteoradionecrosis of the temporal bone. J Otolaryngol. 1979 Oct; 8 (5):396-400.

van Hasselt AC, Gibb AG. Nasopharyngeal Carcinoma, Chinese University Press, Hong Kong, 1991; 105-44.

van Hasselt, A, Woo JKS. Nasopharyngeal carcinoma. Scott Brown's otorhinolaryngology and head and neck surgery, 7th ed., 2008; vol-2: ch188: 2445-74..

Verheij M, Bartelink H. Radiation-induced apoptosis. Cell Tissue Res 2000 Jul; 301 (1):133-42.

Walker DA, Pillow J, Waters KD, et al. Enhanced Cis-platinum ototoxicity in children with brain tumours who have received simultaneous or prior cranial irradiation. Med Pedia Oncol. 1989; 17:48-52.

Wanamaker JR, Kraus DH, Biscotti CV, Eliachar I. Undifferentiated nasopharyngeal carcinoma presenting as a parotid mass. Head Neck. 1994 Nov-Dec; 16(6):589-93.

Wang X, Hu C, Eisbruch A. Organ-sparing radiation therapy for head and neck cancer. Nat Rev Clin Oncol. 2011 Jul 26. doi: 10.1038/nrclinonc.2011;106.

Wei WL., Lund VJ, Howard, DJ. Serious otitis media in malignancies of the nasopharynx and maxilla. Journal of Laryngol and Otol. 1988 Feb; 102(2): 129-32.

Young, YH, Hsieh T. Eustachian tube dysfunction in patients with nasopharyngeal carcinoma, pre- and post- irradiation. Eur Arch Otorhinolaryngol. 1992; 249 (4): 206-08.

Young YH, Lin CY, Lou PJ, Hsu MM. Intracranial relapse of nasopharyngeal carcinoma manifested as sudden deafness.Otol Neurotol. 2001;22:392–96.

Yuen PW, Wei WI. Tympanomastoidectomy for chronic suppurative otitis media of irradiated ears of nasopharyngeal carcinoma patients. J Otolaryngol. 1994 Aug; 23(4):302-04.

Yuh WTC, Mayr-Yuh NA, Koci TM, Simon JH, Nelson KL, Zyroff J, Jinkins JR. Metastatic lesions involving the cerebellopontine angle. AJNR Am J Neuroradiol. 1993 Jan-Feb; 14(1):99–106.

Zhou Y, Tang A, Li J, Chen P, Mao R. The damaged types of eustachian tube function in the patients of nasopharyngeal carcinoma after radiotherapy. Lin Chuang Er Bi Yan Hou Ke Za Zhi. 2003 Aug; 17(8):464-65.

10

Update on Medical Therapies of Nasopharyngeal Carcinoma

Soumaya Labidi, Selma Aissi, Samia Zarraa,
Said Gritli, Majed Ben Mrad,
Farouk Benna and Hamouda Boussen
Faculty of Medicine of Tunis,
University of Tunis
Tunisia

1. Introduction

Nasopharyngeal carcinoma (NPC) is a common head and neck cancer in most of the countries of the Mediterranean Area (MA) and North Africa (NA). Its incidence is variable from <1 in sporadic areas to 2-7/100000 in NA and MA to 20-30/100000 in Southern China and Southeast Asia (Boussen et al,2010; Lee et al, 1992). It's different from other head and neck cancers due to its particular epidemiology, natural history and therapeutic considerations (Boussen et al, 2010; Lee et al, 1992).

It's highly radiosensitive and chemosensitive. Loco-regional radiotherapy (RT) remains the primary treatment for early stage disease (T1-T2, N0, N1), while combined chemotherapy-radiotherapy became the gold therapeutic standard in locally advanced disease i.e T3-T4, N2-N3 (Boussen et al, 2010; Lee et al, 1992; Baujat et al, 2006). Combined treatment leads to a significant improvement on overall and disease-free survivals, but NPC remains at a high metastatic risk, requiring the search for new salvage therapeutic protocols (Boussen et al, 2010; Lee et al, 1992: Xu et al, 2010). This paper will focus on recent data on epidemiology and progresses on medical therapies in NPC.

2. Transitional epidemiology of NPC

NPC represents 2 to 5% of all cancers in males, it is second to laryngeal cancer in most of the Mediterranean countries ant its incidence varying from 1 in Lebanon, Egypt, Greece, Turkey to 2-5/100000 in North Africa (NA), where it's characterized by a bimodal age repartition with a first peak at adolescence (Boussen et al, 2010; Ben Abdallah M, 2010). This high frequency of children and adolescents affected by NPC in Tunisia open the discussion to reach the maximum cure rate with minimal late aftereffects (Boussen et al, 2010). Endemic NPC is highly frequent in south-east Asia with an incidence > 20/100000 compared to NA (Tse et al, 2006). During the last 10 years, authors from Singapore reported a decrease of NPC incidence especially for UCNT type. This epidemiologic transition could be attributed to a socio-economic level increase as well as diet modification, such as salted fish (rich in nitrosamines) consumption decrease (Tse et al, 2006). The same trend have been observed

(Sun et al,2005) from 1992 to 2002 for the incidence Rates of NPC among Chinese Americans Living in Los Angeles County and the San Francisco Metropolitan Area with a decrease of 37% for men by 37% and only 1% in women(7). Conversely, male and female NPC world age-standardized incidence reported to be 27.5/105 and 11.3/105 respectively, seems to be stable from 1970-2007 in the Chinese endemic area of Zhongshan (Wei et al, 2010). In Tunisia (Ben Abdallah M,2010), we are observing, like in Singapore, a decreasing incidence of NPC and a projection from the North Tunisia cancer registry for 2024 suggests a significant drop of NPC incidence, while breast and colon cancer will clearly increase.

3. Staging and classification

During the last 20 years, NPC natural history became more known in term of loco-regional extension as well as metastatic disease with technical improvements of flexible nasofibroscopes and modern imagery, such as magnetic resonance imagery and Pet-scan(Chan et al,2011). This better definition of loco-regional disease extension leads to successive actualizations (1997, 2002 then 2009), of the more used TNM UICC anatomo-clinical classification, more adapted to discriminate between the different T and N prognostic stages and eventually to adjust therapeutic protocols according to risk group (Union for International Cancer Control,2009).

T1 Nasopharynx, oropharynx or nasal cavity (**was T2a***) without parapharyngeal extension

T2 Parapharyngeal extension (**was T2b***)

T2a Tumour extends to oropharynx and/or nasal cavity without parapharyngeal extension

T2b Tumour with parapharyngeal extension

T3 Bony structures of skull base and/or paranasal sinuses

T4 Intracranial, cranial nerves, hypopharynx, orbit, infratemporal fossa/masticator space

N1 Unilateral **cervical**, unilateral or bilateral retropharyngeal lymph nodes, above supraclavicular fossa; < 6 cm

N2 Bilateral **cervical** above supraclavicular fossa; < 6 cm

N3 Metastasis in lymph node(s), >6 cm in dimension (N3a) or in the supraclavicular fossa (N3b)>6 cm

7th TNM classification of UICC (International Union against Cancer, 2009)-AJCC, American Joint Committee on Cancer. *Recent modification

4. Chemotherapy

Systemic chemotherapy (CT) in NPC is indicated because disease is confined to nasopharynx in < 10% of cases (Lee et al; 1992), while parapharyngeal extension, skull base and intracranial involvement are reported in 80% and 25 to 35% and pathologic cervical nodes are present in 75 to 90% of patients, increasing the risk of initial metastases in advanced stages (Lee et al;1992; Sham et al,1991; Teo et al,1992). CT have been used since the eighties in palliative intent with few devoted phase II trials and the most active agents are cisplatin, 5-fluorouracil (5-FU), doxorubicin, epirubicin, bleomycin, mitoxantrone, methotrexate and vinca alkaloids or more recently ifosfamide or gemcitabine(Bensouda et al,2011;Boussen et al,2010;You et al,2011). CT have been used from the nineties as adjuvant then primary CT(PCT) in NPC(Bachouchi et al,1990) confirming the chemosensitivity of NPC with a high rate of radiologic/endoscopic objective responses to PCT (Bachouchi et al,1990; Ekenel et al,2011).

5. Radiotherapy

RT remains is the mainstay of of NPC treatment due to its radiosensibility (Boussen et al, 2010; Chan et al, 2010; Lee et al, 1992). Loco-regional RT targets primary tumor, its regional extension and both neck sides (levels Ib–V, and retropharyngeal nodes). Consensual dose is around 70 Gy with dose-fractions of 1.8 to 2Gy, indicated for sterilization of bulky tumor volume and 50–60 Gy or 46–60 Gy for areas at high risk (Lee et al, 1992; Chan et al, 2010).

6. Concomitant CT-RT

The results of concurrent chemoradiotherapy (CCRT) Intergroup study 0099, made gradually this combined approach as a standard in the treatment of patients with stage III and IV NPC (Al Sarraf et al, 1998; Chan et al, 2010). Within the randomized other studies, several meta-analysis and a pooled data analysis reported a significant improvement of survival in NPC patients treated by CTRT versus RT alone (Baujat et al, 2006). The NPC meta-analysis had shown the superiority of concomitant scheme vs neoadjuvant chemotherapy. It concerned 1753 patients with N1> 2cm, N2> 3cm, N3, T4, PS 0- 1, WHO 2-3 and a mean age of 46 years. The follow-up was < 5 years for 2 trials (299 pts), 5-9 years for 6 (1454 pts) and a median follow-up of 6 years for the whole population. Delivered radiotherapy were for tumor: 65-74 Gy, for N0 : 50-66 Gy and for N+ 60-76 Gy, by using a "classical" technique and a boost for residual N associated to concomitant cisplatin-based CT in all trials. Authors reported a benefit of concomitant scheme by increasing 5-year OS from 56% to 62% and EFS from 42% to 52% significantly better than neoadjuvant chemotherapy. Recently a meta-analysis focused on South East Asian phase III trials of CT-RT from the NPC endemic area. 1608 patients were collected from seven trials (Zhang L et al, 2010) and they reported Risk ratios (RRs) of 0.63 (95% CI, 0.50 to 0.80), 0.76 (95% CI, 0.61 to 0.93) and 0.74 (95% CI, 0.62 to 0.89) for 2, 3 and 5 years OS respectively in favor of the CCRT group. Concerning the 3-years absolute number of locoregional recurrence rate (LRR), a significant overall benefit in favor of the addition of chemotherapy was found with RR of 0.67 (95% CI, 0.49 to 0.91). A significant decrease of metastatic risk was also observed in term of 3-years absolute number of distant metastasis rate (DMR) with a RR of 0.71. The RRs were larger than that detected in the previously reported meta-analysis (including both endemic and non-endemic), and authors concluded that "the relative benefit of CCRT in endemic population might be less than that from previous meta-analyses".

6.1 CT Protocols of concomitant CT-RT

The schemes used for CTRT are mainly based on "Al Sarraf" schedule with Cisplatin 100mg/m2, every 3 weeks on D1,22,43 or weekly Cisplatin at 40mg/m2(Chan Scheme), who's the most frequently used in MA and NA, while radiotherapy doses is usually ≥66Gy (1.8-2Gy/Fx/d, 5Fx/wk) for primary nasopharyngeal tumor and its extensions + additional boosts to the parapharyngeal space, the primary or nodal sites not exceeding 20Gy. Since 10 years, CCRT is now recognized and applied as the better therapeutic approach for locally advanced NPC (Al Sarraf,1998 ; Chan et al,2010).

6.2 Acute and late toxicities of CT-RT

CT-RT compared to PCT, however increased significantly acute grade 3-4 toxicity at the end of combined treatment i.e mucositis, radiodermitis, dysphagia and consequently severe weight loss (WL) in most of the open or randomized studies (Table 1). This acute toxicity reduced considerably the compliance of weekly concomitant cisplatin, that was administered during the 6 weeks of CT-Rt in 94%,88%,74%,35%,7% and 3% for weeks 1 to 6 in Hui study (Hui et al,2009). The frequency of severe WL > 5-10% is probably underestimated by many authors and requires sometimes nasal tube feeding or parenteral nutrition as well as delay in the planned protocol. In a Chinese study (Qiu et al, 2011), of patients treated by CT-RT for NPC, 56% had at baseline, a mean 5% WL evaluated at 6.9 Kg after CT-RT (range 2.1-12.6 kg). Xerostomia is one of the most frequent sequelae after salivary gland irradiation and Intensity-Modulated RT permits to reach a high tumor control rate, but also to reduce severity and frequency of xerostomia (Lee et al, 2009).

Author/year	Hui/2010			Lee/2010		Zheng/2010
After PCT	An	---		--		1.7%
	Neutr	97%		--		6.8%
	Thr	--		--		--
	N/V	8.8%		--		5.1%
After CT-RT						
	An	8.8	19.2	19	1	39%
	Neutr	26.4	15.3	32%	1%	35.6%
	Thr			2%	0%	
	Mucos	23.5	7.7	61%	48%	---
	N/V	8.8	7.7	18%	1%	47.1%
	WL			27%	27%	
	Rad			20%	16%	
Late toxicities						
	Dys	---	3.8%	1%	0%	3.4%
	Xer	32.4	30.8%	---	---	91.5%
	Skin	11.8	19.2%	4%	5%	
	Subc	20.6	11.5%			
	HL	8.8	11.5%	6%	---	3.4%
	Otit			21	15%	3.5%
	Hypoth			8%	6%	6.8%
	SC	5.9	3.8%			

Table 1. Acute and late toxicities after CT-RT.

Despite many technical advances in RT, late toxicities i.e mainly xerostomia, cervical subcutaneous fibrosis, trismus, hearing loss of less frequently second cancers are observed decreasing the Quality of Life of long-term survivors from NPC, specially those treated in childhood or adolescence (Boussen et al,2010; Xiao et al,2011).

6.3 What next after concomitant CT-RT?

After the era of exclusive CT-RT, appeard the next generation protocols associating PCT followed by CT-RT (Fountzilas et al, 2011, Hui et al, 2009). PCT protocols included "classical" 5FU-cisplatin, anthracyclin-cisplatin or more recently taxanes-cisplatin associations (Table 2). Hui and al, reported their results on 65 patients treated cisplatin-docetaxel (DC) protocol followed by CCRT vs CCRT alone. They observed a significant survival benefit at 2 years for the DC arm (93% vs 76%, p = .013). Others studies including also taxanes, showed a benefit for overall and disease-free survival of patients treated for NPC in MA are currently varying from 66 to 94% and 63 to 88.2% (table 3). Many of these studies have a short Follw-up, but OS and DFS rates seems to be promising probably better than those reported in exclusive CT-RT. In Tunisia, a prospective GORTEC French trial is ongoing, comparing 2 cycles of primary TPF followed by chemoradiotherapy vs CCRT with weekly cisplatin (40mg/m2) in advanced(N2-3, T3-4).

Author/year	Nb	CT	RT	ORPCT	ORCT-RT	OS/DFS
Zheng/2010	60	Ned/FU Ned Conc	IMRT 70/55-60	-----	95.3%	3 yr 85.5/75%
Fountzilas	72	CPE-CRT	66-70/50-66	70%	83%	3 yr 66.6/64.5
2011	69	CRT	--------	-----	85%	3 yr 71.8/63.5
Hui	34	DC-CRT	70/50-60	76,5%	97.1%	3 yr 94.1/88.2%
2009	31	CRT	70/50-60	----	100%	3 yr 69.2/63%

CPE :Cisplatin-Paclitaxel-Epirubicin, DC : Docetaxel-cisplatin, CRT : Concomitant chemo-radiotherapy, Ned : Nedaplatin.

Table 2. Therapeutics results of open or randomized studies of PCT followed by CT-RT.

7. Tumor volume in NPC: A new prognostic factor?

Instead of the classical T,N,Age,Sex and histologic type, prognostic value of Primary Tumor Volume(PTV), measured by CT-scan have been explored for NPC in 112 patients with Stage I-IVB NPC treated by IMRT (Chen et al, 2011). The mean PTV was 33.9 ± 28.7 ml and classified from V1 to V4 (from 15.65 to 50,5ml). It impacted on 5-year overall survival who varies from 88.5, 83.3, 82.4 to 54.5% for V1 to V4 from, showing that V1-V4 are clearly separated from V4 (p = 0.014). Cox proportional hazards regression model analysis showed that a PTV >50 ml was an independent risk factor for radiotherapy (risk ratio = 3.485, P = 0.025). In 56 Turkish patients with locally advanced NPC, PTV have been calculated by measuring tumor diameters by CT and MR film hardcopies computed as an ellipsoid ($V=4/3 \pi \cdot d1 \cdot d2 \cdot d3$) to obtain the diameter-based volume(Sarisahin et al, 2011). They reported in the monovariate analysis, that primary tumor volume have a significant predictive value on DFS and DMFS, if tumor volume < 20ml, DFS was 60% vs 0% if > 60ml(p=0.007). The residual tumor volume (RTV) at first control after treatment was also found to be a significant prognostic factor on LRRFS (p=0.03). However Nasopharyngeal PTV alone is missing the volume of satellite cervical nodes that have probably an important prognostic value.

8. Recurrent/metastatic disease

NPC failures are mainly metastatic, to bones, lungs and liver and loco-regional relapses became more rare due to the high loco-regional control rate obtained by loco-regional RT (Leung et al,2005; Cvitkovic et al,1993). In metastatic situations, NPC remains chemosensitive to cisplatin, adriamycin, 5Fluorouracil or more recently taxanes, gemcitabine or oral capecitabine(Boussen et al,1991,2010;You et al,2011;Bensouda et al,2011). Prolonged survival after palliative CT and/or RT could be observed in patients with bone metastases in case of bone MTS only and less than 4 sites involved (Fandi et al,2000;Cao et al,2011). In isolated bone metastases, prolonged responses under biphosphonates plus CT have been also reported, with a significant reduction of skeletal events and better (11.5 vs 5.5 months, $P < 0.001$) progression-free survival and overall survival (23.5 vs. 17.5 months, $P < 0.001$) of combined vs chemotherapy alone group. (Jin et al,2011). Even in case of lung MTS disease, different prognostic groups could be identified according to size and numbers of metastatic nodules (Cao X et al, 2011).

9. Effective screening for NPC?

Some efforts have been done oriented for early detection in relatives of patients considered at high risk for NPC, according to their viral DNA and anti-EBV profile (Baizig et al,2011;Liu et al,2011). Sophisticated endoscopic technique have been also tested to detect easily early stages of NPC (Lin et al,2011, Lin et al,2011).

10. Conclusion

NPC is a very interesting within the other head and neck cancers, occurring in young patients non-smokers/non drinkers and significant improvement of therapeutic results have been reached during the last 30 years, 5 years-OS increasing from 20-30% to more than 75% with the recent protocols of CT-RT or PCT followed by CT-RT that included taxanes (Boussen et al, 2010, Chan et al,2010). Overexpression of EGRF, present in more than 70% of NPC leads to the use of Cetuximab as adjuvant concomitant or maintenance therapy (Yang Y et al, 2011). Anti-angiogenesis therapies like Pazopanib have been also tested without proven efficacy(Lim et al,2011). The significant survival improvement made NPC a more curable disease and efforts were made to reduce late sequelae specially in children and adolescents and to affect minimally quality of life after combined chemo-radiotherapy (Fang et al,2011;Marucci et al,2011;Shueng et al,2011).

11. References

Al-Sarraf M, LeBlanc M, Giri PG et al. (1998).Chemoradiotherapy versus radiotherapy in patients with advanced nasopharyngeal cancer: phase III randomized Intergroup study 0099. *J Clin Oncol*,16,1310–1317.

Bachouchi M, Cvitkovic E, Azli N et al. (1990). High complete response in advanced nasopharyngeal carcinoma with bleomycin, epirubicin, and cisplatin before radiotherapy. *J Natl Cancer Inst* 1990,82,7,(April 1990):616-20.

Baizig NM, Morand P, Seigneurin JM, Boussen H et al. (2011).Complementary determination of Epstein-Barr virus DNA load and serum markers for nasopharyngeal carcinoma screening and early detection in individuals at risk in Tunisia. *Eur Arch Otorhinolaryngol* (Jul 2011).

Baujat B, Audry H, Bourhis J et al. (2006). MAC-NPC Collaborative Group. Chemotherapy in locally advanced nasopharyngeal carcinoma: an individual patient data meta-analysis of eight randomized trials and 1753 patients. *Int J Radiat Oncol Biol Phys*,64,1, (January 2006),47-56.

Ben Abdallah M. (2010). North Tunisia Cancer Registry. Data for 2003-2007. Institut Salah Azaiz. Tunis.

Bensouda Y, Kaikani W, Ahbeddou N et al. (2011). Treatment for metastatic nasopharyngeal carcinoma. *Eur Ann Otorhinolaryngol Head Neck Dis*,128,2,(Apr 2011),79-85.

Boussen H, Cvitkovic E, Wendling JL, Azli N, Bachouchi M, Mahjoubi R, Kalifa C, Wibault P, Schwaab G, Armand JP. (1991). Chemotherapy of metastatic and/or recurrent undifferentiated nasopharyngeal carcinoma with cisplatin, bleomycin, and fluorouracil. *J Clin Oncol* 9,9,(Sep 1991),1675-81.

Boussen H, Bouaouina N, Daldoul O, Benna F, Gritli S, Ladgham A. (2010). Update on medical therapies of nasopharyngeal carcinomas. *Bull Cancer*,97,4,(April 2010),417-26.

Cao X, Han Y, He L, Xiang J, Wen Z.(2011). Risk subset of the survival for nasopharyngeal carcinoma patients with bone metastases: who will benefit from combined treatment? *Oral Oncol*,47,8,(August 2011),747-52.

Chan AT, Teo PM, Ngan RK et al. (2002). Concurrent chemotherapy-radiotherapy compared with radiotherapy alone in locoregionally advanced nasopharyngeal carcinoma: progression-free survival analysis of a phase III randomized trial. *J Clin Oncol*,20,2038–2044.

Chan ATC, Grégoire V, Lefebvre JL, Licitra L, Felip E(2010).Nasopharyngeal cancer: EHNS–ESMO ESTRO Clinical Practice Guidelines for diagnosis, treatment and follow-up;. *Ann Oncol*,21,(suppl 5): v187-v189.

Chen C, Fei Z, Pan J, Bai P, Chen L et al. (2011). Significance of primary tumor volume and T-stage on prognosis in nasopharyngeal carcinoma treated with intensity-modulated radiation therapy. *Jpn J Clin Oncol*,41,537-42.

Chan SC, Chang JT, Lin CY et al(2011). , Ng SH, Wang HM, Liao CT, Chang CJ, Lin SY, Yen TC. Clinical utility of 18F-FDG PET parameters in patients with advanced nasopharyngeal carcinoma: predictive role for different survival endpoints and impact on prognostic stratification. *Nucl Med Commun*, (August 2011).

Cvitkovic E, Bachouchi M, Boussen H, Busson P, Rousselet G, Mahjoubi R, Flores P, Tursz T, Armand JP, Azli N.(1993). Leukemoid reaction, bone marrow invasion, fever of unknown origin, and metastatic pattern in the natural history of advanced undifferentiated carcinoma of nasopharyngeal type: a review of 255 consecutive cases. *J Clin Oncol*,11,12,(Dec 1993),2434-42.

Ekenel M, Keskin S, Basaran M, Ozdemir C, Meral R, Altun M, Aslan I, Bavbek SE. Induction chemotherapy with docetaxel and cisplatin is highly effective for locally advanced nasopharyngeal carcinoma. *Oral Oncol* 2011 Jul;47(7):660-4.

Fandi A, Bachouchi M, Azli N, Taamma A, Boussen H, Wibault P, Eschwege F, Armand JP, Simon J, Cvitkovic E.(2000). Long-term disease-free survivors in metastatic undifferentiated carcinoma of nasopharyngeal type. *J Clin Oncol* 18,6,(Mar 2000),1324-30.

Fang FM, Tsai WL, Lee TF, Liao KC, Chen HC, Hsu HC.(2010). Multivariate analysis of quality of life outcome for nasopharyngeal carcinoma patients after treatment. Radiother Oncol,97,2, (Nov 2010),263-9.

Fountzilas G, Ciuleanu E, Bobos M et al. (2011). Induction chemotherapy followed by concomitant radiotherapy and weekly cisplatin versus the same concomitant chemoradiotherapy in patients with nasopharyngeal carcinoma: a randomized phase II study conducted by the Hellenic Cooperative Oncology Group (HeCOG) with biomarker evaluation. *Ann Oncol* Apr 27.

Gao F, Wee J, Wong HB, Machin D. (2010). Quality-of-life-adjusted survival analysis of concurrent chemo radiotherapy for locally advanced (nonmetastatic) nasopharyngeal cancer. *Int J Radiat Oncol Biol Phys*,78,454-60.

Hui EP, Ma BB, Leung SF et al. (2009). Randomized phase II trial of concurrent cisplatin radiotherapy with or without neoadjuvant docetaxel and cisplatin in advanced nasopharyngeal carcinoma. *J Clin Oncol* 2009;27:242-9.

Jin Y, An X, Cai YC, Cao Y, Cai XY, Xia Q, Tan YT, Jiang WQ, Shi YX. Zoledronic acid combined with chemotherapy bring survival benefits to patients with bone metastases from nasopharyngeal carcinoma. *J Cancer Res Clin Oncol* 2011 Aug 13.

Lee N, Harris J, Garden AS et al.(2009). Intensity-modulated radiation therapy with or without chemotherapy for nasopharyngeal carcinoma: radiation therapy oncology group phase II trial 0225. *J Clin Oncol* 27,22,(August 2009),3684-90.

Lee AW, Poon YF, Foo W et al. (1992). Retrospective analysis of 5037 patients with nasopharyngeal carcinoma treated during 1976-1985: overall survival and patterns of failure. *Int J Radiat Oncol Biol Phys*,23,2,261-70.

Lee AW, Tung SY, Chua DT et al. (2010). Randomized trial of radiotherapy plus concurrent-adjuvant chemotherapy vs radiotherapy alone for regionally advanced nasopharyngeal carcinoma. J Natl Cancer Inst,102,15,(Aug 2010),1188-98.

Leung TW, Tung SY, Sze WK et al.(2005) Treatment results of 1070 patients with nasopharyngeal carcinoma: an analysis of survival and failure patterns. *Head Neck*,27,555-65.

Lim WT, Ng QS, Ivy P et al. (2011). Tan A Phase II Study of Pazopanib in Asian Patients with Recurrent/Metastatic Nasopharyngeal Carcinoma. *Clin Cancer Res*,17,16,(Aug 2011),5481-9.

Lin B, Bergholt MS, Lau DP, Huang Z. (2011). Diagnosis of early stage nasopharyngeal carcinoma using ultraviolet autofluorescence excitation-emission matrix spectroscopy and parallel factor analysis. *Analyst,136,19*,(Oct 2011),3896-903.

Lin YC, Wang WH. Narrow-band imaging for detecting early recurrent nasopharyngeal carcinoma. (2011). *Head Neck*,33,4,(April 2011)591-4.

Liu Y, Huang Q, Liu W et al. (2011). Establishment of VCA and EBNA1 IgA-based combination by enzyme-linked immunosorbent assay as preferred screening method for nasopharyngeal carcinoma: A two-stage design with a preliminary performance study and a Mass screening in southern china. *Int J Cancer*,(Aug 2011).

Marucci L, Marzi S, Sperduti I, Giovinazzo G, Pinnarò P, Benassi M, Strigari L.(2011).Influence of intensity-modulated radiation therapy technique on xerostomia and related quality of life in patients treated with intensity modulated radiation therapy for nasopharyngeal cancer. *Head Neck*,(Mar2011).

Qiu C, Yang N, Tian G, Liu H. (2011). Weight loss during radiotherapy for nasopharyngeal carcinoma: a prospective study from northern china. *Nutr Cancer*,63,6,(Aug-Sep 2011),873-9.

Sham JS, Choy D.(1991). Prognostic value of paranasopharyngeal extension of nasopharyngeal carcinoma on local control and short-term survival. *Head Neck*,13,298-310

Shueng PW, Shen BJ, Wu LJ, Liao LJ, Hsiao CH, Lin YC, Cheng PW, Lo WC, Jen YM, Hsieh CH. (2011). Concurrent image-guided intensity modulated radiotherapy and chemotherapy following neoadjuvant chemotherapy for locally advanced nasopharyngeal carcinoma. *Radiat Oncol*,13,6(August 2011),95.

Sun LM, Epplein M, Li CI, Vaughan TL, Weiss NS. (2005). Trends in the Incidence Rates of Nasopharyngeal Carcinoma among Chinese Americans Living in Los Angeles County and the San Francisco Metropolitan Area, 1992–2002. *Am. J. Epidemiol*,162,12,(December 2005),1174-1178.

Teo P, Shiu W, Leung SF, Lee WY(1992). Prognostic factors in nasopharyngeal carcinoma investigated by computer tomography--an analysis of 659 patients. *Radiother Oncol*,23,79-93

Tse LA, Yu ITS , Mang OWK, Wong SL.(2006). Incidence rate trends of histological subtypes of nasopharyngeal carcinoma in Hong Kong. *Br J Cancer*,95,9,(Nov 2006),1269–1273.

Wei K, Xu Y, Liu J, Zhang W, Liang Z. (2010). No incidence trends and no change in pathological proportions of nasopharyngeal carcinoma in Zhongshan in 1970-2007. *Asian Pac J Cancer Prev*,11,6,1595-9.

Xiao WW, Huang SM, Han F, Wu SX, Lu LX, Lin CG, Deng XW, Lu TX, Cui NJ, Zhao C. (2011). Local control, survival, and late toxicities of locally advanced nasopharyngeal carcinoma treated by simultaneous modulated accelerated radiotherapy combined with cisplatin concurrent chemotherapy: long-term results of a phase 2 study. *Cancer*,117,9,(May 2011),1874-83.

Xu L, Pan J, Wu J, Pan C, Zhang Y, Lin S, Yang L, Chen C, Zhang C, Zheng W, Lin S, Ni X, Kong FM.(2010). Factors associated with overall survival in 1706 patients with nasopharyngeal carcinoma: significance of intensive neoadjuvant chemotherapy and radiation break. *Radiother Oncol.* ,96,1,(July 2010),94-9.

TNM Classification of malignant tumors. 7th edition. Union for International Cancer Control. .(2009). Geneva. http://www.uicc.org/node/7735.

Xiao WW, Huang SM, Han F et al. (2011). Local control, survival, and late toxicities of locally advanced nasopharyngeal carcinoma treated by simultaneous modulated accelerated radiotherapy combined with cisplatin concurrent chemotherapy: long-term results of a phase 2 study. *Cancer* 2011 May 1;117(9):1874-83.

Yang Y, Xuan J, Yang Z, Han A, Xing L, Yue J, Hu M, Yu J. (2011). The expression of epidermal growth factor receptor and Ki67 in primary and relapse nasopharyngeal cancer: a micro-evidence for anti-EGFR targeted maintenance therapy. *Med Oncol*,2011 Jul 23.

You B, Le Tourneau C, Chen EX et al. A Phase II Trial of Erlotinib as Maintenance Treatment After Gemcitabine Plus Platinum-based Chemotherapy in Patients With Recurrent and/or Metastatic Nasopharyngeal Carcinoma. (2011). *Am J Clin Oncol* 2011 Feb 22.

Zhang L, Zhao C, Ghimire B et al. (2010). The role of concurrent chemoradiotherapy in the treatment of locoregionally advanced nasopharyngeal carcinoma among endemic population: a meta-analysis of the phase III randomized trials. *BMC Cancer*,(October 2010),10,558.

Zheng J, Wang G, Yang GY, Wang D, Luo X, Chen C, Zhang Z, Li Q, Xu W, Li Z, Wang D. Induction chemotherapy with nedaplatin with 5-FU followed by intensity-modulated radiotherapy concurrent with chemotherapy for locoregionally advanced nasopharyngeal carcinoma. *Jpn J Clin Oncol*,40,5(May 2010),425-31.

11

Potential Therapeutic Molecular Targets for Nasopharyngeal Carcinoma

Shih-Shun Chen
Department of Medical Laboratory Science and Biotechnology, Central Taiwan University of Science and Technology, Taichung, Taiwan

1. Introduction

Nasopharyngeal carcinoma (NPC) is the leading cause of death in Southeast Asian populations, especially among Chinese people (338). The specific type of NPC is defined by the World Health Organization and classified histologically as either type I (keratinizing squamous cell carcinoma), type II (non-keratinizing squamous cell carcinoma), or type III (undifferentiated carcinoma) (263). Etiologic factors associated with NPC development are classified according to three determinants, including genetic susceptibility, Epstein-Barr virus (EBV) infection, and environmental exposure to carcinogens (45, 337). Evidence has indicated that EBV infection is implicated in the development of type II and III and is observed particularly in Asia (50, 61, 205, 230). EBV infection is generally not detected in type I NPC patients, especially in non-endemic areas (221, 342). Potential risk factors significantly associated with the initiation and development of type I NPC are cigarette smoking and alcohol consumption (35, 225, 295, 301). However, increasing evidence indicates that EBV appears to be the predominant risk factor associated with the initiation and development of NPC, regardless of histological type (17, 20, 300). In particular, EBV infection is an important event in the early stage of the NPC carcinogenesis process before tumor formation (101). Clinically, NPC exhibits a high incidence of lymph node spread and distant metastasis that is correlated with a poor prognosis, even when employing radiation therapy and chemotherapy (43, 260, 326). In the search for new substances with anti-tumoral effects, many natural compounds from dietary plants, such as herb and fruit extracts, have been shown to inhibit NPC proliferation, invasion, metastasis, and angiogenesis both *in vitro* and *in vivo*. This review summarizes the molecular mechanisms of EBV infection in NPC development as well as the role of natural compounds in the regulation of multiple cellular pathways and their clinical importance for the prevention and treatment of NPC.

2. The molecular mechanisms of EBV infection and the effects on NPC growth and metastasis

Virus binding to the surface of a target cell is a major determinant of cellular tropism and is a critical step in viral pathogenesis. This early event initiates the virus replication cycle by the attachment of the virus to specific receptor (s) and leads to the release of the viral genome into the cytoplasm of the target cell. It is believed that EBV infection is initiated by the interaction of the viral envelope glycoprotein gp350 with the complement receptor 2 (CR2/CD21) of the primary B cell surface membrane (11, 70, 219). The inefficient infection of epithelial cells by EBV is ascribed mainly to the lack of CD21 expression (17). RNA transcripts of the *CD21* gene have been found in the tonsillar epithelial cells of healthy patients by real-time quantitative polymerase chain reaction (PCR), although CD21 protein is not detected in these cells (125). A recent study has demonstrated that EBV-binding to the surface CD21 protein of CD11b-positive memory B cells (but not CD11b-negative naïve B cells) triggers co-capping of virus and integrins on B cells and activation of the adhesion molecules, which can induce the conjugation of EBV-loaded B cells and epithelial cells *via* the capped adhesion molecules while providing efficient virus transfer from B cells to infect epithelial cells (264). Memory B cells are regarded as professional antigen-presenting cells capable of priming T cells, which are responsible for the secretory IgA response and protective humoral immunity to virus. The anatomical localization of memory B cells from human tonsils preferentially colonize the tonsil epithelium, which is a potential site of viral entry, implying that transfer infection of normal epithelial cells may contribute to the EBV-induced tumorigenesis (191). Immunohistochemical analysis of CD21 in samples derived from healthy patients, non-tumoral nasopharyngeal mucosa patients, and NPC patients of different histological types with EBV infection has demonstrated a loss of CD21 expression in all NPC samples analyzed after EBV infection (18). A study of CD21 expression using a sensitive ribonuclease protection assay has demonstrated that a weak transcription signal of the *CD21* gene can be detected in the transplanted EBV-associated NPC tumors of nude mice, thereby suggesting that CD21 is expressed at low levels in EBV-positive NPC cells (11). These data suggest that EBV-induced immunophenotypic modulation of CD21 expression may be associated with NPC malignancy (18).

During EBV latency, NPC cells express a well-defined set of latent genes, including latent membrane proteins (LMP1, LMP2A, and LMP2B) and EBV-determined nuclear antigens (EBNA1 and EBNA2) (16, 84, 323). LMP1, an integral membrane protein encoded by the *BNLF1* gene (115), is the major transforming protein of the virus based on its ability to alter the phenotypic properties of epithelial cells and induce the expression of matrix metalloproteinase 9 (MMP-9), which is thought to contribute to tumor progression, invasiveness, and metastasis of NPC (58, 138, 334). Although low levels of LMP1 protein expression have been detected in NPC biopsies (68, 335), the *LMP1* gene transcripts detected by RT-PCR are present in approximately 95% of nasopharyngeal swab specimens from NPC patients (183). Expression of the *LMP1* gene was especially observed in early stage NPCs and pre-invasive lesions but not in late stage NPCs, therefore suggesting that its expression may initiate the development and progression of NPC (230). When the *LMP1* gene was expressed at high levels, it was toxic to human B-lymphoid cell lines, mouse embryonic fibroblast BALB/3T3 cells, a human osteosarcoma 143/EBNA-1 cell line expressing the EBV *EBNA-1* gene, and the human Larynx carcinoma HEp-2 cell line (93). Stable low-level expression of LMP1 is closely associated with the induction of anchorage-dependent growth and an invasive phenotype in mouse epithelial cells (294). Results have shown that LMP1-derived LALLFWL peptides are able to inhibit the proliferation of T cells and the cytotoxic function of NK cells (63). Studies have also indicated that EBV-infected NPC cells can use the exosome pathway for viral immune escape (134, 140). Moreover, LMP1 was shown to colocalize with the major histocompatibility complex (MHC) class II and be presented on the exosome (71). LMP1-containing exosomes derived from an EBV-positive lymphoblastoid cell line (LCL) were also capable of reducing T cell proliferation (71). LMP1 exerts immunosuppressive activity and can modulate the cytotoxic effects of innate immune cells, which are thought to allow cancer cells to evade the immune system (297). Exposure of cells to exosomes containing LMP1 prepared from EBV-infected NPC cells leads to the activation of the extracellular signal-regulated protein kinase (ERK) and phosphatidylinositol 3-kinase/protein kinase B (PI3K/Akt) pathways in epithelial, endothelial, and fibroblast cells. Moreover, the data presented showed that LMP1 could also induce epidermal growth factor receptor (EGFR) expression in EBV-negative epithelial cells and that purified exosomes from treated cells contained high levels of EGFR (207). Incorporation of cancer cell-secreted EGFR-containing membrane microvesicles by endothelial cells can induce the endothelial cell expression of EGFR and lead to the activation of the mitogen-activated protein kinase (MAPK) and Akt pathways as well as subsequent increased expression of vascular endothelial growth factor (VEGF) (4). These results support the concept that LMP1 plays a role in the modulation of the tumor microenvironment and immune evasion of EBV.

LMP1 also displays pleiotropic effects on the induction of the cell surface adhesion molecule CD23 (303), upregulation of the anti-apoptotic genes *Bcl-2* and *A20* (99, 149), and stimulation of interleukin-6 (IL-6) and -8 production (64, 65). LMP1 operates as a constitutively activated tumor necrosis factor receptor (TNFR) by functionally mimicking CD40, thereby utilizing TNFR-associated factor (TRAF) adaptor proteins to induce signaling pathways in a ligand-independent manner (241). LMP1-regulated IL-6 production in epithelial cells, which is regulated *via* a nuclear factor-kappa B (NF-κB) pathway involving TRAF, is similar to those mediated by the CD40 (65). IL-6 production and cell survival have also been shown to be regulated by p38 MAPK activity in LMP1-expressing epithelial cells (59, 64). Recent studies have demonstrated that activation of the p38 MAPK signaling pathway can promote LMP1 expression, suggesting that LMP1 upregulation by p38 MAPK signaling may contribute to cell survival during the early stage of EBV infection (126). Moreover, LMP1 expression has a significant anti-differentiation effect on human epithelial cells by inducing CD40, CD54, IL-6, and IL-8 expression (57). The serum levels of IL-6 are usually found to be elevated in NPC patients (46). The role that IL-6 plays in the regulation of the growth and invasion of cancer cells has been well demonstrated in various cancer cells such as human melanoma (194), human ductal breast carcinoma (253), renal cell carcinoma (289), ovarian carcinoma cells (243), human oral squamous carcinoma cells (270), head and neck cancer cells (281), human chondrosarcoma cells (286), and human pancreatic cancer cells (112). Ectopic expression of LMP1 in epithelial cells has been shown to result in increased MMP-9 expression (334). The promoter region of MMP-9 contains various *cis*-acting elements, including potential binding sites for NF-κB and activator protein-1 (AP-1) (334). NF-κB is critically involved in tumor progression through transcriptional regulation of invasion related factors, such as MMP-9 and VEGF (3). NF-κB overexpression can protect cancer cells against apoptosis induced by death receptors, thereby promoting the proliferation of cancer cells. Furthermore, constitutive activation of NF-κB has been detected in various tumor cells (224). The involvement of the MAPK pathways in NF-κB activation has been demonstrated to play an important role in tumorigenesis (60). Furthermore, p38 MAPK activity has been reported to be associated with anti-apoptosis (220), cell proliferation (103), and cancer invasion (271). Collectively, the regulation of IL-6 and MMP-9 production *via* the LMP1-TRAF-p38-MAPK-NF-κB pathway may have implications for the tumorigenesis and metastasis of NPC.

Dissociation or dissemination of cells from primary cancer to distant organs has been characterized by the loss of function or expression of epithelial cell adhesion molecules (148, 162). E-cadherin is a homophilic adhesion molecule expressed predominantly in epithelial tissues, which acts as an invasion suppressor and was found to be downregulated in most carcinomas (48). Reduced expression of E-cadherin has been observed in the advanced stages of NPC, therefore suggesting its association with cancer metastasis and poor prognosis (347). Significantly decreased expression levels of E-cadherin regulated by LMP1 have been shown to be associated with a higher invasive capability in human epithelial cells (67). LMP1 induces the downregulation of E-*cadherin* gene expression in NPC cell lines, which was shown by activation of DNA methyltransferases (292). The recent generation of transgenic mice has demonstrated that LMP1 overexpression antagonizes Wingless (WNT)/β-catenin signaling through inhibition of the Wilms' tumor gene on the X chromosome (WTX) and subsequent promotion of epithelial dysplasia of the nasopharynx and oropharynx but not tumorigenesis; downregulation of E-cadherin expression was also observed in these mice (240). The study has indicated that a reduction in WTX expression caused by LMP1 is associated with epithelial dysplasia *via* regulation of the WNT/β-catenin pathway and E-cadherin expression.

LMP1 also has effects on inhibition of p53-mediated apoptosis in stable epithelial cells expressing the *A20* gene (78). Another study has indicated that LMP1 can activate MAPK kinases to modulate p53 phosphorylation (167). The *p53* gene mutation rate was significantly lower in NPC than in other cancers (192, 238, 282). Dominant-negative mutations in the DNA-binding domain of the *p53* gene are rarely detected in NPC (107). An immunohistochemical study has shown significant p53 overexpression in approximately 82% of primary nasopharyngeal biopsy specimens (2). These results indicate that inhibition of p53-mediated apoptosis by LMP1 was probably responsible for p53 overexpression and the lack of *p53* gene mutations in EBV-positive NPC.

The *LMP2* transcription unit generates two alternatively spliced mRNAs that encode two functionally distinct proteins, LMP2A and LMP2B, which differ at their amino terminus (336). Only LMP2A has a 119-amino-acid amino-terminal cytoplasmic domain (79). This domain contains eight tyrosine residues with two of the tyrosines forming an immunoreceptor tyrosine-based activation motif (24, 193, 248). Immunohistochemical analysis of paraffin-embedded NPC biopsy samples with the LMP2A monoclonal antibody has shown that LMP2A mainly localizes to the tumor cell membrane and is expressed in invasive tumor front cells (142). Amino-terminal tyrosine phosphorylation of LMP2A has been shown to be necessary for association with Lyn and Syk protein-tyrosine kinases (210). In addition, tyrosine phosphorylation of LMP2A in epithelial cells can be triggered by cell adhesion to extracellular matrix proteins *via* the C-terminal Src kinase (257). *LMP2A* mRNA has been detected in all NPC specimens (21), whereas protein expression could be detected in only approximately 46% of these specimens (102). Stable expression of LMP2A in squamous epithelial cells was shown to promote cell spreading and migration in the extracellular matrix that required tyrosine kinase activity (5). Similarly, using primary epithelial cells from tonsil tissue that overexpress LMP2A, an increase in cell invasion and extracellular matrix receptor integrin-α-6 (ITGα6) has been demonstrated, therefore suggesting that LMP2 expression may contribute to the invasive process of NPC cells (233). Functional studies have indicated that LMP2 can induce the activation of PI3K/Akt, Syk tyrosine kinase, NF-κB, signal transducer and activators of transcription (STAT), and β-catenin pathways, thereby resulting in the inhibition of cell differentiation and the induction of cell migration in epithelial cells (196, 212, 256, 279, 284). A recent report has demonstrated that the ectopic expression of LMP2A in NPC cells induces epithelial-mesenchymal transition and increases the self-renewal capacity of cancer stem-like cells, which supports the concept that LMP2A functions as a potential inducer of tumor initiation and cellular invasiveness in NPC cells (142).

EBNA1 is a DNA-binding nuclear phosphoprotein that consists of two major functional domains, a carboxy-terminal DNA-binding domain and an amino-terminal chromosome tethering domain (159, 305). Both domains are separated by a glycine-alanine repeat sequence (GAr) that has been identified as a *cis*-acting inhibitor of MHC-class I-restricted antigen presentation (161). It has been recently shown that the GAr suppresses the presentation of MHC-class I-restricted antigen through the entire mRNA direct targeting of the mRNA translation initiation process (7). These results suggest that EBNA1 interferes with virus-encoded protein presentation by the MHC-class I-restricted pathway. Furthermore, EBNA1 expression is able to induce growth inhibition by inducing G_2/M phase arrest in human squamous epithelial cell lines (but not epithelial cell lines of glandular origin) (128). These results further indicate that the induction of the cytotoxicity effects in human squamous epithelial cells by EBNA1 is associated with EBNA1 degradation and processing. This leads to the endogenous degradation of EBNA1 in human squamous epithelial cells resulting from a specific cytotoxic T lymphocyte response (128), which suggests the possibility of the efficient EBV infection in malignant squamous epithelial cells but not in normal epithelial cells.

The dimerization and DNA-binding domains of EBNA1 have previously been shown to be located at the carboxy-terminal domain, amino acids 459 to 487 (36). The DNA-binding domain is essential for EBNA1 binding to the origin of plasmid replication (*ori*P), which is required for the replication and maintenance of the episomal EBV genome (237). The phosphorylation of EBNA1 is crucial for its transcriptional activity and the stability of EBV plasmids in virus-infected cells (62). The formation of the *ori*P-EBNA1 complex is also required for transactivation of the EBV C promoter (Cp), which is involved in the rearrangement of chromatin structure induced by EBNA1 (339). Moreover, recruitment of the histone H2B deubiquitylating complex to the *ori*P can be regulated by EBNA1 (254). EBNA1 has also been reported to upregulate LMP1 promoter activity (81). The effect of EBNA1 in promoting tumorigenesis has been found to increase genomic instability and DNA damage by inducing production of reactive oxygen species (ROS) (89). Stable complex formation between EBNA1 and the nucleosome assembly proteins, NAP1 and TAF-I, can affect cellular DNA replication (309). The EBNA1 portion of the EBNA1-binding protein 2 complex was shown to promote its interaction with mitotic chromosomes (218). A recent study has demonstrated that high-level expression of the EBNA1 protein in NPC cells interferes with mitotic segregation (275).

EBNA1 enhances the activity of the AP-1 transcription factor by binding to the promoter regions of c-Jun and activating transcription factor 2 (222). Elevated expression of the AP-1 targets IL-8, VEGF, and hypoxia-inducible factor-1alpha, has been observed in EBNA1-expressing NPC cells (222). EBNA1 also induces EBV-encoded RNA (EBER) expression through the induction of EBER-associated cellular transcription factors, ATF-2 and c-Myc, in an EBV-infected human adenocarcinoma cell line derived from nasopharynx (226). EBNA1 expression also influences the expression of genes involved in the dysregulation of oncogenic pathways in epithelial 293 cell lines (25) and decreases the expression levels and nuclear localization of phosphate-NF-κB in NPC cell lines (296). Survivin is a member of the family of inhibitors of apoptosis protein (IAP). It is expressed in a number of human cancer cells but not in normal adult tissue (6). The anti-apoptotic function of survivin involves its ability to block the activity of caspase-3 and caspase-7 (269, 285). Dysregulation of survivin expression in NPC cells affects cell viability and induces apoptosis (266, 333). More recent studies have demonstrated that EBNA1 forms a complex with SP1 or SP1-like protein at the *cis*-element of the survivin promoter and thereby regulates survivin expression. Results have further demonstrated an increase in resistance to apoptosis through upregulation of survivin expression by EBNA1 (197). Thus, EBNA1 may regulate multiple cellular signaling pathways to control cell proliferation and survival, thereby promoting the development of NPC.

EBNA2 is a nuclear phosphoprotein lacking sequence-specific DNA-binding activity. It was found to associate with the chromatin and nuclear matrix (32) and has been identified previously as a transcriptional regulator of the expression of cellular and EBV genes including *AML-2* (*RUNX3*), *CD21*, *CD23*, c-*MYC*, *EBI-1*, *Hes-1*, *LMP1*, and *LMP2A* (19, 44, 51, 80, 85, 130, 152, 255, 278, 303, 304). Their mechanism of regulation is suggested by the binding of EBNA2 with cellular transcription factors RBPJ, CBF-2/AUF1 or Spi-1/PU.1 to specific response elements of each promoter (137). Recent work has demonstrated that human endogenous retrovirus K nuclear protein NP9 can bind to EBNA2 and negatively regulate the EBNA2-mediated activation of the EBV viral C- and LMP2A promoters (88). The carboxy-terminal acidic activation domain of EBNA2 is required for direct interaction with the CSL family of DNA-binding protein (CBF1) and participates in EBNA2-mediated gene transcription (306). EBNA2 has been shown to be able to functionally replace the intracellular region of Notch in the regulation of gene expression of B cells by targeting CBF1 and localizing the coactivators p300, PCAF, and CBP to the promoter (109, 122, 250, 280, 306, 321). In normal cells, CBF-1 is bound by Notch to regulate the expression of cellular genes involved in cell proliferation (14, 187). Lee *et al.* have demonstrated that like Notch, EBNA2 can block orphan nuclear receptor Nur77-mediated apoptosis through interaction between its amino acids 123–147 conserved domain and Nur77 (158). Although Notch signaling functions have been linked to a variety of cellular processes such as adhesion, differentiation, cell proliferation, apoptosis, epithelial to mesenchymal transition, migration, and angiogenesis, Notch can also function as an oncogene or a tumor suppressor in cancer development (14). The biological effect of Notch signaling depends on the type and fate of the cell (244). An immunocytochemical study of NPC biopsies using antibodies against the activated form of Notch1 and Hes-1 have demonstrated that Notch signaling is activated in human primary NPC cells (345). High expression levels of both Notch and Notch ligand (Jagged1) were detected in human head and neck and breast cancer samples, and patients harboring these tumors showed poor prognosis (174, 246). Recent studies have indicated that activation of Notch signaling contributes to the survival and proliferation of several types of cancer entities, such as human non-small cell lung cancer (40), human tongue carcinoma (343), human leukemia cells (164), human gastric cancer (332), and human colon adenocarcinoma (247). These findings suggest that EBNA2 mimics the effects of Notch, thereby upregulating Notch signaling activity to maintain cell proliferation and survival of NPC.

3. The inhibitory mechanisms of natural compounds against NPC survival and metastasis signaling

The prognosis of NPC is based on the size of the tumor and the spread of the cancer to the lymph nodes or to other organs. Traditionally, this type of cancer is treated either with surgery, radiotherapy, chemotherapy, immunotherapy, or other methods. The main treatment of NPC is radiotherapy, usually given in combination with chemotherapy drugs (315). However, NPC exhibits a high incidence of lymph node spread and distant metastasis that is correlated with a poor prognosis, even during the use of radiation therapy and chemotherapy (43, 260, 326). The currently available chemotherapy agents for cancer treatment are usually toxic to normal cells, often resulting in adverse side effects such as temporary hair loss, nausea and vomiting. The use of chemopreventative agents is now regarded as a promising strategy against cancer development (10). Cancer development and progression is a complex process that involves the dysregulation of multiple signaling pathways and molecular changes. These events may contribute to tumor growth, invasion, metastasis, and immune evasion (27). In the search for new substances with anti-tumoral effects, many natural, dietary, or synthetic substances have been shown to inhibit carcinogenesis *in vitro* and *in vivo* through the targeting of specific proteins or modulating signal transduction pathways (133).

Aloe-emodin (AE; 1,8-dihydroxy-3-(hydroxymethyl)-anthraquinone), which is isolated from the rhizomes of *Rheum palmatum*, has been shown to inhibit cell growth and induce apoptosis *in vitro* in several cancer cell lines, such as human cervical carcinoma HeLa (91), rat C6 glioma carcinoma (209), human hepatoma HepG2 (147, 180), human neuroblastoma SJ-N-KP and SK-N-BE(2c) (232), human lung squamous carcinoma CH27 (155), and human lung non-small cell carcinoma H460 cell lines (331). Animal studies using severe combined immune deficiency (SCID) mice have shown that AE selectively inhibited the growth of human neuroectodermal tumors but not normal fibroblasts and hematopoietic progenitor cells (231). The results of a recent *in vitro* study have shown that high concentrations (up to 100 μM) of AE exhibit low cytotoxicity in normal human fibroblasts WI-38, Detroit 551, and MRC-5 cells (178), which are consistent with evidence provided by other reports in other normal cells including the proximal tubule-derived opossum kidney OK cell line, the human keratinocyte HACAT cell line, the human airway epithelial BEAS-2B cell line (195), and rat primary astrocytes (209). AE also inhibited the proliferation of both human umbilical vein endothelial and bovine aortic endothelial cells (28). These results suggest that the effect of AE is highly specific for cancer cells and endothelial cells, thereby supporting the concept that AE could be a potent cancer chemotherapeutic and anti-angiogenic agent. Apoptosis is a physiological mechanism involved in the elimination of malignant or cancer cells without eliciting damage to normal cells or surrounding tissues. Thus, the induction of apoptosis exclusively in target cells is an attractive approach for anticancer therapy (133). It is now recognized that the mitochondria play a crucial role in the regulation of cell death, which seems to be the main target for apoptosis induction in response to a variety of stress stimuli, such as growth factor withdrawal and chemopreventative components (133). Bcl-2 and Bcl-X_L have been well characterized as important regulators of apoptosis in response to a wide range of stimuli, including chemopreventative components (1, 272). In addition, the ability of Bcl-2 and Bcl-X_L to suppress the mitochondrial-mediated pathway of apoptosis is well known (86, 87, 310). Overexpression of either Bcl-2 or Bcl-X_L in tumor cells has been shown to be associated with poor prognosis in many human cancers (52) and contributes to the development of resistance to chemotherapy and radiation treatment (127, 261). Although EBV LMP1 can block apoptosis in B cells by upregulating Bcl-2 expression (99), knockdown of *Bcl-X_L* by siRNA has been shown to induce apoptosis in NPC cells (166), thereby suggesting that Bcl-X_L is an important effector of resistance to apoptosis in NPC cells. A recent *in vitro* NPC cell study has shown that increasing levels of cyclin B1 bound to cyclin-dependent kinase 2 contributes to 60 μM AE-induced G_2/M phase cell cycle arrest (178). AE (60 μM)-induced apoptosis of NPC-TW076 and NPC-TW039 cells was mediated by elevated Bax and decreased Bcl-X_L expression, which was confirmed by ectopic expression of Bcl-X_L, although it was not observed in Bcl-2 or small interfering RNA (siRNA)-mediated attenuation of Bax suppressing AE-induced apoptotic cell death (178). The reduction of mitochondrial membrane potential and the increase in cellular Ca^{2+} content, ROS production, and apoptosis induced by AE were attenuated by treatment with either cyclosporin A or the caspase-8 inhibitor Z-IETD-FMK. Further analysis has shown that suppression of caspase-8 with the specific inhibitor Z-IETD-FMK inhibited AE-induced activation of Bax, the cleavage of Bid, the translocation of tBid to the mitochondria, and the release of cytochrome *c*, apoptosis-inducing factor and endonuclease G from the mitochondria, and subsequent apoptosis. These results indicate that caspase-8-mediated activation of the mitochondrial death pathway plays a critical role in 60 μM AE-induced apoptosis of NPC cells (178). A more recent investigation has revealed that 40 μM AE significantly inhibits NPC cell growth through cell cycle arrest at the S-G_2/M phase, which is associated with increased levels of cyclin B1 bound to Cdk1 but not the apoptotic process (179). Gene silencing of MMP-2 mediated by siRNA inhibits NPC cell invasion, thereby demonstrating the involvement of MMP-2 in the NPC invasion process (179). Using siRNA against p38 MAPK, the p38 MAPK inhibitor SB203580, NF-κB inhibitors N-*p*-tosyl-L-phenylalanine chloromethyl ketone and pyrrolidine dithiocarbamate, transient ectopic expression of wild type NF-κB, a MMP-2 promoter activity assay, and an NF-κB-dependent reporter assay it has been further demonstrated that 40 μM AE inhibits the invasion of NPC cells by reducing the expression of MMP-2, likely through the inhibition of the p38 MAPK-NF-κB pathway, and that NF-κB activity is involved in regulating the expression of MMP-2 and VEGF through the p38 MAPK-dependent pathway (179). The reason that NPC cells are more sensitive to 60 μM than 40 μM AE for the induction of apoptosis remains unclear. AE was found to induce DNA single-strand breaks and nuclear condensation through the generation of ROS, leading to apoptosis in the human lung non-small cell carcinoma H460 cell line (156). Previous studies have also reported that the release of the nuclear protein nucleophosmin from the nucleus to the cytosol is associated with AE-induced cell apoptosis (157). These observations led to the speculation that nuclear DNA might be a target of AE during AE-induced apoptotic cell death. The results from another group have shown that AE displayed an affinity for nuclear DNA; disrupted chromatin structure and DNA template function were detected in susceptible cell lines upon treatment with a high dose of AE (214). The participation of ROS in cancer cell apoptosis stimulated by chemotherapeutic agents through the induction of DNA damage has been investigated for several decades (154). Oxidative damage to DNA is a result of the interaction of DNA with ROS. AE contains a quinone structure that was predicted to have the ability to induce ROS production, which may play a role in the induction of cancer cell apoptosis (156). Consistent with the data presented by Lee *et al.* (156), an increase in intracellular ROS levels was observed when apoptosis was induced in NPC cells using 60 μM AE (178). However, apoptosis, DNA damage, and increases in ROS levels were not detected in the same cells treated with 40 μM AE, therefore suggesting that different concentrations of AE could differentially modulate the expression of cellular genes that are involved in cell growth, apoptosis, and cell invasion in different types of cancer cells (179).

Berberine (2,3-Methylenedioxy-9,10-dimethoxyprotoberberine chloride), is an isoquinoline plant alkaloid isolated from the roots, rhizomes, and stem bark of *Hydrastis Canadensis, Coptis chinensis, Berberis aquifolium, Berberis vulgaris, Berberis aristata,* and *Berberis thunbergii* (143). It is traditionally used in China to treat gastrointestinal diseases such as dysentery and diarrhea. Clinical studies conducted in 1985 and 1987 have shown that berberine is considered to be a non-toxic alkaloid and is useful for the treatment of bacterial diarrhea (136, 242). Berberine also has anti-fungal (76), anti-human immunodeficiency virus (HIV) infection (53), and anti-protozoan properties (131). Berberine-induced apoptosis of cancer cells likely involves the enhanced activities of the mitochondria-dependent signaling events or Fas/FasL signaling as implied by the loss of mitochondrial membrane potential ($\Delta\psi_m$) and the release of cytochrome *c* in human colonic carcinoma SW620 (118), promonocytic U937 (121), leukemia HL-60 (169), and oral cancer HSC-3 cell lines (170); the decrease of Bcl-X_L and Bcl-2 expression in human epidermoid carcinoma A431 cell lines (204); and the generation of ROS and activation of FasL in human colonic carcinoma SW620 cell lines (111). Other signaling pathways have also been shown to be required for berberine-induced apoptosis, including the JNK/p38 MAPK (111), p53-dependent ATF3 (235), ER stress (172), and NF-κB pathways (227). In addition to apoptosis induction, berberine has also shown potent anti-angiogenic effects on the inhibition of tumor-induced angiogenesis and MMP-1, -2, and -9 expression (313). Berberine inhibits the invasion of human lung cancer A549 cells *in vitro* by decreasing the production of the urokinase-plasminogen activator and MMP-2 (234). The inhibition of cell invasion by berberine through downregulation of MMP-2 and -9 expression was also observed in human breast cancer MDA-MB-231 (139), gastric cancer SNU-5 (173), glioma U-87 (184), and tongue squamous carcinoma SSC-4 cell lines (106). Moreover, oral administration of berberine in mice significantly inhibited the spontaneous mediastinal lymph node metastasis of Lewis lung carcinoma into the lung parenchyma (211). In NPC cells, berberine inhibits the intracranial invasion of tumors in nude mice injected with NPC 5-8F cells through the induction of NM23-H1 expression (190). Other investigations have also found that berberine exerts a potent *in vitro* anti-invasive effect on the NPC 5-8F cell line through the reduction of filopodia formation (287). Significant inhibition of tumor metastasis to the lymph nodes and a decrease in Ezrin phosphorylation at threonine 567 (Thr^{567}) in metastatic samples were observed in nude mice injected *via* intravenous (tail vein) injection with NPC 5-8F cell lines and treated with berberine. The authors further demonstrated that berberine-induced reduction in filopodia formation was associated with decreased Rho kinase-mediated Ezrin phosphorylation at Thr^{567} (287).

Curcumin (1,7-bis(4-hydroxy-3-methoxyphenyl)-1,6-heptadiene-3,5-dione) is a polyphenol isolated from the rhizomes of *Curcuma longa,* which has demonstrated low toxicity in humans (299). It has been shown to inhibit cell growth and induce apoptosis *in vitro* in several cancer cell lines, such as breast cancer; human basal cell carcinoma BCC-1/KMC (123); biliary cancer KKU100, KKU-M156 and KKU-M213 (239); colon cancer HT-29 and HCT116 (124, 129, 314); esophageal adenocarcinoma OE33 (95); hepatoma HepG2 (26, 124, 308); myeloid leukemia U937 and HL60 (252); liposarcoma SW872 (307); lung adenocarcinoma A549 (38, 39, 340, 341); lung squamous carcinoma H520 (258); medulloblastoma MED (8); neuroblastoma Lan-5, SK-N-SH, and Kelly (77); esophageal cancer OE21 and OE33 (223); prostate carcinoma PC3 (105); salivary adenoid cystic carcinoma SACC-83 (283); and small cell lung cancer NCI-H446 and PC-9 cell lines (249, 322, 328). *In vitro* cell culture studies have shown that curcumin can also suppress the migration and invasion of human cancer cell lines, such as breast carcinoma MDA-MB-231 and MDA-MB-468 (217, 277); colon cancer HCT116 (213, 311); gastric cancer BGC823 (23); glioblastoma A-172, MZ-18, MZ-54, MZ-256, and MZ-304 (259); hepatocellular carcinoma SK-Hep-1 (175); lung adenocarcinoma A549 and CL1-5 (33, 182); medulloblastoma MED (8, 34); and prostate cancer PC-3 cell lines (100). Animal studies using SCID mice have shown that curcumin selectively inhibits the growth of human breast, colon, gastric, liver, ovarian, and brain cancers but not normal tissues (144). Curcumin also induces apoptosis and cell growth arrest in cancer cells by modulating the expression of cell cycle regulatory factors, inhibiting the transcriptional regulation of NF-κB, and activating the activities of caspases (144). In addition, curcumin blocks angiogenesis and metastasis by modulating the signaling pathways involved in the expression of growth factors and cell adhesion molecules (144). Although the anti-cancer mechanisms of curcumin that are involved in the modulation of signal transducer and activator pathways to interrupt the process of carcinogenesis are diverse (144, 317), it exhibits potential as an anti-cancer chemotherapeutic agent for the treatment of many human cancers. Curcumin's inhibitory effect on NPC cell migration has been demonstrated to increase the expression of E-cadherin (320). Conversely, curcumin exerts an apoptotic effect on NPC cells through the decrease in the relative ratio of Bcl-2 to Bax, dysfunction of the mitochondria, cytochrome *c* release, and the activation of caspase-9 and caspase-3, therefore indicating that the mitochondrial death pathway is involved in the curcumin-induced apoptosis of NPC cells (145).

Epigallocatechin gallate (EGCG), also known as epigallocatechin 3-gallate, is a polyphenol isolated from green tea leaves (329). EGCG has been reported to possess several biochemical and pharmacological properties, which include anti-HIV and HCV infection activity (49, 94, 318, 325), reduction of Sjögren's syndrome in murine models (83, 110), prevention of Alzheimer's and Parkinson's diseases (203), anti-obesity effects on mice and humans (41, 319), anti-oxidant activity (75, 104, 293, 348), and anti-neoplastic activity (135, 262). The cancer-preventive effects of EGCG have been proposed to suppress the transformative, hyperproliferative, and inflammatory processes that are involved in carcinogenesis (288). The anti-oxidant activity of EGCG is thought to play an important role in the induction of apoptotic signaling pathways in cancer cells (104, 151), such as human hepatoma Hepa1c1c7 (151), cervical cancer HeLa (274), chondrosarcoma (330), lung cancer H1299 (165), and glioblastoma T98G and U87MG cell lines (56). EGCG displays anti-oxidant activity due to the presence of phenolic groups in the molecule that are sensitive to oxidation (151, 215). However, the molecular targets of EGCG in the inhibition of cancer growth, metastasis, and angiogenesis are diverse. EGCG also affects various signaling pathways (273). Yan *et al.* have showed that EGCG inhibits the growth of NPC CNE-LMP1 cell lines by suppressing

LMP-1-induced NF-κB activity *via* the inhibition of inhibitory protein IkappaBα phosphorylation (327). LMP-1-promoted activator protein-1 (AP-1) transcriptional activity, the nuclear translocation of JNK, the phosphorylation of c-Jun, promoter activity and phosphorylation of EGFR, and cyclin D expression in NPC CNE-LMP1 cell lines were also suppressed by EGCG (327, 346), thereby suggesting that EGCG suppresses LMP-1-mediated NPC cell growth through the inhibition of AP-1 and NF-κB signaling pathways.

Osajin (5-hydroxy-3-(4-hydroxyphenyl)-8,8-dimethyl-6-(3-methylbut-2-enyl) pyrano[2,3-h]chromen-4-one;5-Hydroxy-3-(4-hydroxyphenyl)-8,8-dimethyl-6-(3-methyl-2-butenyl)-4H,8H-benzo[1,2-b:3,4-b']dipyran-4-one) is a prenylated isoflavone originally isolated from the fruit of *Maclura pomifera* (302). The biological activity of osajin is thought to have anti-oxidant properties that can attenuate the myocardial dysfunction provoked by ischemia reperfusion in rats (72). It has been shown to inhibit the growth of six types of human cancer cell lines *in vitro*, including renal carcinoma ACHN, lung adenocarcinoma NCI-H23, prostate cancer PC-3, breast cancer MDA-MB-231, melanoma LOX-IMVI, and colon carcinoma HCT-15 cell lines (276). Osajin has demonstrated low toxicity in human hepatocytes compared with human cancer cell lines (276). However, the mechanism of growth inhibition in human cancer cells by osajin is not clear. A recent study has shown that the activation of the death receptor Fas/FasL, mitochondrial death, and endoplasmic reticulum (ER) stress signaling pathways are involved in the apoptosis of NPC cells induced by osajin (114).

Resveratrol (3,4,5-trihydroxy-trans-stilbene), a polyphenol phytoalexin, is widely present in foods such as grapes, berries, peanuts, and other plant sources. It has been shown to possess diverse biochemical and physiological functions, including anti-aging (9), anti-platelet aggregation (201, 312), anti-inflammatory (268), cardioprotection (15, 116, 119), and estrogenic properties (160). Experimental results from animal models have revealed that the anti-inflammatory properties of resveratrol control the development of arthritis (66), pancreatitis (198, 199), and colitis (153). Although resveratrol is a poor ROS scavenger *in vitro*, it behaves as a potent anti-oxidant due to its ability to increase the synthesis of nitric oxide *in vivo* (22, 54, 96, 324). During the last decade, resveratrol has been shown to have strong anti-carcinogenic activity in a wide range of human cancer cell lines, such as anaplastic large-cell lymphoma SR-786 (141), breast cancer MCF-7 and MDA MB231 (267), chronic myeloid leukemia K562 (132), colon cancer HT-29 (298), diffuse large B cell lymphoma DLBCL (117), glioblastoma A172 and T98G (171), glioma U87 (69), hepatocellular carcinoma Huh-7 (168), leukemia HL-60 (163), leukemic monocyte lymphoma U937 (90), lung adenocarcinoma ASTC-a-1 (344), medullary thyroid cancer (291), melanoma YUZAZ6 and M14 (290), neuroblastoma B65 (236), non-small cell lung cancer A549 (188, 189), and prostate cancer LNCaP cell lines (37). Resveratrol also been shown to suppress the growth of cancer *in vivo* such as colon (55, 316), hepatocellular (13), lung (200), mammary (31), and skin cancer (82). *In vitro* and *in vivo* studies have led to several clinical trials to evaluate resveratrol's potential for cancer chemoprevention and chemotherapy, including the prevention and treatment of colon cancer (12, 228, 229). The anti-cancer activity of resveratrol has been attributed to the induction of apoptotic cell death *via* its anti-proliferation and anti-invasion properties (216, 228). Its mechanism of action and molecular targets are diverse (216, 228). In human NPC TWP4 cells, treatment with resveratrol induced apoptosis and was associated with the induction of multiple apoptotic pathways, including death receptor, mitochondria, and ER stress pathways (113). Chow *et al.* have suggested that ΔNp63 is a molecular target of resveratrol-induced apoptosis in NPC-TW076 and NPC-TW039 cell lines (47).

Rhein (4, 5-dihydroxyanthraquinone-2-carboxylic acid), a major constituent in the rhizome of *rhubarb*, shows anti-oxidant and free radical scavenging effects similar to AE, which has been shown to play an important role in the inhibition of carcinogenesis (202). In addition to the inhibitory effects on the process of hepatic fibrosis in rats (92), synthesis of aggrecan and tissue inhibitor of metalloproteinases-1 in cultured human chondrocytes (251), activation of the MEK/ERK pathway induced by IL-1β in chondrocytes cultured in hypoxia (206), and fungal infection of plants (349), rhein also protects the dysfunction of human umbilical endothelium ECV-304 cell lines induced by transforming growth factor β1 through the inhibition of plasminogen activator inhibitor-1 (350). *In vivo* experimental results have shown that rhein has the ability to suppress the growth of tumor cells in rat liver (208). The anti-angiogenic property of rhein has been characterized in a zebrafish model (97, 98). Interestingly, rhein lysinate showed a synergistic increase in the anti-tumor activity of Taxol in mice (185, 186). It has also been shown to influence cell growth and apoptosis in several human cancer cell lines such as cervical cancer Ca Ski (120), colon adenocarcinoma CaCo-2 (245), glioma U-373MG (74), hepatocellular carcinoma BEL-7402 (265), hepatoblastoma HepG2 (146), lung cancer A549 (108), promyelocytic leukemia HL-60 (181), and human tongue SSC-4 cancer cell lines (42, 150). Moreover, rhein can inhibit the uptake and glycolysis of glucose and protein synthesis in cancer cells (29, 30, 73). Although it has been reported that increased expression of p53, p21, and CD96 may be responsible for the apoptosis of human hepatoblastoma HepG2 cell lines induced by rhein in a similar manner to AE (146), the molecular mechanisms by which rhein influences cell growth and apoptosis of cancer cells differ from AE. In NPC-TW076 and -TW039 cells, rhein induces apoptotic cell death *via* the ER stress and Ca^{2+}-dependent mitochondrial death pathways. The induction of ER stress by rhein correlated with the augmented expression of glucose-regulated protein 78, PKR-like ER kinase, activating transcription factor 6 and CCAAT/enhancer-binding protein homologous protein as well as the cleavage of procaspase-12 (176). In addition, NPC cells exposed to rhein have demonstrated a dramatic increase in mitochondrial dysfunction, including the loss of $\Delta\psi_m$ and the release of cytochrome *c* and apoptosis-inducing factor (176). Lin *et al.* have further demonstrated that rhein inhibits the invasion of NPC cells by suppressing the expression of MMP-9 and VEGF *via* the NF-κB signaling pathway (177).

4. Conclusion

Although numerous studies have attempted to define the initiation and development of NPC, the exact mechanism remains controversial. The understanding of the signaling pathways and regulatory mechanisms leading to NPC carcinogenesis will provide sufficient information for the identification of potent chemopreventive agents against NPC. Based on the studies discussed here, there is strong evidence that the anti-NPC activities of AE, berberine, curcumin, osajin, resveratrol, and rhein involve the inhibition of cell growth and metastasis as well as the induction of apoptosis through modulation of multiple signaling pathways and molecular factors. Further studies should attempt to analyze other active components or chemotherapeutic agents and integrate with *in vivo* studies and clinical trials to evaluate the applicability of these natural compounds in NPC prevention and treatment.

5. References

[1] Adams, J. M., and S. Cory. 2007. The Bcl-2 apoptotic switch in cancer development and therapy. Oncogene 26:1324-37.

[2] Agaoglu, F. Y., Y. Dizdar, O. Dogan, C. Alatli, I. Ayan, N. Savci, S. Tas, N. Dalay, and M. Altun. 2004. P53 overexpression in nasopharyngeal carcinoma. In Vivo 18:555-60.

[3] Aggarwal, B. B. 2004. Nuclear factor-kappaB: the enemy within. Cancer Cell 6:203-8.

[4] Al-Nedawi, K., B. Meehan, R. S. Kerbel, A. C. Allison, and J. Rak. 2009. Endothelial expression of autocrine VEGF upon the uptake of tumor-derived microvesicles containing oncogenic EGFR. Proc Natl Acad Sci U S A 106:3794-9.

[5] Allen, M. D., L. S. Young, and C. W. Dawson. 2005. The Epstein-Barr virus-encoded LMP2A and LMP2B proteins promote epithelial cell spreading and motility. J Virol 79:1789-802.

[6] Altieri, D. C. 2008. New wirings in the survivin networks. Oncogene 27:6276-84.

[7] Apcher, S., C. Daskalogianni, B. Manoury, and R. Fahraeus. 2010. Epstein Barr virus-encoded EBNA1 interference with MHC class I antigen presentation reveals a close correlation between mRNA translation initiation and antigen presentation. PLoS Pathog 6:e1001151.

[8] Bangaru, M. L., S. Chen, J. Woodliff, and S. Kansra. 2010. Curcumin (diferuloylmethane) induces apoptosis and blocks migration of human medulloblastoma cells. Anticancer Res 30:499-504.

[9] Baur, J. A., K. J. Pearson, N. L. Price, H. A. Jamieson, C. Lerin, A. Kalra, V. V. Prabhu, J. S. Allard, G. Lopez-Lluch, K. Lewis, P. J. Pistell, S. Poosala, K. G. Becker, O. Boss, D. Gwinn, M. Wang, S. Ramaswamy, K. W. Fishbein, R. G. Spencer, E. G. Lakatta, D. Le Couteur, R. J. Shaw, P. Navas, P. Puigserver, D. K. Ingram, R. de Cabo, and D. A. Sinclair. 2006. Resveratrol improves health and survival of mice on a high-calorie diet. Nature 444:337-42.

[10] Benner, S. E., and W. K. Hong. 1993. Clinical chemoprevention: developing a cancer prevention strategy. J Natl Cancer Inst 85:1446-7.

[11] Billaud, M., P. Busson, D. Huang, N. Mueller-Lantzch, G. Rousselet, O. Pavlish, H. Wakasugi, J. M. Seigneurin, T. Tursz, and G. M. Lenoir. 1989. Epstein-Barr virus (EBV)-containing nasopharyngeal carcinoma cells express the B-cell activation antigen blast2/CD23 and low levels of the EBV receptor CR2. J Virol 63:4121-8.

[12] Bishayee, A. 2009. Cancer prevention and treatment with resveratrol: from rodent studies to clinical trials. Cancer Prev Res (Phila) 2:409-18.

[13] Bishayee, A., and N. Dhir. 2009. Resveratrol-mediated chemoprevention of diethylnitrosamine-initiated hepatocarcinogenesis: inhibition of cell proliferation and induction of apoptosis. Chem Biol Interact 179:131-44.

[14] Bolos, V., J. Grego-Bessa, and J. L. de la Pompa. 2007. Notch signaling in development and cancer. Endocr Rev 28:339-63.

[15] Bradamante, S., L. Barenghi, F. Piccinini, A. A. Bertelli, R. De Jonge, P. Beemster, and J. W. De Jong. 2003. Resveratrol provides late-phase cardioprotection by means of a nitric oxide- and adenosine-mediated mechanism. Eur J Pharmacol 465:115-23.

[16] Brooks, L., Q. Y. Yao, A. B. Rickinson, and L. S. Young. 1992. Epstein-Barr virus latent gene transcription in nasopharyngeal carcinoma cells: coexpression of EBNA1, LMP1, and LMP2 transcripts. J Virol 66:2689-97.

[17] Burgos, J. S. 2005. Involvement of the Epstein-Barr virus in the nasopharyngeal carcinoma pathogenesis. Med Oncol 22:113-21.

[18] Burgos, J. S., and F. J. Vera-Sempere. 2000. Immunohistochemical absence of CD21 membrane receptor in nasopharyngeal carcinoma cells infected by Epstein-Barr virus in Spanish patients. Laryngoscope 110:2081-4.

[19] Burgstahler, R., B. Kempkes, K. Steube, and M. Lipp. 1995. Expression of the chemokine receptor BLR2/EBI1 is specifically transactivated by Epstein-Barr virus nuclear antigen 2. Biochem Biophys Res Commun 215:737-43.

[20] Busson, P., C. Keryer, T. Ooka, and M. Corbex. 2004. EBV-associated nasopharyngeal carcinomas: from epidemiology to virus-targeting strategies. Trends Microbiol 12:356-60.

[21] Busson, P., R. McCoy, R. Sadler, K. Gilligan, T. Tursz, and N. Raab-Traub. 1992. Consistent transcription of the Epstein-Barr virus LMP2 gene in nasopharyngeal carcinoma. J Virol 66:3257-62.

[22] Cadenas, S., and G. Barja. 1999. Resveratrol, melatonin, vitamin E, and PBN protect against renal oxidative DNA damage induced by the kidney carcinogen KBrO3. Free Radic Biol Med 26:1531-7.

[23] Cai, X. Z., J. Wang, X. D. Li, G. L. Wang, F. N. Liu, M. S. Cheng, and F. Li. 2009. Curcumin suppresses proliferation and invasion in human gastric cancer cells by downregulation of PAK1 activity and cyclin D1 expression. Cancer Biol Ther 8:1360-8.

[24] Cambier, J. C. 1995. New nomenclature for the Reth motif (or ARH1/TAM/ARAM/YXXL). Immunol Today 16:110.

[25] Canaan, A., I. Haviv, A. E. Urban, V. P. Schulz, S. Hartman, Z. Zhang, D. Palejev, A. B. Deisseroth, J. Lacy, M. Snyder, M. Gerstein, and S. M. Weissman. 2009. EBNA1 regulates cellular gene expression by binding cellular promoters. Proc Natl Acad Sci U S A 106:22421-6.

[26] Cao, J., Y. Liu, L. Jia, H. M. Zhou, Y. Kong, G. Yang, L. P. Jiang, Q. J. Li, and L. F. Zhong. 2007. Curcumin induces apoptosis through mitochondrial hyperpolarization and mtDNA damage in human hepatoma G2 cells. Free Radic Biol Med 43:968-75.

[27] Carbone, M., and H. I. Pass. 2004. Multistep and multifactorial carcinogenesis: when does a contributing factor become a carcinogen? Semin Cancer Biol 14:399-405.

[28] Cardenas, C., A. R. Quesada, and M. A. Medina. 2006. Evaluation of the anti-angiogenic effect of aloe-emodin. Cell Mol Life Sci 63:3083-9.

[29] Castiglione, S., M. Fanciulli, T. Bruno, M. Evangelista, C. Del Carlo, M. G. Paggi, A. Chersi, and A. Floridi. 1993. Rhein inhibits glucose uptake in Ehrlich ascites tumor cells by alteration of membrane-associated functions. Anticancer Drugs 4:407-14.

[30] Castiglione, S., M. G. Paggi, A. Delpino, M. Zeuli, and A. Floridi. 1990. Inhibition of protein synthesis in neoplastic cells by rhein. Biochem Pharmacol 40:967-73.

[31] Chatterjee, M., S. Das, M. Janarthan, H. K. Ramachandran, and M. Chatterjee. 2011. Role of 5-lipoxygenase in resveratrol mediated suppression of 7,12-

dimethylbenz(alpha)anthracene-induced mammary carcinogenesis in rats. Eur J Pharmacol 668:99-106.

[32] Chau, C. M., and P. M. Lieberman. 2004. Dynamic chromatin boundaries delineate a latency control region of Epstein-Barr virus. J Virol 78:12308-19.

[33] Chen, H. W., J. Y. Lee, J. Y. Huang, C. C. Wang, W. J. Chen, S. F. Su, C. W. Huang, C. C. Ho, J. J. Chen, M. F. Tsai, S. L. Yu, and P. C. Yang. 2008. Curcumin inhibits lung cancer cell invasion and metastasis through the tumor suppressor HLJ1. Cancer Res 68:7428-38.

[34] Chen, H. W., S. L. Yu, J. J. Chen, H. N. Li, Y. C. Lin, P. L. Yao, H. Y. Chou, C. T. Chien, W. J. Chen, Y. T. Lee, and P. C. Yang. 2004. Anti-invasive gene expression profile of curcumin in lung adenocarcinoma based on a high throughput microarray analysis. Mol Pharmacol 65:99-110.

[35] Chen, L., L. Gallicchio, K. Boyd-Lindsley, X. G. Tao, K. A. Robinson, T. K. Lam, J. G. Herman, L. E. Caulfield, E. Guallar, and A. J. Alberg. 2009. Alcohol consumption and the risk of nasopharyngeal carcinoma: a systematic review. Nutr Cancer 61:1-15.

[36] Chen, M. R., J. M. Middeldorp, and S. D. Hayward. 1993. Separation of the complex DNA binding domain of EBNA-1 into DNA recognition and dimerization subdomains of novel structure. J Virol 67:4875-85.

[37] Chen, Q., S. Ganapathy, K. P. Singh, S. Shankar, and R. K. Srivastava. 2010. Resveratrol induces growth arrest and apoptosis through activation of FOXO transcription factors in prostate cancer cells. PLoS One 5:e15288.

[38] Chen, Q., Y. Wang, K. Xu, G. Lu, Z. Ying, L. Wu, J. Zhan, R. Fang, Y. Wu, and J. Zhou. 2010. Curcumin induces apoptosis in human lung adenocarcinoma A549 cells through a reactive oxygen species-dependent mitochondrial signaling pathway. Oncol Rep 23:397-403.

[39] Chen, Q. Y., J. G. Shi, Q. H. Yao, D. M. Jiao, Y. Y. Wang, H. Z. Hu, Y. Q. Wu, J. Song, J. Yan, and L. J. Wu. 2012. Lysosomal membrane permeabilization is involved in curcumin-induced apoptosis of A549 lung carcinoma cells. Mol Cell Biochem. 359:389-98.

[40] Chen, Y., D. Li, H. Liu, H. Xu, H. Zheng, F. Qian, W. Li, C. Zhao, Z. Wang, and X. Wang. 2011. Notch-1 signaling facilitates survivin expression in human non-small cell lung cancer cells. Cancer Biol Ther 11:14-21.

[41] Chen, Y. K., C. Cheung, K. R. Reuhl, A. B. Liu, M. J. Lee, Y. P. Lu, and C. S. Yang. 2011. Effects of Green Tea Polyphenol (-)-Epigallocatechin-3-gallate on a Newly Developed High-fat/Western-style Diet-induced Obesity and Metabolic Syndrome in Mice. J Agric Food Chem 59:11862-71.

[42] Chen, Y. Y., S. Y. Chiang, J. G. Lin, J. S. Yang, Y. S. Ma, C. L. Liao, T. Y. Lai, N. Y. Tang, and J. G. Chung. 2010. Emodin, aloe-emodin and rhein induced DNA damage and inhibited DNA repair gene expression in SCC-4 human tongue cancer cells. Anticancer Res 30:945-51.

[43] Cheng, S. H., J. J. Jian, S. Y. Tsai, K. L. Yen, N. M. Chu, K. Y. Chan, T. D. Tan, J. C. Cheng, S. Y. Leu, C. Y. Hsieh, and A. T. Huang. 2000. Long-term survival of

nasopharyngeal carcinoma following concomitant radiotherapy and chemotherapy. Int J Radiat Oncol Biol Phys 48:1323-30.
[44] Chiaramonte, R., E. Calzavara, A. Basile, P. Comi, and G. V. Sherbet. 2002. Notch signal transduction is not regulated by SEL1L in leukaemia and lymphoma cells in culture. Anticancer Res 22:4211-4.
[45] Chou, J., Y. C. Lin, J. Kim, L. You, Z. Xu, B. He, and D. M. Jablons. 2008. Nasopharyngeal carcinoma--review of the molecular mechanisms of tumorigenesis. Head Neck 30:946-63.
[46] Chow, K. C., S. H. Chiou, S. P. Ho, M. H. Tsai, C. L. Chen, L. S. Wang, and K. H. Chi. 2003. The elevated serum interleukin-6 correlates with the increased serum butyrate level in patients with nasopharyngeal carcinoma. Oncol Rep 10:813-9.
[47] Chow, S. E., J. S. Wang, S. F. Chuang, Y. L. Chang, W. K. Chu, W. S. Chen, and Y. W. Chen. 2010. Resveratrol-induced p53-independent apoptosis of human nasopharyngeal carcinoma cells is correlated with the downregulation of DeltaNp63. Cancer Gene Ther 17:872-82.
[48] Christofori, G., and H. Semb. 1999. The role of the cell-adhesion molecule E-cadherin as a tumour-suppressor gene. Trends Biochem Sci 24:73-6.
[49] Ciesek, S., T. von Hahn, C. C. Colpitts, L. M. Schang, M. Friesland, J. Steinmann, M. P. Manns, M. Ott, H. Wedemeyer, P. Meuleman, T. Pietschmann, and E. Steinmann. 2011. The green tea polyphenol epigallocatechin-3-gallate (EGCG) inhibits hepatitis C virus (HCV) entry. Hepatology 54:1947-55.
[50] Cohen, J. I. 2000. Epstein-Barr virus infection. N Engl J Med 343:481-92.
[51] Cordier-Bussat, M., M. Billaud, A. Calender, and G. M. Lenoir. 1993. Epstein-Barr virus (EBV) nuclear-antigen-2-induced up-regulation of CD21 and CD23 molecules is dependent on a permissive cellular context. Int J Cancer 53:153-60.
[52] Cory, S., and J. M. Adams. 2002. The Bcl2 family: regulators of the cellular life-or-death switch. Nat Rev Cancer 2:647-56.
[53] Cos, P., T. De Bruyne, N. Hermans, S. Apers, D. V. Berghe, and A. J. Vlietinck. 2004. Proanthocyanidins in health care: current and new trends. Curr Med Chem 11:1345-59.
[54] Csiszar, A., N. Labinskyy, S. Olson, J. T. Pinto, S. Gupte, J. M. Wu, F. Hu, P. Ballabh, A. Podlutsky, G. Losonczy, R. de Cabo, R. Mathew, M. S. Wolin, and Z. Ungvari. 2009. Resveratrol prevents monocrotaline-induced pulmonary hypertension in rats. Hypertension 54:668-75.
[55] Cui, X., Y. Jin, A. B. Hofseth, E. Pena, J. Habiger, A. Chumanevich, D. Poudyal, M. Nagarkatti, P. S. Nagarkatti, U. P. Singh, and L. J. Hofseth. 2010. Resveratrol suppresses colitis and colon cancer associated with colitis. Cancer Prev Res (Phila) 3:549-59.
[56] Das, A., N. L. Banik, and S. K. Ray. 2010. Flavonoids activated caspases for apoptosis in human glioblastoma T98G and U87MG cells but not in human normal astrocytes. Cancer 116:164-76.
[57] Dawson, C. W., A. G. Eliopoulos, S. M. Blake, R. Barker, and L. S. Young. 2000. Identification of functional differences between prototype Epstein-Barr virus-

encoded LMP1 and a nasopharyngeal carcinoma-derived LMP1 in human epithelial cells. Virology 272:204-17.

[58] Dawson, C. W., A. B. Rickinson, and L. S. Young. 1990. Epstein-Barr virus latent membrane protein inhibits human epithelial cell differentiation. Nature 344:777-80.

[59] Dawson, C. W., G. Tramountanis, A. G. Eliopoulos, and L. S. Young. 2003. Epstein-Barr virus latent membrane protein 1 (LMP1) activates the phosphatidylinositol 3-kinase/Akt pathway to promote cell survival and induce actin filament remodeling. J Biol Chem 278:3694-704.

[60] Dhillon, A. S., S. Hagan, O. Rath, and W. Kolch. 2007. MAP kinase signalling pathways in cancer. Oncogene 26:3279-90.

[61] Dickson, R. I., and A. D. Flores. 1985. Nasopharyngeal carcinoma: an evaluation of 134 patients treated between 1971-1980. Laryngoscope 95:276-83.

[62] Duellman, S. J., K. L. Thompson, J. J. Coon, and R. R. Burgess. 2009. Phosphorylation sites of Epstein-Barr virus EBNA1 regulate its function. J Gen Virol 90:2251-9.

[63] Dukers, D. F., P. Meij, M. B. Vervoort, W. Vos, R. J. Scheper, C. J. Meijer, E. Bloemena, and J. M. Middeldorp. 2000. Direct immunosuppressive effects of EBV-encoded latent membrane protein 1. J Immunol 165:663-70.

[64] Eliopoulos, A. G., N. J. Gallagher, S. M. Blake, C. W. Dawson, and L. S. Young. 1999. Activation of the p38 mitogen-activated protein kinase pathway by Epstein-Barr virus-encoded latent membrane protein 1 coregulates interleukin-6 and interleukin-8 production. J Biol Chem 274:16085-96.

[65] Eliopoulos, A. G., M. Stack, C. W. Dawson, K. M. Kaye, L. Hodgkin, S. Sihota, M. Rowe, and L. S. Young. 1997. Epstein-Barr virus-encoded LMP1 and CD40 mediate IL-6 production in epithelial cells via an NF-kappaB pathway involving TNF receptor-associated factors. Oncogene 14:2899-916.

[66] Elmali, N., O. Baysal, A. Harma, I. Esenkaya, and B. Mizrak. 2007. Effects of resveratrol in inflammatory arthritis. Inflammation 30:1-6.

[67] Fahraeus, R., W. Chen, P. Trivedi, G. Klein, and B. Obrink. 1992. Decreased expression of E-cadherin and increased invasive capacity in EBV-LMP-transfected human epithelial and murine adenocarcinoma cells. Int J Cancer 52:834-8.

[68] Fahraeus, R., H. L. Fu, I. Ernberg, J. Finke, M. Rowe, G. Klein, K. Falk, E. Nilsson, M. Yadav, P. Busson, and et al. 1988. Expression of Epstein-Barr virus-encoded proteins in nasopharyngeal carcinoma. Int J Cancer 42:329-38.

[69] Filippi-Chiela, E. C., E. S. Villodre, L. L. Zamin, and G. Lenz. 2011. Autophagy interplay with apoptosis and cell cycle regulation in the growth inhibiting effect of resveratrol in glioma cells. PLoS One 6:e20849.

[70] Fingeroth, J. D., J. J. Weis, T. F. Tedder, J. L. Strominger, P. A. Biro, and D. T. Fearon. 1984. Epstein-Barr virus receptor of human B lymphocytes is the C3d receptor CR2. Proc Natl Acad Sci U S A 81:4510-4.

[71] Flanagan, J., J. Middeldorp, and T. Sculley. 2003. Localization of the Epstein-Barr virus protein LMP 1 to exosomes. J Gen Virol 84:1871-9.

[72] Florian, T., J. Necas, L. Bartosikova, J. Klusakova, V. Suchy, E. B. Naggara, E. Janostikova, and T. Bartosik. 2006. Effects of prenylated isoflavones osajin and

pomiferin in premedication on heart ischemia-reperfusion. Biomed Pap Med Fac Univ Palacky Olomouc Czech Repub 150:93-100.
[73] Floridi, A., S. Castiglione, C. Bianchi, and A. Mancini. 1990. Effect of rhein on the glucose metabolism of Ehrlich ascites tumor cells. Biochem Pharmacol 40:217-22.
[74] Floridi, A., F. P. Gentile, T. Bruno, S. Castiglione, M. Zeuli, and M. Benassi. 1990. Growth inhibition by rhein and lonidamine of human glioma cells in vitro. Anticancer Res 10:1633-6.
[75] Frei, B., and J. V. Higdon. 2003. Antioxidant activity of tea polyphenols in vivo: evidence from animal studies. J Nutr 133:3275S-84S.
[76] Freile, M. L., F. Giannini, G. Pucci, A. Sturniolo, L. Rodero, O. Pucci, V. Balzareti, and R. D. Enriz. 2003. Antimicrobial activity of aqueous extracts and of berberine isolated from Berberis heterophylla. Fitoterapia 74:702-5.
[77] Freudlsperger, C., J. Greten, and U. Schumacher. 2008. Curcumin induces apoptosis in human neuroblastoma cells via inhibition of NFkappaB. Anticancer Res 28:209-14.
[78] Fries, K. L., W. E. Miller, and N. Raab-Traub. 1996. Epstein-Barr virus latent membrane protein 1 blocks p53-mediated apoptosis through the induction of the A20 gene. J Virol 70:8653-9.
[79] Fruehling, S., R. Swart, K. M. Dolwick, E. Kremmer, and R. Longnecker. 1998. Tyrosine 112 of latent membrane protein 2A is essential for protein tyrosine kinase loading and regulation of Epstein-Barr virus latency. J Virol 72:7796-806.
[80] Fujiwara, S., Y. Nitadori, H. Nakamura, T. Nagaishi, and Y. Ono. 1999. Epstein-barr virus (EBV) nuclear protein 2-induced disruption of EBV latency in the Burkitt's lymphoma cell line Akata: analysis by tetracycline-regulated expression. J Virol 73:5214-9.
[81] Gahn, T. A., and B. Sugden. 1995. An EBNA-1-dependent enhancer acts from a distance of 10 kilobase pairs to increase expression of the Epstein-Barr virus LMP gene. J Virol 69:2633-6.
[82] George, J., M. Singh, A. K. Srivastava, K. Bhui, P. Roy, P. K. Chaturvedi, and Y. Shukla. 2011. Resveratrol and Black Tea Polyphenol Combination Synergistically Suppress Mouse Skin Tumors Growth by Inhibition of Activated MAPKs and p53. PLoS One 6:e23395.
[83] Gillespie, K., I. Kodani, D. P. Dickinson, K. U. Ogbureke, A. M. Camba, M. Wu, S. Looney, T. C. Chu, H. Qin, F. Bisch, M. Sharawy, G. S. Schuster, and S. D. Hsu. 2008. Effects of oral consumption of the green tea polyphenol EGCG in a murine model for human Sjogren's syndrome, an autoimmune disease. Life Sci 83:581-8.
[84] Glickman, J. N., J. G. Howe, and J. A. Steitz. 1988. Structural analyses of EBER1 and EBER2 ribonucleoprotein particles present in Epstein-Barr virus-infected cells. J Virol 62:902-11.
[85] Gordadze, A. V., C. W. Onunwor, R. Peng, D. Poston, E. Kremmer, and P. D. Ling. 2004. EBNA2 amino acids 3 to 30 are required for induction of LMP-1 and immortalization maintenance. J Virol 78:3919-29.
[86] Green, D. R., and J. C. Reed. 1998. Mitochondria and apoptosis. Science 281:1309-12.
[87] Gross, A., J. M. McDonnell, and S. J. Korsmeyer. 1999. BCL-2 family members and the mitochondria in apoptosis. Genes Dev 13:1899-911.

[88] Gross, H., S. Barth, T. Pfuhl, V. Willnecker, A. Spurk, V. Gurtsevitch, M. Sauter, B. Hu, E. Noessner, N. Mueller-Lantzsch, E. Kremmer, and F. A. Grasser. 2011. The NP9 protein encoded by the human endogenous retrovirus HERV-K(HML-2) negatively regulates gene activation of the Epstein-Barr virus nuclear antigen 2 (EBNA2). Int J Cancer 129:1105-15.

[89] Gruhne, B., R. Sompallae, D. Marescotti, S. A. Kamranvar, S. Gastaldello, and M. G. Masucci. 2009. The Epstein-Barr virus nuclear antigen-1 promotes genomic instability via induction of reactive oxygen species. Proc Natl Acad Sci U S A 106:2313-8.

[90] Guha, P., A. Dey, R. Sen, M. Chatterjee, S. Chattopadhyay, and S. K. Bandyopadhyay. 2011. Intracellular GSH depletion triggered mitochondrial Bax translocation to accomplish resveratrol-induced apoptosis in the U937 cell line. J Pharmacol Exp Ther 336:206-14.

[91] Guo, J. M., B. X. Xiao, Q. Liu, S. Zhang, D. H. Liu, and Z. H. Gong. 2007. Anticancer effect of aloe-emodin on cervical cancer cells involves G2/M arrest and induction of differentiation. Acta Pharmacol Sin 28:1991-5.

[92] Guo, M. Z., X. S. Li, D. M. Shen, X. Q. Guan, H. R. Xu, and J. Gao. 2003. [Effect of Rhein on the development of hepatic fibrosis in rats]. Zhonghua Gan Zang Bing Za Zhi 11:26-9.

[93] Hammerschmidt, W., B. Sugden, and V. R. Baichwal. 1989. The transforming domain alone of the latent membrane protein of Epstein-Barr virus is toxic to cells when expressed at high levels. J Virol 63:2469-75.

[94] Hamza, A., and C. G. Zhan. 2006. How can (-)-epigallocatechin gallate from green tea prevent HIV-1 infection? Mechanistic insights from computational modeling and the implication for rational design of anti-HIV-1 entry inhibitors. J Phys Chem B 110:2910-7.

[95] Hartojo, W., A. L. Silvers, D. G. Thomas, C. W. Seder, L. Lin, H. Rao, Z. Wang, J. K. Greenson, T. J. Giordano, M. B. Orringer, A. Rehemtulla, M. S. Bhojani, D. G. Beer, and A. C. Chang. 2010. Curcumin promotes apoptosis, increases chemosensitivity, and inhibits nuclear factor kappaB in esophageal adenocarcinoma. Transl Oncol 3:99-108.

[96] Hattori, R., H. Otani, N. Maulik, and D. K. Das. 2002. Pharmacological preconditioning with resveratrol: role of nitric oxide. Am J Physiol Heart Circ Physiol 282:H1988-95.

[97] He, Z. H., M. F. He, S. C. Ma, and P. P. But. 2009. Anti-angiogenic effects of rhubarb and its anthraquinone derivatives. J Ethnopharmacol 121:313-7.

[98] He, Z. H., R. Zhou, M. F. He, C. B. Lau, G. G. Yue, W. Ge, and P. P. But. 2011. Anti-angiogenic effect and mechanism of rhein from Rhizoma Rhei. Phytomedicine 18:470-8.

[99] Henderson, S., M. Rowe, C. Gregory, D. Croom-Carter, F. Wang, R. Longnecker, E. Kieff, and A. Rickinson. 1991. Induction of bcl-2 expression by Epstein-Barr virus latent membrane protein 1 protects infected B cells from programmed cell death. Cell 65:1107-15.

[100] Herman, J. G., H. L. Stadelman, and C. E. Roselli. 2009. Curcumin blocks CCL2-induced adhesion, motility and invasion, in part, through down-regulation of CCL2 expression and proteolytic activity. Int J Oncol 34:1319-27.

[101] Herrmann, K., and G. Niedobitek. 2003. Epstein-Barr virus-associated carcinomas: facts and fiction. J Pathol 199:140-5.

[102] Heussinger, N., M. Buttner, G. Ott, E. Brachtel, B. Z. Pilch, E. Kremmer, and G. Niedobitek. 2004. Expression of the Epstein-Barr virus (EBV)-encoded latent membrane protein 2A (LMP2A) in EBV-associated nasopharyngeal carcinoma. J Pathol 203:696-9.

[103] Hideshima, T., M. Akiyama, T. Hayashi, P. Richardson, R. Schlossman, D. Chauhan, and K. C. Anderson. 2003. Targeting p38 MAPK inhibits multiple myeloma cell growth in the bone marrow milieu. Blood 101:703-5.

[104] Higdon, J. V., and B. Frei. 2003. Tea catechins and polyphenols: health effects, metabolism, and antioxidant functions. Crit Rev Food Sci Nutr 43:89-143.

[105] Hilchie, A. L., S. J. Furlong, K. Sutton, A. Richardson, M. R. Robichaud, C. A. Giacomantonio, N. D. Ridgway, and D. W. Hoskin. 2010. Curcumin-induced apoptosis in PC3 prostate carcinoma cells is caspase-independent and involves cellular ceramide accumulation and damage to mitochondria. Nutr Cancer 62:379-89.

[106] Ho, Y. T., J. S. Yang, T. C. Li, J. J. Lin, J. G. Lin, K. C. Lai, C. Y. Ma, W. G. Wood, and J. G. Chung. 2009. Berberine suppresses in vitro migration and invasion of human SCC-4 tongue squamous cancer cells through the inhibitions of FAK, IKK, NF-kappaB, u-PA and MMP-2 and -9. Cancer Lett 279:155-62.

[107] Hoe, S. L., E. S. Lee, A. S. Khoo, and S. C. Peh. 2009. p53 and nasopharyngeal carcinoma: a Malaysian study. Pathology 41:561-5.

[108] Hsia, T. C., J. S. Yang, G. W. Chen, T. H. Chiu, H. F. Lu, M. D. Yang, F. S. Yu, K. C. Liu, K. C. Lai, C. C. Lin, and J. G. Chung. 2009. The roles of endoplasmic reticulum stress and Ca2+ on rhein-induced apoptosis in A-549 human lung cancer cells. Anticancer Res 29:309-18.

[109] Hsieh, J. J., and S. D. Hayward. 1995. Masking of the CBF1/RBPJ kappa transcriptional repression domain by Epstein-Barr virus EBNA2. Science 268:560-3.

[110] Hsu, S. D., D. P. Dickinson, H. Qin, J. Borke, K. U. Ogbureke, J. N. Winger, A. M. Camba, W. B. Bollag, H. J. Stoppler, M. M. Sharawy, and G. S. Schuster. 2007. Green tea polyphenols reduce autoimmune symptoms in a murine model for human Sjogren's syndrome and protect human salivary acinar cells from TNF-alpha-induced cytotoxicity. Autoimmunity 40:138-47.

[111] Hsu, W. H., Y. S. Hsieh, H. C. Kuo, C. Y. Teng, H. I. Huang, C. J. Wang, S. F. Yang, Y. S. Liou, and W. H. Kuo. 2007. Berberine induces apoptosis in SW620 human colonic carcinoma cells through generation of reactive oxygen species and activation of JNK/p38 MAPK and FasL. Arch Toxicol 81:719-28.

[112] Huang, C., G. Yang, T. Jiang, G. Zhu, H. Li, and Z. Qiu. 2011. The effects and mechanisms of blockage of STAT3 signaling pathway on IL-6 inducing EMT in human pancreatic cancer cells in vitro. Neoplasma 58:396-405.

[113] Huang, T. T., H. C. Lin, C. C. Chen, C. C. Lu, C. F. Wei, T. S. Wu, F. G. Liu, and H. C. Lai. 2011. Resveratrol induces apoptosis of human nasopharyngeal carcinoma cells via activation of multiple apoptotic pathways. J Cell Physiol 226:720-8.
[114] Huang, T. T., F. G. Liu, C. F. Wei, C. C. Lu, C. C. Chen, H. C. Lin, D. M. Ojcius, and H. C. Lai. 2011. Activation of multiple apoptotic pathways in human nasopharyngeal carcinoma cells by the prenylated isoflavone, osajin. PLoS One 6:e18308.
[115] Hudson, G. S., P. J. Farrell, and B. G. Barrell. 1985. Two related but differentially expressed potential membrane proteins encoded by the EcoRI Dhet region of Epstein-Barr virus B95-8. J Virol 53:528-35.
[116] Hung, L. M., M. J. Su, and J. K. Chen. 2004. Resveratrol protects myocardial ischemia-reperfusion injury through both NO-dependent and NO-independent mechanisms. Free Radic Biol Med 36:774-81.
[117] Hussain, A. R., S. Uddin, R. Bu, O. S. Khan, S. O. Ahmed, M. Ahmed, and K. S. Al-Kuraya. 2011. Resveratrol Suppresses Constitutive Activation of AKT via Generation of ROS and Induces Apoptosis in Diffuse Large B Cell Lymphoma Cell Lines. PLoS One 6:e24703.
[118] Hwang, J. M., H. C. Kuo, T. H. Tseng, J. Y. Liu, and C. Y. Chu. 2006. Berberine induces apoptosis through a mitochondria/caspases pathway in human hepatoma cells. Arch Toxicol 80:62-73.
[119] Imamura, G., A. A. Bertelli, A. Bertelli, H. Otani, N. Maulik, and D. K. Das. 2002. Pharmacological preconditioning with resveratrol: an insight with iNOS knockout mice. Am J Physiol Heart Circ Physiol 282:H1996-2003.
[120] Ip, S. W., Y. S. Weng, S. Y. Lin, D. Mei, N. Y. Tang, C. C. Su, and J. G. Chung. 2007. The role of Ca+2 on rhein-induced apoptosis in human cervical cancer Ca Ski cells. Anticancer Res 27:379-89.
[121] Jantova, S., L. Cipak, and S. Letasiova. 2007. Berberine induces apoptosis through a mitochondrial/caspase pathway in human promonocytic U937 cells. Toxicol In Vitro 21:25-31.
[122] Jarriault, S., C. Brou, F. Logeat, E. H. Schroeter, R. Kopan, and A. Israel. 1995. Signalling downstream of activated mammalian Notch. Nature 377:355-8.
[123] Jee, S. H., S. C. Shen, C. R. Tseng, H. C. Chiu, and M. L. Kuo. 1998. Curcumin induces a p53-dependent apoptosis in human basal cell carcinoma cells. J Invest Dermatol 111:656-61.
[124] Jiang, M. C., H. F. Yang-Yen, J. J. Yen, and J. K. Lin. 1996. Curcumin induces apoptosis in immortalized NIH 3T3 and malignant cancer cell lines. Nutr Cancer 26:111-20.
[125] Jiang, R., X. Gu, C. O. Nathan, and L. Hutt-Fletcher. 2008. Laser-capture microdissection of oropharyngeal epithelium indicates restriction of Epstein-Barr virus receptor/CD21 mRNA to tonsil epithelial cells. J Oral Pathol Med 37:626-33.
[126] Johansson, P., A. Jansson, U. Ruetschi, and L. Rymo. 2010. The p38 signaling pathway upregulates expression of the Epstein-Barr virus LMP1 oncogene. J Virol 84:2787-97.
[127] Johnstone, R. W., A. A. Ruefli, and S. W. Lowe. 2002. Apoptosis: a link between cancer genetics and chemotherapy. Cell 108:153-64.

[128] Jones, R. J., L. J. Smith, C. W. Dawson, T. Haigh, N. W. Blake, and L. S. Young. 2003. Epstein-Barr virus nuclear antigen 1 (EBNA1) induced cytotoxicity in epithelial cells is associated with EBNA1 degradation and processing. Virology 313:663-76.
[129] Jung, K. H., and J. W. Park. 2011. Suppression of mitochondrial NADP(+)-dependent isocitrate dehydrogenase activity enhances curcumin-induced apoptosis in HCT116 cells. Free Radic Res 45:431-8.
[130] Kaiser, C., G. Laux, D. Eick, N. Jochner, G. W. Bornkamm, and B. Kempkes. 1999. The proto-oncogene c-myc is a direct target gene of Epstein-Barr virus nuclear antigen 2. J Virol 73:4481-4.
[131] Kaneda, Y., M. Torii, T. Tanaka, and M. Aikawa. 1991. In vitro effects of berberine sulphate on the growth and structure of Entamoeba histolytica, Giardia lamblia and Trichomonas vaginalis. Ann Trop Med Parasitol 85:417-25.
[132] Kartal, M., G. Saydam, F. Sahin, and Y. Baran. 2011. Resveratrol triggers apoptosis through regulating ceramide metabolizing genes in human K562 chronic myeloid leukemia cells. Nutr Cancer 63:637-44.
[133] Kelloff, G. J. 2000. Perspectives on cancer chemoprevention research and drug development. Adv Cancer Res 78:199-334.
[134] Keryer-Bibens, C., C. Pioche-Durieu, C. Villemant, S. Souquere, N. Nishi, M. Hirashima, J. Middeldorp, and P. Busson. 2006. Exosomes released by EBV-infected nasopharyngeal carcinoma cells convey the viral latent membrane protein 1 and the immunomodulatory protein galectin 9. BMC Cancer 6:283.
[135] Khan, N., F. Afaq, M. Saleem, N. Ahmad, and H. Mukhtar. 2006. Targeting multiple signaling pathways by green tea polyphenol (-)-epigallocatechin-3-gallate. Cancer Res 66:2500-5.
[136] Khin Maung, U., K. Myo, W. Nyunt Nyunt, K. Aye, and U. Tin. 1985. Clinical trial of berberine in acute watery diarrhoea. Br Med J (Clin Res Ed) 291:1601-5.
[137] Kieff, E., and A. E. Rickinson. 2007. Epstein-Barr virus and its replication. Fields Virology 2:2603–2654.
[138] Kim, K. R., T. Yoshizaki, H. Miyamori, K. Hasegawa, T. Horikawa, M. Furukawa, S. Harada, M. Seiki, and H. Sato. 2000. Transformation of Madin-Darby canine kidney (MDCK) epithelial cells by Epstein-Barr virus latent membrane protein 1 (LMP1) induces expression of Ets1 and invasive growth. Oncogene 19:1764-71.
[139] Kim, S., J. H. Choi, J. B. Kim, S. J. Nam, J. H. Yang, J. H. Kim, and J. E. Lee. 2008. Berberine suppresses TNF-alpha-induced MMP-9 and cell invasion through inhibition of AP-1 activity in MDA-MB-231 human breast cancer cells. Molecules 13:2975-85.
[140] Klibi, J., T. Niki, A. Riedel, C. Pioche-Durieu, S. Souquere, E. Rubinstein, S. Le Moulec, J. Guigay, M. Hirashima, F. Guemira, D. Adhikary, J. Mautner, and P. Busson. 2009. Blood diffusion and Th1-suppressive effects of galectin-9-containing exosomes released by Epstein-Barr virus-infected nasopharyngeal carcinoma cells. Blood 113:1957-66.
[141] Ko, Y. C., C. L. Chang, H. F. Chien, C. H. Wu, and L. I. Lin. 2011. Resveratrol enhances the expression of death receptor Fas/CD95 and induces differentiation and apoptosis in anaplastic large-cell lymphoma cells. Cancer Lett 309:46-53.

[142] Kong, Q. L., L. J. Hu, J. Y. Cao, Y. J. Huang, L. H. Xu, Y. Liang, D. Xiong, S. Guan, B. H. Guo, H. Q. Mai, Q. Y. Chen, X. Zhang, M. Z. Li, J. Y. Shao, C. N. Qian, Y. F. Xia, L. B. Song, Y. X. Zeng, and M. S. Zeng. 2010. Epstein-Barr virus-encoded LMP2A induces an epithelial-mesenchymal transition and increases the number of side population stem-like cancer cells in nasopharyngeal carcinoma. PLoS Pathog 6:e1000940.

[143] Kulkarni, S. K., and A. Dhir. 2010. Berberine: a plant alkaloid with therapeutic potential for central nervous system disorders. Phytother Res 24:317-24.

[144] Kunnumakkara, A. B., P. Anand, and B. B. Aggarwal. 2008. Curcumin inhibits proliferation, invasion, angiogenesis and metastasis of different cancers through interaction with multiple cell signaling proteins. Cancer Lett 269:199-225.

[145] Kuo, C. L., S. Y. Wu, S. W. Ip, P. P. Wu, C. S. Yu, J. S. Yang, P. Y. Chen, S. H. Wu, and J. G. Chung. 2011. Apoptotic death in curcumin-treated NPC-TW 076 human nasopharyngeal carcinoma cells is mediated through the ROS, mitochondrial depolarization and caspase-3-dependent signaling responses. Int J Oncol 39:319-28.

[146] Kuo, P. L., Y. L. Hsu, L. T. Ng, and C. C. Lin. 2004. Rhein inhibits the growth and induces the apoptosis of Hep G2 cells. Planta Med 70:12-6.

[147] Kuo, P. L., T. C. Lin, and C. C. Lin. 2002. The antiproliferative activity of aloe-emodin is through p53-dependent and p21-dependent apoptotic pathway in human hepatoma cell lines. Life Sci 71:1879-92.

[148] Lafrenie, R. M., M. R. Buchanan, and F. W. Orr. 1993. Adhesion molecules and their role in cancer metastasis. Cell Biophys 23:3-89.

[149] Laherty, C. D., H. M. Hu, A. W. Opipari, F. Wang, and V. M. Dixit. 1992. The Epstein-Barr virus LMP1 gene product induces A20 zinc finger protein expression by activating nuclear factor kappa B. J Biol Chem 267:24157-60.

[150] Lai, W. W., J. S. Yang, K. C. Lai, C. L. Kuo, C. K. Hsu, C. K. Wang, C. Y. Chang, J. J. Lin, N. Y. Tang, P. Y. Chen, W. W. Huang, and J. G. Chung. 2009. Rhein induced apoptosis through the endoplasmic reticulum stress, caspase- and mitochondria-dependent pathways in SCC-4 human tongue squamous cancer cells. In Vivo 23:309-16.

[151] Lambert, J. D., and R. J. Elias. 2010. The antioxidant and pro-oxidant activities of green tea polyphenols: a role in cancer prevention. Arch Biochem Biophys 501:65-72.

[152] Larcher, C., B. Kempkes, E. Kremmer, W. M. Prodinger, M. Pawlita, G. W. Bornkamm, and M. P. Dierich. 1995. Expression of Epstein-Barr virus nuclear antigen-2 (EBNA2) induces CD21/CR2 on B and T cell lines and shedding of soluble CD21. Eur J Immunol 25:1713-9.

[153] Larrosa, M., M. J. Yanez-Gascon, M. V. Selma, A. Gonzalez-Sarrias, S. Toti, J. J. Ceron, F. Tomas-Barberan, P. Dolara, and J. C. Espin. 2009. Effect of a low dose of dietary resveratrol on colon microbiota, inflammation and tissue damage in a DSS-induced colitis rat model. J Agric Food Chem 57:2211-20.

[154] Lau, A. T., Y. Wang, and J. F. Chiu. 2008. Reactive oxygen species: current knowledge and applications in cancer research and therapeutic. J Cell Biochem 104:657-67.

[155] Lee, H. Z., S. L. Hsu, M. C. Liu, and C. H. Wu. 2001. Effects and mechanisms of aloe-emodin on cell death in human lung squamous cell carcinoma. Eur J Pharmacol 431:287-95.

[156] Lee, H. Z., C. J. Lin, W. H. Yang, W. C. Leung, and S. P. Chang. 2006. Aloe-emodin induced DNA damage through generation of reactive oxygen species in human lung carcinoma cells. Cancer Lett 239:55-63.

[157] Lee, H. Z., C. H. Wu, and S. P. Chang. 2005. Release of nucleophosmin from the nucleus: Involvement in aloe-emodin-induced human lung non small carcinoma cell apoptosis. Int J Cancer 113:971-6.

[158] Lee, J. M., K. H. Lee, M. Weidner, B. A. Osborne, and S. D. Hayward. 2002. Epstein-Barr virus EBNA2 blocks Nur77- mediated apoptosis. Proc Natl Acad Sci U S A 99:11878-83.

[159] Leight, E. R., and B. Sugden. 2000. EBNA-1: a protein pivotal to latent infection by Epstein-Barr virus. Rev Med Virol 10:83-100.

[160] Levenson, A. S., B. D. Gehm, S. T. Pearce, J. Horiguchi, L. A. Simons, J. E. Ward, 3rd, J. L. Jameson, and V. C. Jordan. 2003. Resveratrol acts as an estrogen receptor (ER) agonist in breast cancer cells stably transfected with ER alpha. Int J Cancer 104:587-96.

[161] Levitskaya, J., M. Coram, V. Levitsky, S. Imreh, P. M. Steigerwald-Mullen, G. Klein, M. G. Kurilla, and M. G. Masucci. 1995. Inhibition of antigen processing by the internal repeat region of the Epstein-Barr virus nuclear antigen-1. Nature 375:685-8.

[162] Li, D. M., and Y. M. Feng. 2011. Signaling mechanism of cell adhesion molecules in breast cancer metastasis: potential therapeutic targets. Breast Cancer Res Treat 128:7-21.

[163] Li, G., S. He, L. Chang, H. Lu, H. Zhang, H. Zhang, and J. Chiu. 2011. GADD45alpha and annexin A1 are involved in the apoptosis of HL-60 induced by resveratrol. Phytomedicine 18:704-9.

[164] Li, G. H., Y. Z. Fan, X. W. Liu, B. F. Zhang, D. D. Yin, F. He, S. Y. Huang, Z. J. Kang, H. Xu, Q. Liu, Y. L. Wu, X. L. Niu, L. Zhang, L. Liu, M. W. Hao, H. Han, and Y. M. Liang. 2010. Notch signaling maintains proliferation and survival of the HL60 human promyelocytic leukemia cell line and promotes the phosphorylation of the Rb protein. Mol Cell Biochem 340:7-14.

[165] Li, G. X., Y. K. Chen, Z. Hou, H. Xiao, H. Jin, G. Lu, M. J. Lee, B. Liu, F. Guan, Z. Yang, A. Yu, and C. S. Yang. 2010. Pro-oxidative activities and dose-response relationship of (-)-epigallocatechin-3-gallate in the inhibition of lung cancer cell growth: a comparative study in vivo and in vitro. Carcinogenesis 31:902-10.

[166] Li, J. X., K. Y. Zhou, K. R. Cai, T. Liang, X. D. Tang, and Y. F. Zhang. 2005. [Knockdown of bcl-xL expression with RNA interference induces nasopharyngeal carcinoma cells apoptosis]. Zhonghua Er Bi Yan Hou Tou Jing Wai Ke Za Zhi 40:347-51.

[167] Li, L., L. Guo, Y. Tao, S. Zhou, Z. Wang, W. Luo, D. Hu, Z. Li, L. Xiao, M. Tang, W. Yi, S. W. Tsao, and Y. Cao. 2007. Latent membrane protein 1 of Epstein-Barr virus regulates p53 phosphorylation through MAP kinases. Cancer Lett 255:219-31.

[168] Liao, P. C., L. T. Ng, L. T. Lin, C. D. Richardson, G. H. Wang, and C. C. Lin. 2010. Resveratrol arrests cell cycle and induces apoptosis in human hepatocellular carcinoma Huh-7 cells. J Med Food 13:1415-23.

[169] Lin, C. C., S. T. Kao, G. W. Chen, H. C. Ho, and J. G. Chung. 2006. Apoptosis of human leukemia HL-60 cells and murine leukemia WEHI-3 cells induced by berberine through the activation of caspase-3. Anticancer Res 26:227-42.

[170] Lin, C. C., J. S. Yang, J. T. Chen, S. Fan, F. S. Yu, J. L. Yang, C. C. Lu, M. C. Kao, A. C. Huang, H. F. Lu, and J. G. Chung. 2007. Berberine induces apoptosis in human HSC-3 oral cancer cells via simultaneous activation of the death receptor-mediated and mitochondrial pathway. Anticancer Res 27:3371-8.

[171] Lin, H., W. Xiong, X. Zhang, B. Liu, W. Zhang, Y. Zhang, J. Cheng, and H. Huang. 2011. Notch-1 activation-dependent p53 restoration contributes to resveratrol-induced apoptosis in glioblastoma cells. Oncol Rep 26:925-30.

[172] Lin, J. P., J. S. Yang, N. W. Chang, T. H. Chiu, C. C. Su, K. W. Lu, Y. T. Ho, C. C. Yeh, D. Mei, H. J. Lin, and J. G. Chung. 2007. GADD153 mediates berberine-induced apoptosis in human cervical cancer Ca ski cells. Anticancer Res 27:3379-86.

[173] Lin, J. P., J. S. Yang, C. C. Wu, S. S. Lin, W. T. Hsieh, M. L. Lin, F. S. Yu, C. S. Yu, G. W. Chen, Y. H. Chang, and J. G. Chung. 2008. Berberine induced down-regulation of matrix metalloproteinase-1, -2 and -9 in human gastric cancer cells (SNU-5) in vitro. In Vivo 22:223-30.

[174] Lin, J. T., M. K. Chen, K. T. Yeh, C. S. Chang, T. H. Chang, C. Y. Lin, Y. C. Wu, B. W. Su, K. D. Lee, and P. J. Chang. 2010. Association of high levels of Jagged-1 and Notch-1 expression with poor prognosis in head and neck cancer. Ann Surg Oncol 17:2976-83.

[175] Lin, L. I., Y. F. Ke, Y. C. Ko, and J. K. Lin. 1998. Curcumin inhibits SK-Hep-1 hepatocellular carcinoma cell invasion in vitro and suppresses matrix metalloproteinase-9 secretion. Oncology 55:349-53.

[176] Lin, M. L., S. S. Chen, Y. C. Lu, R. Y. Liang, Y. T. Ho, C. Y. Yang, and J. G. Chung. 2007. Rhein induces apoptosis through induction of endoplasmic reticulum stress and Ca2+-dependent mitochondrial death pathway in human nasopharyngeal carcinoma cells. Anticancer Res 27:3313-22.

[177] Lin, M. L., J. G. Chung, Y. C. Lu, C. Y. Yang, and S. S. Chen. 2009. Rhein inhibits invasion and migration of human nasopharyngeal carcinoma cells in vitro by down-regulation of matrix metalloproteinases-9 and vascular endothelial growth factor. Oral Oncol 45:531-7.

[178] Lin, M. L., Y. C. Lu, J. G. Chung, Y. C. Li, S. G. Wang, G. S. N, C. Y. Wu, H. L. Su, and S. S. Chen. 2010. Aloe-emodin induces apoptosis of human nasopharyngeal carcinoma cells via caspase-8-mediated activation of the mitochondrial death pathway. Cancer Lett 291:46-58.

[179] Lin, M. L., Y. C. Lu, J. G. Chung, S. G. Wang, H. T. Lin, S. E. Kang, C. H. Tang, J. L. Ko, and S. S. Chen. 2010. Down-regulation of MMP-2 through the p38 MAPK-NF-kappaB-dependent pathway by aloe-emodin leads to inhibition of nasopharyngeal carcinoma cell invasion. Mol Carcinog 49:783-97.

[180] Lin, M. L., Y. C. Lu, H. L. Su, H. T. Lin, C. C. Lee, S. E. Kang, T. C. Lai, J. G. Chung, and S. S. Chen. 2011. Destabilization of CARP mRNAs by aloe-emodin contributes to caspase-8-mediated p53-independent apoptosis of human carcinoma cells. J Cell Biochem 112:1176-91.

[181] Lin, S., M. Fujii, and D. X. Hou. 2003. Rhein induces apoptosis in HL-60 cells via reactive oxygen species-independent mitochondrial death pathway. Arch Biochem Biophys 418:99-107.

[182] Lin, S. S., K. C. Lai, S. C. Hsu, J. S. Yang, C. L. Kuo, J. P. Lin, Y. S. Ma, C. C. Wu, and J. G. Chung. 2009. Curcumin inhibits the migration and invasion of human A549 lung cancer cells through the inhibition of matrix metalloproteinase-2 and -9 and Vascular Endothelial Growth Factor (VEGF). Cancer Lett 285:127-33.

[183] Lin, S. Y., N. M. Tsang, S. C. Kao, Y. L. Hsieh, Y. P. Chen, C. S. Tsai, T. T. Kuo, S. P. Hao, I. H. Chen, and J. H. Hong. 2001. Presence of Epstein-Barr virus latent membrane protein 1 gene in the nasopharyngeal swabs from patients with nasopharyngeal carcinoma. Head Neck 23:194-200.

[184] Lin, T. H., H. C. Kuo, F. P. Chou, and F. J. Lu. 2008. Berberine enhances inhibition of glioma tumor cell migration and invasiveness mediated by arsenic trioxide. BMC Cancer 8:58.

[185] Lin, Y. J., and Y. S. Zhen. 2009. Rhein lysinate suppresses the growth of breast cancer cells and potentiates the inhibitory effect of Taxol in athymic mice. Anticancer Drugs 20:65-72.

[186] Lin, Y. J., Y. Z. Zhen, B. Y. Shang, and Y. S. Zhen. 2009. Rhein lysinate suppresses the growth of tumor cells and increases the anti-tumor activity of Taxol in mice. Am J Chin Med 37:923-31.

[187] Liu, J. P., L. Cassar, A. Pinto, and H. Li. 2006. Mechanisms of cell immortalization mediated by EB viral activation of telomerase in nasopharyngeal carcinoma. Cell Res 16:809-17.

[188] Liu, P. L., J. R. Tsai, A. L. Charles, J. J. Hwang, S. H. Chou, Y. H. Ping, F. Y. Lin, Y. L. Chen, C. Y. Hung, W. C. Chen, Y. H. Chen, and I. W. Chong. 2010. Resveratrol inhibits human lung adenocarcinoma cell metastasis by suppressing heme oxygenase 1-mediated nuclear factor-kappaB pathway and subsequently downregulating expression of matrix metalloproteinases. Mol Nutr Food Res 54 Suppl 2:S196-204.

[189] Liu, P. L., J. R. Tsai, C. C. Chiu, J. J. Hwang, S. H. Chou, C. K. Wang, S. J. Wu, Y. L. Chen, W. C. Chen, Y. H. Chen, and I. W. Chong. 2010. Decreased expression of thrombomodulin is correlated with tumor cell invasiveness and poor prognosis in nonsmall cell lung cancer. Mol Carcinog 49:874-81.

[190] Liu, S. J., Y. M. Sun, D. F. Tian, Y. C. He, L. Zeng, Y. He, C. Q. Ling, and S. H. Sun. 2008. Downregulated NM23-H1 expression is associated with intracranial invasion of nasopharyngeal carcinoma. Br J Cancer 98:363-9.

[191] Liu, Y. J., C. Barthelemy, O. de Bouteiller, C. Arpin, I. Durand, and J. Banchereau. 1995. Memory B cells from human tonsils colonize mucosal epithelium and directly present antigen to T cells by rapid up-regulation of B7-1 and B7-2. Immunity 2:239-48.

[192] Lo, K. W., and D. P. Huang. 2002. Genetic and epigenetic changes in nasopharyngeal carcinoma. Semin Cancer Biol 12:451-62.

[193] Longnecker, R., B. Druker, T. M. Roberts, and E. Kieff. 1991. An Epstein-Barr virus protein associated with cell growth transformation interacts with a tyrosine kinase. J Virol 65:3681-92.

[194] Lu, C., C. Sheehan, J. W. Rak, C. A. Chambers, N. Hozumi, and R. S. Kerbel. 1996. Endogenous interleukin 6 can function as an in vivo growth- stimulatory factor for advanced-stage human melanoma cells. Clin Cancer Res 2:1417-25.

[195] Lu, G. D., H. M. Shen, M. C. Chung, and C. N. Ong. 2007. Critical role of oxidative stress and sustained JNK activation in aloe-emodin-mediated apoptotic cell death in human hepatoma cells. Carcinogenesis 28:1937-45.

[196] Lu, J., W. H. Lin, S. Y. Chen, R. Longnecker, S. C. Tsai, C. L. Chen, and C. H. Tsai. 2006. Syk tyrosine kinase mediates Epstein-Barr virus latent membrane protein 2A-induced cell migration in epithelial cells. J Biol Chem 281:8806-14.

[197] Lu, J., M. Murakami, S. C. Verma, Q. Cai, S. Haldar, R. Kaul, M. A. Wasik, J. Middeldorp, and E. S. Robertson. 2011. Epstein-Barr Virus nuclear antigen 1 (EBNA1) confers resistance to apoptosis in EBV-positive B-lymphoma cells through up-regulation of survivin. Virology 410:64-75.

[198] Ma, Q., M. Zhang, Z. Wang, Z. Ma, and H. Sha. 2011. The beneficial effect of resveratrol on severe acute pancreatitis. Ann N Y Acad Sci 1215:96-102.

[199] Ma, Z. H., Q. Y. Ma, L. C. Wang, H. C. Sha, S. L. Wu, and M. Zhang. 2005. Effect of resveratrol on peritoneal macrophages in rats with severe acute pancreatitis. Inflamm Res 54:522-7.

[200] Malhotra, A., P. Nair, and D. K. Dhawan. 2010. Modulatory effects of curcumin and resveratrol on lung carcinogenesis in mice. Phytother Res 24:1271-7.

[201] Malinowska, J., and B. Olas. 2011. Response of blood platelets to resveratrol during a model of hyperhomocysteinemia. Platelets 22:277-83.

[202] Malterud, K. E., T. L. Farbrot, A. E. Huse, and R. B. Sund. 1993. Antioxidant and radical scavenging effects of anthraquinones and anthrones. Pharmacology 47 Suppl 1:77-85.

[203] Mandel, S. A., T. Amit, O. Weinreb, L. Reznichenko, and M. B. Youdim. 2008. Simultaneous manipulation of multiple brain targets by green tea catechins: a potential neuroprotective strategy for Alzheimer and Parkinson diseases. CNS Neurosci Ther 14:352-65.

[204] Mantena, S. K., S. D. Sharma, and S. K. Katiyar. 2006. Berberine inhibits growth, induces G1 arrest and apoptosis in human epidermoid carcinoma A431 cells by regulating Cdki-Cdk-cyclin cascade, disruption of mitochondrial membrane potential and cleavage of caspase 3 and PARP. Carcinogenesis 27:2018-27.

[205] Marks, J. E., J. L. Phillips, and H. R. Menck. 1998. The National Cancer Data Base report on the relationship of race and national origin to the histology of nasopharyngeal carcinoma. Cancer 83:582-8.

[206] Martin, G., P. Bogdanowicz, F. Domagala, H. Ficheux, and J. P. Pujol. 2003. Rhein inhibits interleukin-1 beta-induced activation of MEK/ERK pathway and DNA binding of NF-kappa B and AP-1 in chondrocytes cultured in hypoxia: a potential

mechanism for its disease-modifying effect in osteoarthritis. Inflammation 27:233-46.

[207] Meckes, D. G., Jr., K. H. Shair, A. R. Marquitz, C. P. Kung, R. H. Edwards, and N. Raab-Traub. 2010. Human tumor virus utilizes exosomes for intercellular communication. Proc Natl Acad Sci U S A 107:20370-5.

[208] Miccadei, S., R. Pulselli, and A. Floridi. 1993. Effect of lonidamine and rhein on the phosphorylation potential generated by respiring rat liver mitochondria. Anticancer Res 13:1507-10.

[209] Mijatovic, S., D. Maksimovic-Ivanic, J. Radovic, D. Miljkovic, L. Harhaji, O. Vuckovic, S. Stosic-Grujicic, M. Mostarica Stojkovic, and V. Trajkovic. 2005. Anti-glioma action of aloe emodin: the role of ERK inhibition. Cell Mol Life Sci 62:589-98.

[210] Miller, C. L., A. L. Burkhardt, J. H. Lee, B. Stealey, R. Longnecker, J. B. Bolen, and E. Kieff. 1995. Integral membrane protein 2 of Epstein-Barr virus regulates reactivation from latency through dominant negative effects on protein-tyrosine kinases. Immunity 2:155-66.

[211] Mitani, N., K. Murakami, T. Yamaura, T. Ikeda, and I. Saiki. 2001. Inhibitory effect of berberine on the mediastinal lymph node metastasis produced by orthotopic implantation of Lewis lung carcinoma. Cancer Lett 165:35-42.

[212] Morrison, J. A., A. J. Klingelhutz, and N. Raab-Traub. 2003. Epstein-Barr virus latent membrane protein 2A activates beta-catenin signaling in epithelial cells. J Virol 77:12276-84.

[213] Mudduluru, G., J. N. George-William, S. Muppala, I. A. Asangani, R. Kumarswamy, L. D. Nelson, and H. Allgayer. 2011. Curcumin regulates miR-21 expression and inhibits invasion and metastasis in colorectal cancer. Biosci Rep 31:185-97.

[214] Mueller, S. O., and H. Stopper. 1999. Characterization of the genotoxicity of anthraquinones in mammalian cells. Biochim Biophys Acta 1428:406-14.

[215] Mukhtar, H., and N. Ahmad. 2000. Tea polyphenols: prevention of cancer and optimizing health. Am J Clin Nutr 71:1698S-702S; discussion 1703S-4S.

[216] Namasivayam, N. 2011. Chemoprevention in experimental animals. Ann N Y Acad Sci 1215:60-71.

[217] Narasimhan, M., and S. Ammanamanchi. 2008. Curcumin blocks RON tyrosine kinase-mediated invasion of breast carcinoma cells. Cancer Res 68:5185-92.

[218] Nayyar, V. K., K. Shire, and L. Frappier. 2009. Mitotic chromosome interactions of Epstein-Barr nuclear antigen 1 (EBNA1) and human EBNA1-binding protein 2 (EBP2). J Cell Sci 122:4341-50.

[219] Nemerow, G. R., R. Wolfert, M. E. McNaughton, and N. R. Cooper. 1985. Identification and characterization of the Epstein-Barr virus receptor on human B lymphocytes and its relationship to the C3d complement receptor (CR2). J Virol 55:347-51.

[220] Nemoto, S., J. Xiang, S. Huang, and A. Lin. 1998. Induction of apoptosis by SB202190 through inhibition of p38beta mitogen-activated protein kinase. J Biol Chem 273:16415-20.

[221] Niedobitek, G., M. L. Hansmann, H. Herbst, L. S. Young, D. Dienemann, C. A. Hartmann, T. Finn, S. Pitteroff, A. Welt, I. Anagnostopoulos, and et al. 1991. Epstein-Barr virus and carcinomas: undifferentiated carcinomas but not squamous

cell carcinomas of the nasopharynx are regularly associated with the virus. J Pathol 165:17-24.
[222] O'Neil, J. D., T. J. Owen, V. H. Wood, K. L. Date, R. Valentine, M. B. Chukwuma, J. R. Arrand, C. W. Dawson, and L. S. Young. 2008. Epstein-Barr virus-encoded EBNA1 modulates the AP-1 transcription factor pathway in nasopharyngeal carcinoma cells and enhances angiogenesis in vitro. J Gen Virol 89:2833-42.
[223] O'Sullivan-Coyne, G., G. C. O'Sullivan, T. R. O'Donovan, K. Piwocka, and S. L. McKenna. 2009. Curcumin induces apoptosis-independent death in oesophageal cancer cells. Br J Cancer 101:1585-95.
[224] Orlowski, R. Z., and A. S. Baldwin, Jr. 2002. NF-kappaB as a therapeutic target in cancer. Trends Mol Med 8:385-9.
[225] Ou, S. H., J. A. Zell, A. Ziogas, and H. Anton-Culver. 2007. Epidemiology of nasopharyngeal carcinoma in the United States: improved survival of Chinese patients within the keratinizing squamous cell carcinoma histology. Ann Oncol 18:29-35.
[226] Owen, T. J., J. D. O'Neil, C. W. Dawson, C. Hu, X. Chen, Y. Yao, V. H. Wood, L. E. Mitchell, R. J. White, L. S. Young, and J. R. Arrand. 2010. Epstein-Barr virus-encoded EBNA1 enhances RNA polymerase III-dependent EBER expression through induction of EBER-associated cellular transcription factors. Mol Cancer 9:241.
[227] Pandey, M. K., B. Sung, A. B. Kunnumakkara, G. Sethi, M. M. Chaturvedi, and B. B. Aggarwal. 2008. Berberine modifies cysteine 179 of IkappaBalpha kinase, suppresses nuclear factor-kappaB-regulated antiapoptotic gene products, and potentiates apoptosis. Cancer Res 68:5370-9.
[228] Patel, K. R., V. A. Brown, D. J. Jones, R. G. Britton, D. Hemingway, A. S. Miller, K. P. West, T. D. Booth, M. Perloff, J. A. Crowell, D. E. Brenner, W. P. Steward, A. J. Gescher, and K. Brown. 2010. Clinical pharmacology of resveratrol and its metabolites in colorectal cancer patients. Cancer Res 70:7392-9.
[229] Patel, K. R., E. Scott, V. A. Brown, A. J. Gescher, W. P. Steward, and K. Brown. 2011. Clinical trials of resveratrol. Ann N Y Acad Sci 1215:161-9.
[230] Pathmanathan, R., U. Prasad, R. Sadler, K. Flynn, and N. Raab-Traub. 1995. Clonal proliferations of cells infected with Epstein-Barr virus in preinvasive lesions related to nasopharyngeal carcinoma. N Engl J Med 333:693-8.
[231] Pecere, T., M. V. Gazzola, C. Mucignat, C. Parolin, F. D. Vecchia, A. Cavaggioni, G. Basso, A. Diaspro, B. Salvato, M. Carli, and G. Palu. 2000. Aloe-emodin is a new type of anticancer agent with selective activity against neuroectodermal tumors. Cancer Res 60:2800-4.
[232] Pecere, T., F. Sarinella, C. Salata, B. Gatto, A. Bet, F. Dalla Vecchia, A. Diaspro, M. Carli, M. Palumbo, and G. Palu. 2003. Involvement of p53 in specific anti-neuroectodermal tumor activity of aloe-emodin. Int J Cancer 106:836-47.
[233] Pegtel, D. M., A. Subramanian, T. S. Sheen, C. H. Tsai, T. R. Golub, and D. A. Thorley-Lawson. 2005. Epstein-Barr-virus-encoded LMP2A induces primary epithelial cell migration and invasion: possible role in nasopharyngeal carcinoma metastasis. J Virol 79:15430-42.

[234] Peng, P. L., Y. S. Hsieh, C. J. Wang, J. L. Hsu, and F. P. Chou. 2006. Inhibitory effect of berberine on the invasion of human lung cancer cells via decreased productions of urokinase-plasminogen activator and matrix metalloproteinase-2. Toxicol Appl Pharmacol 214:8-15.

[235] Piyanuch, R., M. Sukhthankar, G. Wandee, and S. J. Baek. 2007. Berberine, a natural isoquinoline alkaloid, induces NAG-1 and ATF3 expression in human colorectal cancer cells. Cancer Lett 258:230-40.

[236] Pizarro, J. G., E. Verdaguer, V. Ancrenaz, F. Junyent, F. Sureda, M. Pallas, J. Folch, and A. Camins. 2011. Resveratrol inhibits proliferation and promotes apoptosis of neuroblastoma cells: role of sirtuin 1. Neurochem Res 36:187-94.

[237] Polvino-Bodnar, M., and P. A. Schaffer. 1992. DNA binding activity is required for EBNA 1-dependent transcriptional activation and DNA replication. Virology 187:591-603.

[238] Porter, M. J., J. K. Field, J. C. Lee, S. F. Leung, D. Lo, and C. A. Van Hasselt. 1994. Detection of the tumour suppressor gene p53 in nasopharyngeal carcinoma in Hong Kong Chinese. Anticancer Res 14:1357-60.

[239] Prakobwong, S., S. C. Gupta, J. H. Kim, B. Sung, P. Pinlaor, Y. Hiraku, S. Wongkham, B. Sripa, S. Pinlaor, and B. B. Aggarwal. 2011. Curcumin suppresses proliferation and induces apoptosis in human biliary cancer cells through modulation of multiple cell signaling pathways. Carcinogenesis 32:1372-80.

[240] QingLing, Z., Y. LiNa, L. Li, W. Shuang, Y. YuFang, D. Yi, J. Divakaran, L. Xin, and D. YanQing. 2011. LMP1 antagonizes WNT/beta-catenin signalling through inhibition of WTX and promotes nasopharyngeal dysplasia but not tumourigenesis in LMP1(B95-8) transgenic mice. J Pathol 223:574-83.

[241] Raab-Traub, N. 2002. Epstein-Barr virus in the pathogenesis of NPC. Semin Cancer Biol 12:431-41.

[242] Rabbani, G. H., T. Butler, J. Knight, S. C. Sanyal, and K. Alam. 1987. Randomized controlled trial of berberine sulfate therapy for diarrhea due to enterotoxigenic Escherichia coli and Vibrio cholerae. J Infect Dis 155:979-84.

[243] Rabinovich, A., L. Medina, B. Piura, S. Segal, and M. Huleihel. 2007. Regulation of ovarian carcinoma SKOV-3 cell proliferation and secretion of MMPs by autocrine IL-6. Anticancer Res 27:267-72.

[244] Radtke, F., and K. Raj. 2003. The role of Notch in tumorigenesis: oncogene or tumour suppressor? Nat Rev Cancer 3:756-67.

[245] Raimondi, F., P. Santoro, L. Maiuri, M. Londei, S. Annunziata, F. Ciccimarra, and A. Rubino. 2002. Reactive nitrogen species modulate the effects of rhein, an active component of senna laxatives, on human epithelium in vitro. J Pediatr Gastroenterol Nutr 34:529-34.

[246] Reedijk, M., S. Odorcic, L. Chang, H. Zhang, N. Miller, D. R. McCready, G. Lockwood, and S. E. Egan. 2005. High-level coexpression of JAG1 and NOTCH1 is observed in human breast cancer and is associated with poor overall survival. Cancer Res 65:8530-7.

[247] Reedijk, M., S. Odorcic, H. Zhang, R. Chetty, C. Tennert, B. C. Dickson, G. Lockwood, S. Gallinger, and S. E. Egan. 2008. Activation of Notch signaling in human colon adenocarcinoma. Int J Oncol 33:1223-9.

[248] Reth, M. 1989. Antigen receptor tail clue. Nature 338:383-4.

[249] Saha, A., T. Kuzuhara, N. Echigo, A. Fujii, M. Suganuma, and H. Fujiki. 2010. Apoptosis of human lung cancer cells by curcumin mediated through up-regulation of "growth arrest and DNA damage inducible genes 45 and 153". Biol Pharm Bull 33:1291-9.

[250] Sakai, T., Y. Taniguchi, K. Tamura, S. Minoguchi, T. Fukuhara, L. J. Strobl, U. Zimber-Strobl, G. W. Bornkamm, and T. Honjo. 1998. Functional replacement of the intracellular region of the Notch1 receptor by Epstein-Barr virus nuclear antigen 2. J Virol 72:6034-9.

[251] Sanchez, C., M. Mathy-Hartert, M. A. Deberg, H. Ficheux, J. Y. Reginster, and Y. E. Henrotin. 2003. Effects of rhein on human articular chondrocytes in alginate beads. Biochem Pharmacol 65:377-88.

[252] Sanchez, Y., G. P. Simon, E. Calvino, E. de Blas, and P. Aller. 2010. Curcumin stimulates reactive oxygen species production and potentiates apoptosis induction by the antitumor drugs arsenic trioxide and lonidamine in human myeloid leukemia cell lines. J Pharmacol Exp Ther 335:114-23.

[253] Sansone, P., G. Storci, S. Tavolari, T. Guarnieri, C. Giovannini, M. Taffurelli, C. Ceccarelli, D. Santini, P. Paterini, K. B. Marcu, P. Chieco, and M. Bonafe. 2007. IL-6 triggers malignant features in mammospheres from human ductal breast carcinoma and normal mammary gland. J Clin Invest 117:3988-4002.

[254] Sarkari, F., T. Sanchez-Alcaraz, S. Wang, M. N. Holowaty, Y. Sheng, and L. Frappier. 2009. EBNA1-mediated recruitment of a histone H2B deubiquitylating complex to the Epstein-Barr virus latent origin of DNA replication. PLoS Pathog 5:e1000624.

[255] Schlee, M., T. Krug, O. Gires, R. Zeidler, W. Hammerschmidt, R. Mailhammer, G. Laux, G. Sauer, J. Lovric, and G. W. Bornkamm. 2004. Identification of Epstein-Barr virus (EBV) nuclear antigen 2 (EBNA2) target proteins by proteome analysis: activation of EBNA2 in conditionally immortalized B cells reflects early events after infection of primary B cells by EBV. J Virol 78:3941-52.

[256] Scholle, F., K. M. Bendt, and N. Raab-Traub. 2000. Epstein-Barr virus LMP2A transforms epithelial cells, inhibits cell differentiation, and activates Akt. J Virol 74:10681-9.

[257] Scholle, F., R. Longnecker, and N. Raab-Traub. 1999. Epithelial cell adhesion to extracellular matrix proteins induces tyrosine phosphorylation of the Epstein-Barr virus latent membrane protein 2: a role for C-terminal Src kinase. J Virol 73:4767-75.

[258] Sen, S., H. Sharma, and N. Singh. 2005. Curcumin enhances Vinorelbine mediated apoptosis in NSCLC cells by the mitochondrial pathway. Biochem Biophys Res Commun 331:1245-52.

[259] Senft, C., M. Polacin, M. Priester, V. Seifert, D. Kogel, and J. Weissenberger. 2010. The nontoxic natural compound Curcumin exerts anti-proliferative, anti-migratory, and anti-invasive properties against malignant gliomas. BMC Cancer 10:491.

[260] Sham, J. S., D. Choy, and P. H. Choi. 1990. Nasopharyngeal carcinoma: the significance of neck node involvement in relation to the pattern of distant failure. Br J Radiol 63:108-13.
[261] Shangary, S., and D. E. Johnson. 2003. Recent advances in the development of anticancer agents targeting cell death inhibitors in the Bcl-2 protein family. Leukemia 17:1470-81.
[262] Shankar, S., S. Ganapathy, S. R. Hingorani, and R. K. Srivastava. 2008. EGCG inhibits growth, invasion, angiogenesis and metastasis of pancreatic cancer. Front Biosci 13:440-52.
[263] Shanmugaratnam, K., and L. H. Sobin. 1993. The World Health Organization histological classification of tumours of the upper respiratory tract and ear. A commentary on the second edition. Cancer 71:2689-97.
[264] Shannon-Lowe, C., and M. Rowe. 2011. Epstein-Barr virus infection of polarized epithelial cells via the basolateral surface by memory B cell-mediated transfer infection. PLoS Pathog 7:e1001338.
[265] Shi, P., Z. Huang, and G. Chen. 2008. Rhein induces apoptosis and cell cycle arrest in human hepatocellular carcinoma BEL-7402 cells. Am J Chin Med 36:805-13.
[266] Shi, W., C. Bastianutto, A. Li, B. Perez-Ordonez, R. Ng, K. Y. Chow, W. Zhang, I. Jurisica, K. W. Lo, A. Bayley, J. Kim, B. O'Sullivan, L. Siu, E. Chen, and F. F. Liu. 2006. Multiple dysregulated pathways in nasopharyngeal carcinoma revealed by gene expression profiling. Int J Cancer 119:2467-75.
[267] Shi, Y., S. Yang, S. Troup, X. Lu, S. Callaghan, D. S. Park, Y. Xing, and X. Yang. 2011. Resveratrol induces apoptosis in breast cancer cells by E2F1-mediated up-regulation of ASPP1. Oncol Rep 25:1713-9.
[268] Shigematsu, S., S. Ishida, M. Hara, N. Takahashi, H. Yoshimatsu, T. Sakata, and R. J. Korthuis. 2003. Resveratrol, a red wine constituent polyphenol, prevents superoxide-dependent inflammatory responses induced by ischemia/reperfusion, platelet-activating factor, or oxidants. Free Radic Biol Med 34:810-7.
[269] Shin, S., B. J. Sung, Y. S. Cho, H. J. Kim, N. C. Ha, J. I. Hwang, C. W. Chung, Y. K. Jung, and B. H. Oh. 2001. An anti-apoptotic protein human survivin is a direct inhibitor of caspase-3 and -7. Biochemistry 40:1117-23.
[270] Shinriki, S., H. Jono, M. Ueda, K. Ota, T. Ota, T. Sueyoshi, Y. Oike, M. Ibusuki, A. Hiraki, H. Nakayama, M. Shinohara, and Y. Ando. 2011. Interleukin-6 signalling regulates vascular endothelial growth factor-C synthesis and lymphangiogenesis in human oral squamous cell carcinoma. J Pathol 225:142-50.
[271] Simon, C., H. Goepfert, and D. Boyd. 1998. Inhibition of the p38 mitogen-activated protein kinase by SB 203580 blocks PMA-induced Mr 92,000 type IV collagenase secretion and in vitro invasion. Cancer Res 58:1135-9.
[272] Simonian, P. L., D. A. Grillot, and G. Nunez. 1997. Bcl-2 and Bcl-XL can differentially block chemotherapy-induced cell death. Blood 90:1208-16.
[273] Singh, B. N., S. Shankar, and R. K. Srivastava. 2011. Green tea catechin, epigallocatechin-3-gallate (EGCG): Mechanisms, perspectives and clinical applications. Biochem Pharmacol 82:1807-21.

[274] Singh, M., R. Singh, K. Bhui, S. Tyagi, Z. Mahmood, and Y. Shukla. 2011. Tea polyphenols induce apoptosis through mitochondrial pathway and by inhibiting nuclear factor-kappaB and Akt activation in human cervical cancer cells. Oncol Res 19:245-57.

[275] Sivachandran, N., N. N. Thawe, and L. Frappier. 2011. Epstein-barr virus nuclear antigen 1 replication and segregation functions in nasopharyngeal carcinoma cell lines. J Virol 85:10425-30.

[276] Son, I. H., I. M. Chung, S. I. Lee, H. D. Yang, and H. I. Moon. 2007. Pomiferin, histone deacetylase inhibitor isolated from the fruits of Maclura pomifera. Bioorg Med Chem Lett 17:4753-5.

[277] Soung, Y. H., and J. Chung. 2011. Curcumin inhibition of the functional interaction between integrin alpha6beta4 and the epidermal growth factor receptor. Mol Cancer Ther 10:883-91.

[278] Spender, L. C., G. H. Cornish, A. Sullivan, and P. J. Farrell. 2002. Expression of transcription factor AML-2 (RUNX3, CBF(alpha)-3) is induced by Epstein-Barr virus EBNA-2 and correlates with the B-cell activation phenotype. J Virol 76:4919-27.

[279] Stewart, S., C. W. Dawson, K. Takada, J. Curnow, C. A. Moody, J. W. Sixbey, and L. S. Young. 2004. Epstein-Barr virus-encoded LMP2A regulates viral and cellular gene expression by modulation of the NF-kappaB transcription factor pathway. Proc Natl Acad Sci U S A 101:15730-5.

[280] Strobl, L. J., H. Hofelmayr, G. Marschall, M. Brielmeier, G. W. Bornkamm, and U. Zimber-Strobl. 2000. Activated Notch1 modulates gene expression in B cells similarly to Epstein-Barr viral nuclear antigen 2. J Virol 74:1727-35.

[281] Su, Y. W., T. X. Xie, D. Sano, and J. N. Myers. 2011. IL-6 stabilizes Twist and enhances tumor cell motility in head and neck cancer cells through activation of casein kinase 2. PLoS One 6:e19412.

[282] Sun, Y., G. Hegamyer, Y. J. Cheng, A. Hildesheim, J. Y. Chen, I. H. Chen, Y. Cao, K. T. Yao, and N. H. Colburn. 1992. An infrequent point mutation of the p53 gene in human nasopharyngeal carcinoma. Proc Natl Acad Sci U S A 89:6516-20.

[283] Sun, Z. J., G. Chen, W. Zhang, X. Hu, Y. Liu, Q. Zhou, L. X. Zhu, and Y. F. Zhao. 2010. Curcumin dually inhibits both mammalian target of rapamycin and nuclear factor-kappaB pathways through a crossed phosphatidylinositol 3-kinase/Akt/IkappaB kinase complex signaling axis in adenoid cystic carcinoma. Mol Pharmacol 79:106-18.

[284] Swart, R., I. K. Ruf, J. Sample, and R. Longnecker. 2000. Latent membrane protein 2A-mediated effects on the phosphatidylinositol 3-Kinase/Akt pathway. J Virol 74:10838-45.

[285] Tamm, I., Y. Wang, E. Sausville, D. A. Scudiero, N. Vigna, T. Oltersdorf, and J. C. Reed. 1998. IAP-family protein survivin inhibits caspase activity and apoptosis induced by Fas (CD95), Bax, caspases, and anticancer drugs. Cancer Res 58:5315-20.

[286] Tang, C. H., C. F. Chen, W. M. Chen, and Y. C. Fong. 2011. IL-6 increases MMP-13 expression and motility in human chondrosarcoma cells. J Biol Chem 286:11056-66.

[287] Tang, F., D. Wang, C. Duan, D. Huang, Y. Wu, Y. Chen, W. Wang, C. Xie, J. Meng, L. Wang, B. Wu, S. Liu, D. Tian, F. Zhu, Z. He, F. Deng, and Y. Cao. 2009. Berberine inhibits metastasis of nasopharyngeal carcinoma 5-8F cells by targeting Rho kinase-mediated Ezrin phosphorylation at threonine 567. J Biol Chem 284:27456-66.

[288] Thawonsuwan, J., V. Kiron, S. Satoh, A. Panigrahi, and V. Verlhac. 2010. Epigallocatechin-3-gallate (EGCG) affects the antioxidant and immune defense of the rainbow trout, Oncorhynchus mykiss. Fish Physiol Biochem 36:687-97.

[289] Thiounn, N., F. Pages, T. Flam, E. Tartour, V. Mosseri, M. Zerbib, P. Beuzeboc, L. Deneux, W. H. Fridman, and B. Debre. 1997. IL-6 is a survival prognostic factor in renal cell carcinoma. Immunol Lett 58:121-4.

[290] Trapp, V., B. Parmakhtiar, V. Papazian, L. Willmott, and J. P. Fruehauf. 2010. Anti-angiogenic effects of resveratrol mediated by decreased VEGF and increased TSP1 expression in melanoma-endothelial cell co-culture. Angiogenesis 13:305-15.

[291] Truong, M., M. R. Cook, S. N. Pinchot, M. Kunnimalaiyaan, and H. Chen. 2010. Resveratrol induces Notch2-mediated apoptosis and suppression of neuroendocrine markers in medullary thyroid cancer. Ann Surg Oncol 18:1506-11.

[292] Tsai, C. N., C. L. Tsai, K. P. Tse, H. Y. Chang, and Y. S. Chang. 2002. The Epstein-Barr virus oncogene product, latent membrane protein 1, induces the downregulation of E-cadherin gene expression via activation of DNA methyltransferases. Proc Natl Acad Sci U S A 99:10084-9.

[293] Tsai, P. Y., S. M. Ka, J. M. Chang, H. C. Chen, H. A. Shui, C. Y. Li, K. F. Hua, W. L. Chang, J. J. Huang, S. S. Yang, and A. Chen. 2011. Epigallocatechin-3-gallate prevents lupus nephritis development in mice via enhancing the Nrf2 antioxidant pathway and inhibiting NLRP3 inflammasome activation. Free Radic Biol Med 51:744-54.

[294] Tsao, S. W., X. Wang, Y. Liu, Y. C. Cheung, H. Feng, Z. Zheng, N. Wong, P. W. Yuen, A. K. Lo, Y. C. Wong, and D. P. Huang. 2002. Establishment of two immortalized nasopharyngeal epithelial cell lines using SV40 large T and HPV16E6/E7 viral oncogenes. Biochim Biophys Acta 1590:150-8.

[295] Tse, L. A., I. T. Yu, O. W. Mang, and S. L. Wong. 2006. Incidence rate trends of histological subtypes of nasopharyngeal carcinoma in Hong Kong. Br J Cancer 95:1269-73.

[296] Valentine, R., C. W. Dawson, C. Hu, K. M. Shah, T. J. Owen, K. L. Date, S. P. Maia, J. Shao, J. R. Arrand, L. S. Young, and J. D. O'Neil. 2010. Epstein-Barr virus-encoded EBNA1 inhibits the canonical NF-kappaB pathway in carcinoma cells by inhibiting IKK phosphorylation. Mol Cancer 9:1.

[297] van Niel, G., I. Porto-Carreiro, S. Simoes, and G. Raposo. 2006. Exosomes: a common pathway for a specialized function. J Biochem 140:13-21.

[298] Vanamala, J., S. Radhakrishnan, L. Reddivari, V. B. Bhat, and A. Ptitsyn. 2011. Resveratrol suppresses human colon cancer cell proliferation and induces apoptosis via targeting the pentose phosphate and the talin-FAK signaling pathways-A proteomic approach. Proteome Sci 9:49.

[299] Vareed, S. K., M. Kakarala, M. T. Ruffin, J. A. Crowell, D. P. Normolle, Z. Djuric, and D. E. Brenner. 2008. Pharmacokinetics of curcumin conjugate metabolites in healthy human subjects. Cancer Epidemiol Biomarkers Prev 17:1411-7.

[300] Vasef, M. A., A. Ferlito, and L. M. Weiss. 1997. Nasopharyngeal carcinoma, with emphasis on its relationship to Epstein-Barr virus. Ann Otol Rhinol Laryngol 106:348-56.

[301] Vaughan, T. L., J. A. Shapiro, R. D. Burt, G. M. Swanson, M. Berwick, C. F. Lynch, and J. L. Lyon. 1996. Nasopharyngeal cancer in a low-risk population: defining risk factors by histological type. Cancer Epidemiol Biomarkers Prev 5:587-93.

[302] Vesela, D., R. Kubinova, J. Muselik, M. Zemlicka, and V. Suchy. 2004. Antioxidative and EROD activities of osajin and pomiferin. Fitoterapia 75:209-11.

[303] Wang, F., C. Gregory, C. Sample, M. Rowe, D. Liebowitz, R. Murray, A. Rickinson, and E. Kieff. 1990. Epstein-Barr virus latent membrane protein (LMP1) and nuclear proteins 2 and 3C are effectors of phenotypic changes in B lymphocytes: EBNA-2 and LMP1 cooperatively induce CD23. J Virol 64:2309-18.

[304] Wang, F., S. F. Tsang, M. G. Kurilla, J. I. Cohen, and E. Kieff. 1990. Epstein-Barr virus nuclear antigen 2 transactivates latent membrane protein LMP1. J Virol 64:3407-16.

[305] Wang, J., S. E. Lindner, E. R. Leight, and B. Sugden. 2006. Essential elements of a licensed, mammalian plasmid origin of DNA synthesis. Mol Cell Biol 26:1124-34.

[306] Wang, L., S. R. Grossman, and E. Kieff. 2000. Epstein-Barr virus nuclear protein 2 interacts with p300, CBP, and PCAF histone acetyltransferases in activation of the LMP1 promoter. Proc Natl Acad Sci U S A 97:430-5.

[307] Wang, L., L. Wang, R. Song, Y. Shen, Y. Sun, Y. Gu, Y. Shu, and Q. Xu. 2011. Targeting sarcoplasmic/endoplasmic reticulum Ca(2)+-ATPase 2 by curcumin induces ER stress-associated apoptosis for treating human liposarcoma. Mol Cancer Ther 10:461-71.

[308] Wang, M., Y. Ruan, Q. Chen, S. Li, Q. Wang, and J. Cai. 2011. Curcumin induced HepG2 cell apoptosis-associated mitochondrial membrane potential and intracellular free Ca(2+) concentration. Eur J Pharmacol 650:41-7.

[309] Wang, S., and L. Frappier. 2009. Nucleosome assembly proteins bind to Epstein-Barr virus nuclear antigen 1 and affect its functions in DNA replication and transcriptional activation. J Virol 83:11704-14.

[310] Wang, X. 2001. The expanding role of mitochondria in apoptosis. Genes Dev 15:2922-33.

[311] Wang, X., Q. Wang, K. L. Ives, and B. M. Evers. 2006. Curcumin inhibits neurotensin-mediated interleukin-8 production and migration of HCT116 human colon cancer cells. Clin Cancer Res 12:5346-55.

[312] Wang, Z., Y. Huang, J. Zou, K. Cao, Y. Xu, and J. M. Wu. 2002. Effects of red wine and wine polyphenol resveratrol on platelet aggregation in vivo and in vitro. Int J Mol Med 9:77-9.

[313] Wartenberg, M., P. Budde, M. De Marees, F. Grunheck, S. Y. Tsang, Y. Huang, Z. Y. Chen, J. Hescheler, and H. Sauer. 2003. Inhibition of tumor-induced angiogenesis and matrix-metalloproteinase expression in confrontation cultures of embryoid

bodies and tumor spheroids by plant ingredients used in traditional chinese medicine. Lab Invest 83:87-98.
[314] Watson, J. L., R. Hill, P. B. Yaffe, A. Greenshields, M. Walsh, P. W. Lee, C. A. Giacomantonio, and D. W. Hoskin. 2010. Curcumin causes superoxide anion production and p53-independent apoptosis in human colon cancer cells. Cancer Lett 297:1-8.
[315] Wei, W. I., and J. S. Sham. 2005. Nasopharyngeal carcinoma. Lancet 365:2041-54.
[316] Weng, Y. L., H. F. Liao, A. F. Li, J. C. Chang, and R. Y. Chiou. 2010. Oral administration of resveratrol in suppression of pulmonary metastasis of BALB/c mice challenged with CT26 colorectal adenocarcinoma cells. Mol Nutr Food Res 54:259-67.
[317] Wilken, R., M. S. Veena, M. B. Wang, and E. S. Srivatsan. 2011. Curcumin: A review of anti-cancer properties and therapeutic activity in head and neck squamous cell carcinoma. Mol Cancer 10:12.
[318] Williamson, M. P., T. G. McCormick, C. L. Nance, and W. T. Shearer. 2006. Epigallocatechin gallate, the main polyphenol in green tea, binds to the T-cell receptor, CD4: Potential for HIV-1 therapy. J Allergy Clin Immunol 118:1369-74.
[319] Wolfram, S., Y. Wang, and F. Thielecke. 2006. Anti-obesity effects of green tea: from bedside to bench. Mol Nutr Food Res 50:176-87.
[320] Wong, T. S., W. S. Chan, C. H. Li, R. W. Liu, W. W. Tang, S. W. Tsao, R. K. Tsang, W. K. Ho, W. I. Wei, and J. Y. Chan. 2010. Curcumin alters the migratory phenotype of nasopharyngeal carcinoma cells through up-regulation of E-cadherin. Anticancer Res 30:2851-6.
[321] Wu, L., J. C. Aster, S. C. Blacklow, R. Lake, S. Artavanis-Tsakonas, and J. D. Griffin. 2000. MAML1, a human homologue of Drosophila mastermind, is a transcriptional co-activator for NOTCH receptors. Nat Genet 26:484-9.
[322] Wu, S. H., L. W. Hang, J. S. Yang, H. Y. Chen, H. Y. Lin, J. H. Chiang, C. C. Lu, J. L. Yang, T. Y. Lai, Y. C. Ko, and J. G. Chung. 2010. Curcumin induces apoptosis in human non-small cell lung cancer NCI-H460 cells through ER stress and caspase cascade- and mitochondria-dependent pathways. Anticancer Res 30:2125-33.
[323] Wu, T. C., R. B. Mann, J. I. Epstein, E. MacMahon, W. A. Lee, P. Charache, S. D. Hayward, R. J. Kurman, G. S. Hayward, and R. F. Ambinder. 1991. Abundant expression of EBER1 small nuclear RNA in nasopharyngeal carcinoma. A morphologically distinctive target for detection of Epstein-Barr virus in formalin-fixed paraffin-embedded carcinoma specimens. Am J Pathol 138:1461-9.
[324] Xia, N., A. Daiber, A. Habermeier, E. I. Closs, T. Thum, G. Spanier, Q. Lu, M. Oelze, M. Torzewski, K. J. Lackner, T. Munzel, U. Forstermann, and H. Li. 2010. Resveratrol reverses endothelial nitric-oxide synthase uncoupling in apolipoprotein E knockout mice. J Pharmacol Exp Ther 335:149-54.
[325] Yamaguchi, K., M. Honda, H. Ikigai, Y. Hara, and T. Shimamura. 2002. Inhibitory effects of (-)-epigallocatechin gallate on the life cycle of human immunodeficiency virus type 1 (HIV-1). Antiviral Res 53:19-34.
[326] Yamashita, S., M. Kondo, and S. Hashimoto. 1985. Squamous cell carcinoma of the nasopharynx. An analysis of failure patterns after radiation therapy. Acta Radiol Oncol 24:315-20.

[327] Yan, Z., T. Yong-Guang, L. Fei-Jun, T. Fa-Qing, T. Min, and C. Ya. 2004. Interference effect of epigallocatechin-3-gallate on targets of nuclear factor kappaB signal transduction pathways activated by EB virus encoded latent membrane protein 1. Int J Biochem Cell Biol 36:1473-81.
[328] Yang, C. L., Y. G. Ma, Y. X. Xue, Y. Y. Liu, H. Xie, and G. R. Qiu. 2011. Curcumin Induces Small Cell Lung Cancer NCI-H446 Cell Apoptosis via the Reactive Oxygen Species-Mediated Mitochondrial Pathway and Not the Cell Death Receptor Pathway. DNA Cell Biol Jun 28. [Epub ahead of print]
[329] Yang, C. S., J. Y. Chung, G. Yang, S. K. Chhabra, and M. J. Lee. 2000. Tea and tea polyphenols in cancer prevention. J Nutr 130:472S-478S.
[330] Yang, W. H., Y. C. Fong, C. Y. Lee, T. R. Jin, J. T. Tzen, T. M. Li, and C. H. Tang. 2011. Epigallocatechin-3-gallate induces cell apoptosis of human chondrosarcoma cells through apoptosis signal-regulating kinase 1 pathway. J Cell Biochem 112:1601-11.
[331] Yeh, F. T., C. H. Wu, and H. Z. Lee. 2003. Signaling pathway for aloe-emodin-induced apoptosis in human H460 lung nonsmall carcinoma cell. Int J Cancer 106:26-33.
[332] Yeh, T. S., C. W. Wu, K. W. Hsu, W. J. Liao, M. C. Yang, A. F. Li, A. M. Wang, M. L. Kuo, and C. W. Chi. 2009. The activated Notch1 signal pathway is associated with gastric cancer progression through cyclooxygenase-2. Cancer Res 69:5039-48.
[333] Yip, K. W., W. Shi, M. Pintilie, J. D. Martin, J. D. Mocanu, D. Wong, C. MacMillan, P. Gullane, B. O'Sullivan, C. Bastianutto, and F. F. Liu. 2006. Prognostic significance of the Epstein-Barr virus, p53, Bcl-2, and survivin in nasopharyngeal cancer. Clin Cancer Res 12:5726-32.
[334] Yoshizaki, T., H. Sato, M. Furukawa, and J. S. Pagano. 1998. The expression of matrix metalloproteinase 9 is enhanced by Epstein-Barr virus latent membrane protein 1. Proc Natl Acad Sci U S A 95:3621-6.
[335] Young, L. S., C. W. Dawson, D. Clark, H. Rupani, P. Busson, T. Tursz, A. Johnson, and A. B. Rickinson. 1988. Epstein-Barr virus gene expression in nasopharyngeal carcinoma. J Gen Virol 69 (Pt 5):1051-65.
[336] Young, L. S., and P. G. Murray. 2003. Epstein-Barr virus and oncogenesis: from latent genes to tumours. Oncogene 22:5108-21.
[337] Yu, M. C., J. H. Ho, R. K. Ross, and B. E. Henderson. 1981. Nasopharyngeal carcinoma in Chinese---salted fish or inhaled smoke? Prev Med 10:15-24.
[338] Yu, M. C., and J. M. Yuan. 2002. Epidemiology of nasopharyngeal carcinoma. Semin Cancer Biol 12:421-9.
[339] Zetterberg, H., C. Borestrom, T. Nilsson, and L. Rymo. 2004. Multiple EBNA1-binding sites within oriPI are required for EBNA1-dependent transactivation of the Epstein-Barr virus C promoter. Int J Oncol 25:693-6.
[340] Zhang, J., Y. Du, C. Wu, X. Ren, X. Ti, J. Shi, F. Zhao, and H. Yin. 2010. Curcumin promotes apoptosis in human lung adenocarcinoma cells through miR-186* signaling pathway. Oncol Rep 24:1217-23.
[341] Zhang, J., T. Zhang, X. Ti, J. Shi, C. Wu, X. Ren, and H. Yin. 2010. Curcumin promotes apoptosis in A549/DDP multidrug-resistant human lung adenocarcinoma cells through an miRNA signaling pathway. Biochem Biophys Res Commun 399:1-6.

[342] Zhang, J. X., H. L. Chen, Y. S. Zong, K. H. Chan, J. Nicholls, J. M. Middeldorp, J. S. Sham, B. E. Griffin, and M. H. Ng. 1998. Epstein-Barr virus expression within keratinizing nasopharyngeal carcinoma. J Med Virol 55:227-33.

[343] Zhang, T. H., H. C. Liu, L. J. Zhu, M. Chu, Y. J. Liang, L. Z. Liang, and G. Q. Liao. 2011. Activation of Notch signaling in human tongue carcinoma. J Oral Pathol Med 40:37-45.

[344] Zhang, W., X. Wang, and T. Chen. 2011. Resveratrol induces mitochondria-mediated AIF and to a lesser extent caspase-9-dependent apoptosis in human lung adenocarcinoma ASTC-a-1 cells. Mol Cell Biochem 354:29-37.

[345] Zhang, Y., J. Peng, H. Zhang, Y. Zhu, L. Wan, J. Chen, X. Chen, R. Lin, H. Li, X. Mao, and K. Jin. 2010. Notch1 signaling is activated in cells expressing embryonic stem cell proteins in human primary nasopharyngeal carcinoma. J Otolaryngol Head Neck Surg 39:157-66.

[346] Zhao, Y., H. Wang, X. R. Zhao, F. J. Luo, M. Tang, and Y. Cao. 2004. [Epigallocatechin-3-gallate interferes with EBV-encoding AP-1 signal transduction pathway]. Zhonghua Zhong Liu Za Zhi 26:393-7.

[347] Zheng, Z., J. Pan, B. Chu, Y. C. Wong, A. L. Cheung, and S. W. Tsao. 1999. Downregulation and abnormal expression of E-cadherin and beta-catenin in nasopharyngeal carcinoma: close association with advanced disease stage and lymph node metastasis. Hum Pathol 30:458-66.

[348] Zhong, Y., and F. Shahidi. 2011. Lipophilized epigallocatechin gallate (EGCG) derivatives as novel antioxidants. J Agric Food Chem 59:6526-33.

[349] Zhou, X., B. Song, L. Jin, D. Hu, C. Diao, G. Xu, Z. Zou, and S. Yang. 2006. Isolation and inhibitory activity against ERK phosphorylation of hydroxyanthraquinones from rhubarb. Bioorg Med Chem Lett 16:563-8.

[350] Zhu, J., Z. Liu, H. Huang, Z. Chen, and L. Li. 2003. Rhein inhibits transforming growth factor beta1 induced plasminogen activator inhibitor-1 in endothelial cells. Chin Med J (Engl) 116:354-9.

12

Nasopharyngeal Cancer – An Expanding Puzzle – Claiming for Answers

E. Breda[1,2], R. Catarino[3] and R. Medeiros[3,4,5]
[1]*Otorrinolaringology Department - Portuguese Institute of Oncology, Porto,*
[2]*Health Sciences Department, University of Aveiro,*
[3]*Molecular Oncology Unit - Portuguese Institute of Oncology, Porto,*
[4]*ICBAS, Abel Salazar Institute for the Biomedical Sciences, Porto,*
[5]*Faculty of Health Sciences of Fernando Pessoa University, Porto,*
Portugal

1. Introduction

1.1 The Nasopharynx (an unusual perspective of a peculiar structure)

Nasopharynx is a peculiar anatomic structure with an essential role in respiratory, digestive and auditory systems. It is located between the respiratory and digestive tracts and its anatomic and physiologic characteristics depend on complex and not totally explained phylogenic, ontogenic and embryologic factors. Some of these factors demonstrated to be relevant not only on the pathogenesis, characteristics and development of nasopharyngeal carcinoma (NPC), but also on therapeutic options and their implications (Breda, Catarino et al. 2008).

In what concerns to phylogenic aspects, it is important to emphasize that either in chordates as even in the first aquatic vertebrates (agnate), the upper aerodigestive and respiratory tracts were associated, providing both the oxygenation and feeding supplies needed in an aquatic environment. However, according to Everett C. Olson (Rainger 1997), the appraisal of the oxygen and nourish requirements requested by the tetrapods, demanded the taking apart of oronasal cavity and the formation of primitive choanae; this was performed by the expansion of the branchial arches and the development of the mandible. Interestingly, this original functional ambivalence persists in mammals, and is visible in their anatomic relationships: nasal cavity is in a dorsal position relatively to the oral cavity but the larynx diverges ventrally from the pharynx.

In humans, as in most mammalians, pharyngeal and most of nasal cavity mucosa are the end result of a unique embryologic origin, depending from the cephalic portion of the primitive gut, a blind ending tube, lined with endodermic tissue, separated from the ectodermic *stomatodeum* by the buccopharyngeal membrane (Beasly 2008). Before the rupture of buccopharyngeal membrane happens, two recesses will form in this region: the Rathke pouch, which will origin the adenohypophysis and the Seesel pouch, representing the primordium of the future nasopharynx (Figure 1).

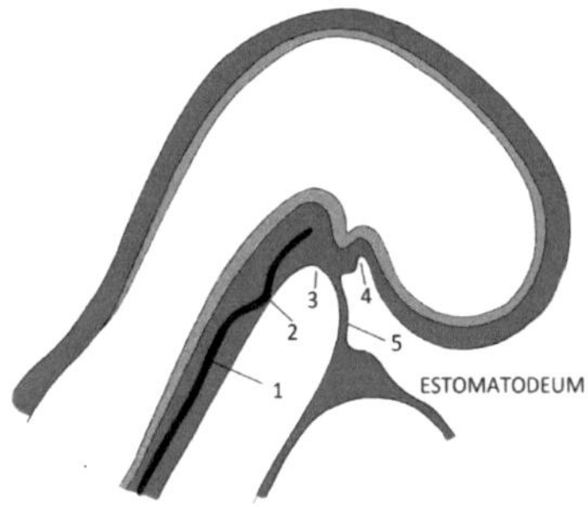

Fig. 1. Human embryo (about 3 weeks): 1 - notocordium; 2 - Tornwaldt pouch origin; 3- Seesel pouch; 4 - Rathke pouch; 5 - buccopharyngeal membrane [Adapted from (Breda, Catarino et al. 2008)].

The muscle and osseous components of nasopharynx will take origin from the viscerocranium (pharyngeal or branchial arches and clefts), and neurocranium (Saddlet 1995). Pharyngeal arches contribute with mesenchymal tissue covered on the outside by surface ectoderm and on the inside by epithelium of endodermal origin. In addition, each arch receives substantial numbers of neural crest cells, which migrate into the arches to contribute to skeletal components of the face (Saddlet 2009). The development of Meckel cartilage is associated with a predominance of sagital craniofacial growth and increase of vertical and anterior-posterior length compared with transversal diameter.

Nasopharyngeal osseous superior and posterior limits (body of the shpenoid bone and the basilar part of occipital bone united in the sphenobasilarsynchondrosis) are derived from the prechordal chondrocranium (cartilages lying in front of the rostral limit of the notochord, which ends at the level of the pituitary gland in the center of the sella turcica, derived from neural crest cells) and the chordal chondrocranium, composed by those cartilages that lie posterior to this limit and arise from occipital sclerotomes formed by paraxial mesoderm (Saddlet 2009).

Intra-uterine increase of supratentorial and craniobasal angles and simultaneous shortness of infratentorial one (Jeffery 2005) contribute also to nasopharyngeal final shape, and these changes could be connected, according to Bull, to the development of occipital lobe, associated with bipedalism (Bull 1969) (Figure 2).

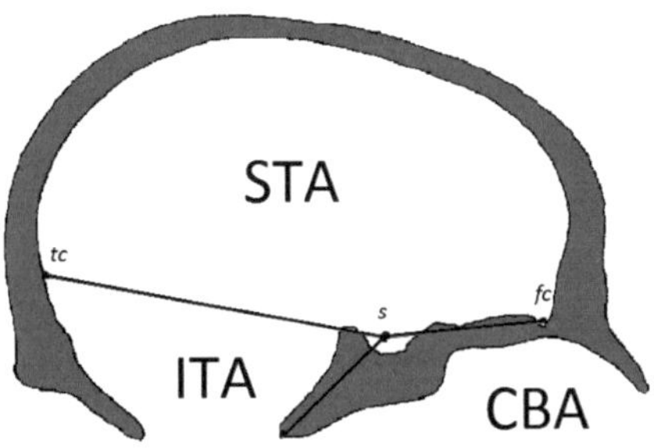

Fig. 2. Ontogenic aspects of cranial morphogenesis: TSA – supratentorial angle; ITA – infratentorial angle;CBA – craniobasal angle; *tc* – cranial attachment of tentorium cerebelli; *s* – sella; *fc* – foramen caecum [Adapted from (Breda, Catarino et al. 2008)].

The nasopharynx is thus the end result of the several factors affecting its development, resulting in a trapezoid tubular about 128° angled structure, with average 4cm to 5,5cm transversal diameter, 2,5cm to 3,5cm anterior-posterior diameter e 4cm high(Snow Jr and Ballenger 2003). It has an anterior opening continuous with the posterior choanae and communicates with the oropharynx inferiorly, through a complex sphincteric mechanism. Superior wall is continuous with the posterior and in lateral walls an apparent Rosenmuller lateral pharyngeal recess posterior to the internal opening of pharyngotympanic tube are the main anatomic evidences.

The nasopharyngeal wall is composed of mucous membrane (with pseudostratified columnar epithelium, *"lamina propria"*, lymphoid tissue and stem cells), pharyngobasilar fascia, muscle layer and buccopharyngeal fascia(Standring 2008).Immediately posterior lie the retropharyngeal lymph nodes, between this and the prevertebral fascia.

When considering local anatomic implications on nasopharyngeal malignancies, the organization and function of lymphoid tissue, the potential oncologic relevance of stem cells and the significance of the cellular structure of the epithelium, muscles and neighboring salivary (minor and major) glands are examples of some topics waiting for answers.

The mucosal immune system of upper aero-digestive tract provides the first line of defense against the ingress of microbial pathogens during the physiological processes of inhalation and ingestion. One of the major components of the mucosal immune system is secretory IgA (S-IgA),which is produced by the mucosal interaction of epithelial cells, IgA-committed B cells, and Th cells(Shikina, Hiroi et al. 2004).

Nasopharynx-associated lymphoid tissue (NALT) plays a pivotal role in the initiation of Ag-specific immune responses at both systemic and mucosal sites, acting acts as an important inductive site for the generation of Ag-specific IgA-committed B cells(Fukuyama, Nagatake et al. 2006). The relationship between NALT system and Epstein-Barr virus (EBV) infection is being studied. There is now increasing evidence that defects in the immune control of EBV infection are linked to EBV associated malignancies, namely Hodgkin's disease and NPC, with the selective loss of EBV specific T cells and induction of local immunosuppressive microenvironment that favors tumor growth (Braz-Silva, Vitale et al. 2011).

In the identification of the malignant population that might be responsible for tumor initiation, the cancer stem cell (CSC) (Clarke, Dick et al. 2006), is other promising scientific advance. CSC is commonly assumed to have developed from a normal tissue stem cell. In normal organs, stem cells are defined as a subset of cells with the capacity of self-renewal to maintain the stem cell reservoir and of differentiation to generate various types of cells in the tissue. By self-renewal, stem cells divide symmetrically and perpetuate themselves by generating daughter cells with identical stem cell abilities of the parent. By differentiation, stem cells give rise to a hierarchy of limitedly proliferative but functional mature cells (Brady, Heilman et al. 2010). Zhang *et al* described for the first time stem cells in mouse nasopharyngeal epithelium; they represent less than 3% of cell population, and they lie mostly in basal and superbasal layers (Zhang, Wu et al. 1982). The polycomb group protein *Bmi*-1 is required for the maintenance and self-renewal of stem cells. The molecular mechanisms underlying the modulation of such stem-like cell populations in NPC remain unclear. However, according to Song *et al* (Song, Li et al. 2009), previous upregulation of

Bmi-1 correlates with invasion of NPC and otherwise a possible mechanism of tumorigenesis involves repression of the *Ink4a-Arf* locus, which encodes the tumor suppressors INK4A and ARF, by direct binding of *Bmi*-1.

Furthermore, there is an ongoing debate over whether CSCs represent a mature tissue stem cell which has undergone malignant change or whether more differentiated cells re-initiate a 'stemness' programme as part of, or following, malignant transformation (Bomken, Fiser et al. 2010).

These and other questions are yet to be answered, namely how to explain the relationship between CSC, NPC and EBV. The recent accomplishment that LMP2A EBV encoded latent protein, induces epithelial–mesenchymal transition and stem-like cell self-renewal in NPC, is a strong evidence of this association (Kong, Hu et al. 2010).

2. The Epstein Barr virus and mechanisms of infection

Many epidemiological studies have been performed concerning NPC and three well-defined etiological factors involved in its pathogenesis have been identified. These include genetic susceptibility, early-age exposure to chemical carcinogens and an association with a latent EBV infection (Chan, Teo et al. 2002; Busson, Keryer et al. 2004).

It is widely accepted that EBV infection plays a major role in the pathogenesis of NPC in endemic areas, although not entirely clear in non-endemic regions (Henle and Henle 1976; Pathmanathan, Prasad et al. 1995). The association between NPC and EBV was initially discovered from serological studies and was later supported by demonstration of EBV DNA and nuclear antigen proteins (EBNA) in NPC tumor cells (zur Hausen, Schulte-Holthausen et al. 1970; Henle and Henle 1976). The notion that EBV plays an important role in the development of NPC is further supported by the observation that early nasopharyngeal lesions (dysplasia or carcinoma-in situ) are already EBV-positive, harbouring latent and clonal viral genomes as well as viral oncoproteins such as latent membrane protein (LMP) (zur Hausen, Schulte-Holthausen et al. 1970; Pathmanathan, Prasad et al. 1995).

In 1958, Denis Burkitt, a British surgeon working in Africa, described a common cancer primarily affecting children in specific regions of Africa (Burkitt 1958). Burkitt believed that a virus might be implicated in cancer development, given the climatic and geographic distribution of the cases (Burkitt 1962). EBV was first identified in 1964 when Anthony Epstein, Yvonne Barr and Bert Achong detected virus-like particles by electron microscopy in a cell line that had been established from a Burkitt's lymphoma biopsy (Epstein, Achong et al. 1964). The causal link between EBV and BL was corroborated by evidence showing that BL patient sera had elevated antibodies to EBV antigens (Henle and Henle 1966) . This group also established a link between primary EBV infection and infectious mononucleosis and, subsequently, the association of EBV with nasopharyngeal carcinoma (Henle, Henle et al. 1968; Henle, Henle et al. 1970; zur Hausen, Schulte-Holthausen et al. 1970).

Nasopharyngeal cancer, particularly when showing histological patterns of non-keratinization (WHO/1978 II or III), is associated with previous EBV infection with sequential immortalization of the virus in the host's B-lymphocytes (Niedobitek, Hansmann et al. 1991).

EBV is a member of the herpesvirus family. As other herpesviruses, EBV is an enveloped virus that contains a DNA core surrounded by an icosahedral nucleocapsid and a tegument. Family members include herpes simplex 1 (HSV-1) and 2 (HSV-2) and varicella-zoster virus (VZV) - alphavirus subfamily; cytomegalovirus (CMV) and human herpesvirus 6 (HHV-6) and 7 (HHV-7) - betaherpesvirus subfamily; and human herpesvirus 8 (HHV-8) and EBV - gammaherpesvirus subfamily. The oncogenic potential of EBV was recognized through the association with numerous human malignancies. In addition to endemic Burkitt's lymphoma and NPC, EBV was later found in Hodgkin's lymphoma cases, post-transplant lymphoproliferative diseases, some T-cell lymphomas and a proportion of gastric carcinomas (Young and Rickinson 2004). Research is currently ongoing to determine the role of EBV-encoded gene products in these different cellular environments in an attempt to understand the role that EBV plays in the pathogenesis of these malignancies.

It is now known that EBV infects 90% of the world's adult population. Although herpesviruses are ubiquitous in nature, humans are the only natural host for EBV. Upon infection, the individual remains a life-long carrier of the virus (Henle and Henle 1976). During acute infection, EBV seems to primarily infect and replicate in the stratified squamous epithelium of the oropharynx, followed by a latent infection of the B lymphocytes. EBV infection of B lymphocytes is thought to occur in the upper aerodigestive tract lymphoid organs and the virus persists in circulating memory B cells (Sixbey, Nedrud et al. 1984; Farrell 1995). Taking in account that EBV infection is a common event in the entire World, the reasons why only some individuals will develop EBV-related malignancies, are interesting aspects yet to clarify.

Much of the known biology of EBV relates to its interaction with B-lymphocytes. This is mainly a result of the ability of EBV to readily infect and transform normal resting B-lymphocytes in vitro, which also confirms the B-lymphotropic nature of this virus. EBV latent gene expression in various EBV-associated malignancies and EBV-derived cell lines has led to the identification of three different and distinct latency patterns. These latency patterns characterize a heterogeneous group of diseases and are based on EBV genome expression arrangements as the result of differential promoter activity influenced by host cell factors (Thompson and Kurzrock 2004; Young and Rickinson 2004). Latency type I is generally associated with Burkitt's lymphoma and is characterized by expression of the EBV-encoded RNAs (EBERs) and the BamHI-A rightward transcripts (BARTs), in addition to EBV nuclear antigen-1 (EBNA1) expression. Latency type II is associated with NPC, gastric cancer and EBV-positive Hodgkin lymphoma and is characterized by expression of EBERs, BARTs, EBNA1 and the latent membrane proteins (LMP1, LMP2A and LMP2B). Latency type III is associated with lymphoblastoid cell lines and post-transplant lymphoproliferative diseases: the full range of latent gene products are expressed, including EBNAs 1, 2, 3A, 3B, 3C and -LP, the expression of all three latent membrane proteins (LMP1, LMP2A and LMP2B) and EBERs and BART RNAs. Although these classifications of latency are useful in characterizing the distinct gene expression patterns, they are by no means completely definitive (Thompson and Kurzrock 2004). In recent years, there has been increasing interest in the presence of different viral and cellular micro-RNAs in EBV-infected B cells and epithelial cells. Future works should investigate the role of EBV-encoded micro-RNAs and its correlation with transcriptional regulation of both the viral and cellular genome.

Analysis of EBV in NPC tumors has revealed the presence of clonal EBV genomes, suggesting that these carcinomas arise from the clonal expansion of a single EBV-infected progenitor cell (Raab-Traub and Flynn 1986). Similar to most EBV-associated malignancies, the exact role of EBV in NPC pathogenesis remains poorly understood. Unlike EBV-associated B cell tumors, where the virus is considered to be an initiating factor in the oncogenic process, virus infection in the context of NPC pathogenesis seems to act as a tumor-promoting agent.

Recent studies investigated circulating tumor-derived EBV DNA in the blood of NPC patients. Using real-time PCR methodology, studies indicate that the level of pre-treatment EBV DNA has prognostic significance. Furthermore, post-treatment EBV DNA levels seem to be correlated with treatment response and overall survival of NPC patients (Lo, Chan et al. 2000; Lo, Leung et al. 2000; Lin, Chen et al. 2001; Chan, Lo et al. 2002). This methodology should be applied in large-scale trials as an approach for early disease diagnosis.

3. Genetic basis of NPC

The identification of genetic changes in pre-malignant lesions and NPC tumors has led to the proposal of a multi-step model for the pathogenesis of NPC. Genome-wide analyses of genetic alterations in NPC have identified consistent genetic losses on several chromosomal arms, including 3p, 9p, 9q, 11q, 14q and 16q. Recurrent chromosomal gains were also identified on chromosomes 1q, 3q, 8q, 12p and 12q (Chan, To et al. 2000; Chan, To et al. 2002; Lo and Huang 2002). The most common genetic change seems to be the loss of chromosome regions on 9p21 and 3p, which is thought to occur early during NPC pathogenesis (Hui, Lo et al. 2002). NPC carcinogenesis seems to develop in a step by step fashion, where the chromosomal alterations, such deletion, tumor suppressor gene inactivation and oncogene promotion, are associated with morphological changes in the cell (Young and Rickinson 2004) (Figure 3).

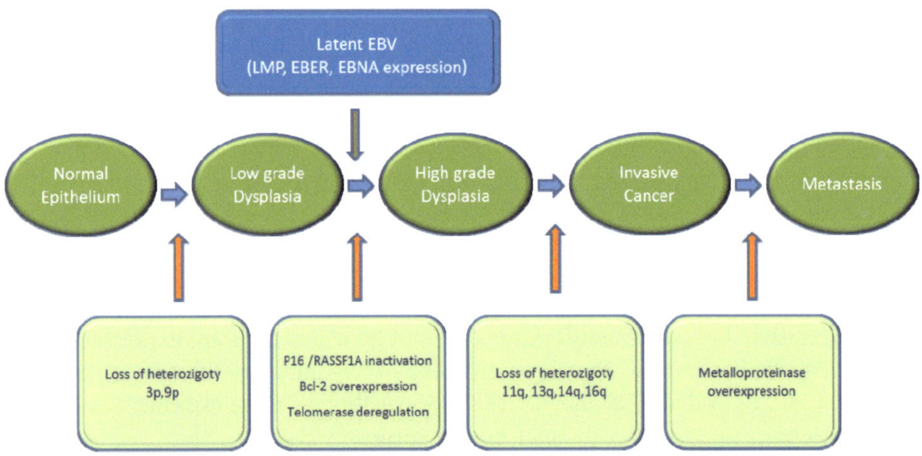

Fig. 3. NPC carcinogenesis scheme.

Although the precise role of these genetic alterations in NPC carcinogenesis remains to be clarified, these genetic changes may predispose nasopharyngeal cells to facilitate latent EBV infection and this seems to be a crucial event in the multi-step progression towards NPC.

The development and progression of NPC involves the accumulation of genetic alterations. Both genetic and epigenetic changes can affect the development of NPC, by altering the function of genes that are critical for proliferation, apoptosis and differentiation.

Host factors previously shown to be associated with NPC development include *HLA* class I and II alleles and polymorphisms of genes responsible for critical cellular functions, as carcinogen metabolism and detoxification, cell cycle control, DNA repair and immune response. Published studies demonstrated that some genetic variations are associated with a higher risk of NPC development (Hildesheim, Anderson et al. 1997; Nazar-Stewart, Vaughan et al. 1999; Cho, Hildesheim et al. 2003; Catarino, Breda et al. 2006; Sousa, Santos et al. 2006). This genetic predisposition to NPC may be modulated by environmental factors and this may have a differential impact in endemic and non-endemic NPC.

Familial clustering of the disease has been widely documented in the Chinese population and several polymorphisms have been associated with NPC development, namely in nitrosamine metabolizing genes cytochrome P450 2A6 (CYP2A6), P450 2E1 (CYP2E1) and P450 2F1 (CYP2F1), Glutathione S- transferase M1 (GSTM1), XRCC1 (codons 194 arg-trp), have been suggested to influence the susceptibility to NPC (Hildesheim and Levine 1993; Pathmanathan, Prasad et al. 1995; Sousa, Santos et al. 2006; Tiwawech, Srivatanakul et al. 2006).

Less in known in non-endemic areas, but it has been suggested that the individual genetic background may influence the onset of NPC, also in these regions. Regarding cell cycle control, some studies investigated the role of polymorphisms in cyclin D1 (CCND1) and TP53 genes in the genetic susceptibility to NPC (Pathmanathan, Prasad et al. 1995; Cho, Hildesheim et al. 2003; Catarino, Pereira et al. 2008). These genetic variants have been associated with increased individual risk of NPC development. Regarding the key regulator of cell cycle, cyclin D1, the study by Catarino et al, demonstrate that individuals carrying the genetic variant present a 2-fold increased risk for the development of NPC, the proportion of cases attributable to the genotype being 14.76% (Catarino, Breda et al. 2006). Moreover, another study indicates that cyclin D1 variants influence the age of onset of oncogenic virus-associated cancers, namely NPC (Catarino, Pereira et al. 2008). The results of this study demonstrate that the waiting time for onset of oncogenic virus-associated neoplasia in patients carrying the cyclin D1 variant was 12 years earlier in comparison with the other patients. Another study by Sousa et al, focus on the polymorphic variants (Arg/Pro) on *TP53* codon 72 in nasopharyngeal cancer development. This study revealed a three-fold risk for carriers of Pro/Pro genotype, suggesting that Pro/Pro genotype represents a stable risk factor for nasopharyngeal carcinoma (Sousa, Santos et al. 2006).

Another study revealed that a MDM2 polymorphism is associated with increased risk to develop NPC adjusted for age and gender, with particular effect in undifferentiated types and early clinical stages. The study also indicates that the median age of onset of NPC was significantly different according to the genetics variants (Sousa, Pando et al. 2011). Regarding the immune response markers, a study revealed an increased frequency of a tumor necrosis factor-alpha (TNF-α) polymorphic variant in patients with NPC. The authors indicate that this variant is associated with a 2-fold increased risk for the development of this disease. Moreover, this effect seems to be stronger in undifferentiated types (Sousa, Breda et al. 2011).

These results performed in low-risk, non-endemic areas indicate that these genetic variations may represent risk markers for NPC and contribute to the definition of genetic susceptibility profiles for the development of this disease. Furthermore, the knowledge of the mechanisms involved in NPC carcinogenesis may help to identify targets for the development of chemoprevention or therapeutic strategies.

4. The Nasopharyngeal Carcinoma (NPC)

4.1 NPC histopathologic classification (final clarification?)

The histopathologic designation of this kind of tumor is matter of debate since the first description of "Primary Carcinoma of Nasopharynx", performed by Chevalier Jackson (1901) based upon the description of 14 cases(Jackson 1901; Van Hasselt and Gibb 1999). From that time on, several designations have been used to designate this tumor, namely lymphoepithelioma, lymphoepitheliomalike carcinoma, lymphoepithelial carcinoma, Schmincke type lymphoepithelioma, Regaud type lymphoepithelioma, transitional cell carcinoma, intermediate cell carcinoma, anaplastic carcinoma, undifferentiated carcinoma with lymphoid stroma, vesicular nucleus cell carcinoma, and so on.

This controversy seems to be solved with the WHO (2003) classification of NPC into three histologic types: keratinizing squamous carcinoma, nonkeratinizing carcinoma and basaloid carcinoma (IARC 2005).

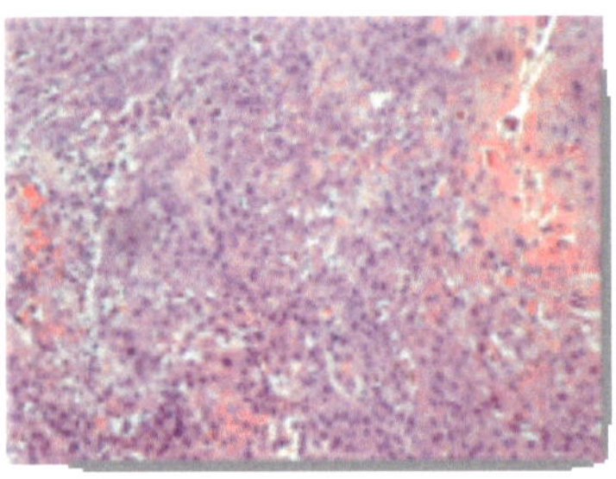

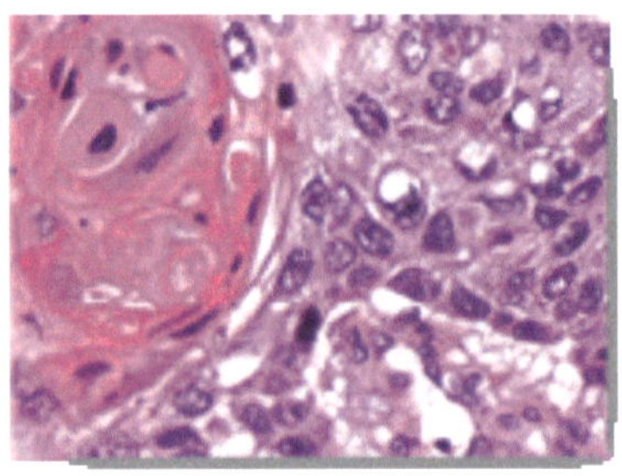

Fig. 4. Keratinizing squamous carcinoma.

In keratinizing squamous carcinoma, the polygonal and stratified tumor cells grow in the form of irregular islands, accompanied by an abundant desmoplastic stroma infiltrated by variable numbers of lymphocytes, plasma cells, neutrophils and eosinophils. The cell borders are distinct and separated by intercellular bridges and possess abundant cytoplasm and small hiperchromatic nucleus. Often keratin pearls can be seen (Figure 4).

Oppositely, the undifferentiated subtype of nonkeratinizing carcinoma is characterized by syncytial-appearing large tumor cells with indistinct cell borders, round to oval vesicular nuclei, and large central nucleoli, scanty cytoplasm. Often immunostaining for cytokeratins (eg MNF116) is needed to demonstrate the epithelial nature of the tumor (Figure 5).

WHO (2003) classification recognizes the behavior similarities between diferentiated and undiferentiated subtypes of nonkeratinizing carcinoma (type II and III of the previous WHO classification-1978) (IARC 2005). Accordingly, there is clinical, histopathologic and immunologic evidence that nasopharyngeal carcinomas constitute two distinct diseases, keratinizing squamous carcinoma in one side and nonkeratinizing carcinoma in the other, this later being linked to previous infection by Epstein-Barr virus.

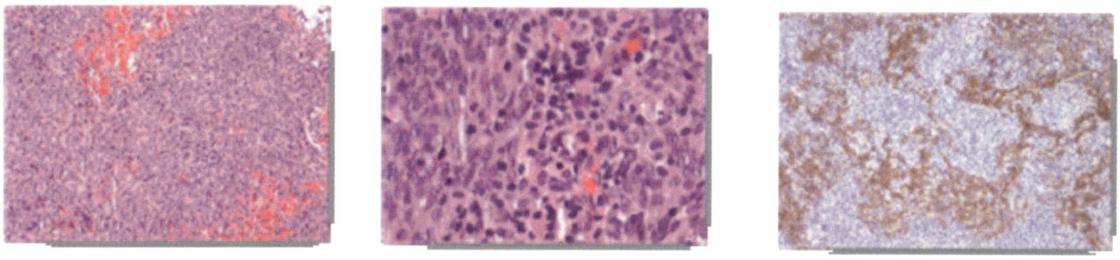

Fig. 5. The undifferentiated subtype of NPC.

However, IARC "WHO Classification of Head and Neck Tumors" (IARC 2005), also describes 6 cases of basaloid squamous cell carcinoma (BSCC) arising as primary tumors of the nasopharynx. These tumors demonstrated to be morphologically identical to the same tumors more commonly occurring in other head and neck sites (larynx, hypopharynx and oropharynx) (Ereno, Gaafar et al. 2008), strongly associated with traditional risk factors, such as tobacco and alcohol abuse.

BSCC of the upper aerodigestive tract was originally described by Wain *et al* (1986) (Wain, Kier et al. 1986), as a rare variant of squamous cell carcinoma, is characterized by clinically aggressive behavior and worse prognosis, independent of tumor stage. Two major histopathologic features define BSCC. Morphologically, BSCC also possess distinct histological features, presenting basaloid tumor cells (solid, lobular, small, crowded cells with scant cytoplasm, hyperchromatic round nuclei, and small cystic spaces containing PAS-or alcian blue-positive myxoid material) in a festooning growth pattern, interspersed by tumor cells with squamous differentiation (Chernock, Lewis et al. 2010).

These histopathologic features are also very similar with those of oropharyngeal human papillomavirus (HPV)-related nonkeratinizing squamous cell carcinoma (NK SCC). This kind of carcinoma occurs predominantly in the tonsillar tissue of the oropharynx, in younger patients and have unique risk factors related to sexual behavior, including multiple partners, early age at first intercourse, and oral sex (Chernock, El-Mofty et al. 2009). The tumor appears to show a lower clinical aggressiveness compared with basaloid squamous cell carcinoma occurring in other head and neck sites (Begum and Westra 2008).

The analogy between viral etiology and histomorphological characteristics of tumor development site (close relationship between epithelium and lymphoid tissue) in HPV-related"basaloid" NK SCC of oropharynx and NPC nonkeratinizing carcinoma EBV-related, seems to be quite obvious, but not completely clarified, and so are their histopathologic patterns.

4.2 NPC commented epidemiologic data

Considering all nasopharyngeal tumors, the probability of being originated in the epithelial lining varies from 75 to 95% in low-risk populations, and all of them are virtually cancers in high-risk population (Parkin DM 2002). NPC is a patchy worldwide malignant disease, characterized by remarkable divergence in incidences among populations of diverse geographic regions and races. It is very common in southern Asia (20-30/100 000 inhabitants/year) (Vasef, Ferlito et al. 1997) and quite rare in western countries (<1/100 000 inhabitants/year) (Parkin DM 2002). Intermediate incidence (8-12/100000 inhabitants/year) occurs in certain African and Mediterranean populations (Cvitkovic, Bachouchi et al. 1991) and also in the Inuits from Greenland and Alaska and Malays from Singapore and Malaysia.

The relative percentage of NPC types according to the WHO classification seems to vary accordingly to the geographic distribution with about 95% rates of nonkeratinizing carcinoma in endemic regions (Wenig 1999) and 75% of keratinizing squamous carcinoma in countries with low prevalence of the disease, as in United States of America (Marks, Phillips et al. 1998). As far as we know, there is no European statistics dealing about this point, and online search at the GLOBACAN, doesn't discriminate these histopathologic types. However detailed studies in a non-endemic European country (Portugal), reveal that in this population the relative rate of nonkeratinizing/keratinizing carcinoma is closer to the findings obtained in endemic countries (Breda, Catarino et al. 2007; d'Espiney Amaro, Montalvao et al. 2009) (Table 1). These findings suggest that studies envisaging the possible rearrangement of the relative weight of the different NPC types in European populations are needed.

Nasopharyngeal Carcinoma in Portugal (age, sex and histopathologic distribution)				
INSTITUTION	N. PATIENTS	AVERAGE AGE (years)	GENDER (%) m/f	WHO TYPE II/III (%)
IPO-PORTO	320	48	67/33	93,75%
IPO-LISBOA	157	53	65/35	88%

Table 1. Nasopharyngeal carcinoma in Portugal

It is also known that nonkeratizing NPC has a male preponderance and occurs earlier in life than head and neck carcinomas (Parkin DM 2002). These aspects are quite intriguing, as none of the commonly cited endogenous and exogenous risk factors for NPC seem to be directly linked to gender or age of cancer development.

Familial clustering has also been frequently reported (Zhang and Zhang 1999), and can be explained by the demonstration of correlation between the HLA haplotype and NPC susceptibility. However, these very interesting findings need also to be better understood.

It has been hypothesized that certain HLA polymorphic antigens have lower efficiency in activating the cytotoxic T cell recognition and host immune response to EBV infection (Lu, Day et al. 1990; Lo, To et al. 2004). In this context, potential role of the MHC class I chain–related A (MICA) gene belonging to the nonclassical HLA family and located 46 kb centromeric to the human leukocyte antigen (HLA)–B gene is of particular interest. MICA is highly polymorphic, with more than 60 alleles (defined by nucleotide substitutions within exons encoding the three alfa-domains) described to date. Each of these variants is characterized by the presence of a variable number of short tandem repeats (STRs) within the exon encoding for the transmembrane region of the molecule(Douik, Ben Chaaben et al. 2009).There are multiple evidences that the MICA*A9 is linked with several of those HLA haplotypes NPC related (HLA-B35, -B38, -B39, -B51, -B58) (Chan, Day et al. 1983; Wu, Hwang et al. 1989; Zhu, Chen et al. 1990; Tian, Boggs et al. 2001).

Wei Tian *et al* (Tian, Zeng et al. 2006) demonstrated a positive association between MICA*A9 and nasopharyngeal carcinoma, only observed in male subjects, and this finding had statistical significance (P=0.0001). This fact is not well explained, but it should be remembered that HLA genes are sex-linked and transmitted in bloc.

Furthermore, a recent study demonstrated the existence of a binding site in the long intron 1 of the MICA gene for NF-kappaB (Molinero, Fuertes et al. 2004). It has been shown that physiologic concentrations of male hormones (androgens) cause prolonged NF-kappaB DNA binding activities, which are diminished by vitamins C and E (Ripple, Henry et al. 1999)and estrogen inhibits NF-kappa B activity (Ghisletti, Meda et al. 2005; Kalaitzidis and Gilmore 2005). These findings are mostly fascinating when we consider that TRAF is activated by the LMP1 latent EBV protein.

The NPC age distribution is also quite different than usual, and seems to vary according to the incidence. It is accepted that in low-risk countries, the NPC incidence rises monotonically with age, but in high-risk regions the age incidence hit the highest point at 55 years(Chang and Adami 2006), showing bimodal age presentation in Northern Africa and India (Bray, Haugen et al. 2008). These results also need an explanation, namely on the influence of some genetic polymorphisms that may influence the age of onset of disease (Catarino, Pereira et al. 2008; Sousa H 2010).

The close relationship between nonkeratinizing NPC and EBV is sustained by *"in-situ"* hybridization studies (Wei and Sham 2005) and occurs both in endemic as in non-endemic countries (Niedobitek, Hansmann et al. 1991; Breda, Catarino et al. 2010). However, infection with EBV is a worldwide phenomenon and other endogenous and exogenous factors must be associated with NPC development. The relative weight of these factors is not yet clearly understood, namely in non-endemic regions.

4.3 NPC stage classification and prognostic evaluation

Whatever its localization, cancer prognosis will conceptually depend on biological aggressiveness of tumor itself, host characteristics and therapeutic options.

The tumor, node, metastasis (TNM) staging system, allows clinicians to categorize tumors of the head and neck region in a specific manner, to assist with the assessment of disease status, prognosis and management (Daniel G. Deschler 2008). The introduction of several clinical staging systems (American Joint Committee on Cancer (AJCC) staging, the International Union Against Cancer (UICC) staging, Ho's staging from Hong Kong, Fuzhou staging from Mainland China, Huang's or Hsu's staging from Taiwan), permitted that TNM staging for NPC remained relatively confused during many years and this was undesirable.

It is accepted that a good TNM classification should fulfill the following criteria:(1) the subgroups defined by T, N, and M that make up a given group within a grouping scheme must have similar survival rates (hazard consistency); (2) the survival rates must differ among the groups (hazard discrimination); (3) the prediction of cure must be high (outcome prediction); and (4) the distribution of patients among the groups must be balanced (Groome, Schulze et al. 2001). The association between the AJCC and UICC staging systems and their succeeding modifications taking into account the criteria previously enunciated, namely with rearrangements on T and N arrays, allowed a better TNM prognostic significance in the most recent classifications (Liu, Tang et al. 2008).

However, NPC TNM classification only takes into account the aggressiveness of the "clinical" tumor; understand all the factors influencing the clinical course of NPC in order to improve the TNM classification (Greene, Page et al. 2002) and anticipate NPC prognosis, is still a challenge, recognized by several authors (Lee, Au et al. 2004; Liu, Tang et al. 2008). Accordingly, other tumor characterystics may confirm relevance on prognosis, suhc as histological types (WHO type II and III versus type I). Furthermore, taking into account the relationship between histological types and EBV, it also seems to be very interesting to know how relevant can be the measurement of EBV related proteins in the patient's serum as a prognostic factor of survival. Plasma EBV-DNA measurement is actually believed to be a more sensitive and specific marker than the serum IgA/VCA titer for the diagnosis and monitoring of patients with NPC (Shao, Li et al. 2004). Even more, plasma EBV-DNA findings provide convincing evidence of their usefulness on the early diagnosis and staging of NPC as well as for monitoring recurrence and metastasis of this tumor. Some studies indicate that high marker level (>500 copies/ml) at 6 weeks after radio(chemo)therapy is a powerful prognosticator of recurrence, whereas pretreatment EBV DNA is a better discriminator of prognosis than conventional TNM classification for stage II NPC (Haddad 2011).

Patient's related prognostic factors are seldom referred in literature. Some authors claim that patients with younger age are associated with improved overall survival. One study involving 2,054 NPC patients from several European countries also showed that overall survival declined with age (Jiong, Berrino et al. 1998), and other series from endemic regions demonstrated similar results (Leung, Tung et al. 2005) (Liu, Tang et al. 2008). However, not always is disentangled age with better performance status and less comorbidity characteristics, more often present in younger patients, which might contribute to better tolerance to radical radio(chemo)therapy, thus resulting in better survival.

The relationship between gender and prognosis is subject to similar doubts (Leung, Tung et al. 2005) (Liu, Tang et al. 2008) with controversial results being described. Again, it is difficult to straighten out gender with lifestyle (including body weight, central adiposity, physical activity, exposure to smoking, fruit and vegetable intake a.s.o. and these aspects still wait for clarification.

4.4 NPC treatment, survival rate and quality of life

Radiation therapy (RT) is considered the mainstay treatment for NPC. Recent retrospective analysis including more than two thousand patients treated by RT alone (mostly using 2D technique) showed that the 5-year overall survival (OS) was 85% for stages I–II (Lee, Sze et al. 2005), corroborating that NPC is highly sensitive to ionizing radiation. However, the same study demonstrated an OS of only 66% for stages III–IVB, with metastatic rate remaining high (25% at 5-years) for patients who achieved locoregional control, and these findings supported the need of some kind of systemic treatment, namely for advanced disease.

The advantages of adding chemotherapy (Ch) to RT had already been accomplished by the Intergroup 0099 study, the first prospectively randomized study to demonstrate an improvement in OS from the addition of concurrent chemotherapy and adjuvant chemotherapy to radiation therapy (when compared with radiation therapy alone), without unacceptably increasing the toxicity of treatment (Al-Sarraf, LeBlanc et al. 1998).

From that time on, several trials confirmed not only that the addition of chemotherapy concurrent with radiation therapy has improved the outcomes of patients with NPC, but also that improvements in radiation treatment technology and the adoption of IMRT (Intensity-Modulated Radiation Therapy) have also improved local control, reducing also the morbidity.

Besides the superior dose conformity delivered to tumor, one of the most important promised advantages of IMRT is the achievement of sufficient sparing of critical normal structures adjacent to treated areas, namely spinal cord, parotid glands, temporomandibular joint, middle and inner ears, skin (in the region of the target volumes), and oral cavity, mandible, glottic larynx, brachial plexus, and esophagus (including postcricoid pharynx) (Brady, Heilman et al. 2010) and such sparing has obvious advantages.

However, even with IMRT, minor salivary glands and both palatal and masticator muscles (medial pterygoid and lateral pterygoid) are often included in target volumes, either gross tumor volume (GTV), clinical target volume (CTV) or planned target volume (PTV). The impact of such distresses on Quality of life (QoL) seems not to be disentangled enough (Bhatia, King et al. 2009; Lee, Harris et al. 2009).

Quality of life refers to the perception of the effects of disease and its impact on the patient's daily functioning; QoL is a multi-dimensional issue, incorporating physical, psychological, social and emotional domains, and it must be self-reported according to the patient's own experiences (List and Stracks 2000). These very important mind and corporal approach is not often mentioned in scientific literature; usually, the endpoint of medical care for cancer patients is focused on the survival rate, local control rate, or complication rate. These endpoints were typically assessed from the physician's points of view and lacked knowledge of patients' mental or emotional well-being. According to Fang and co-workers (Fang, Tsai et al. 2010), in addition to socioeconomic levels, advanced RT techniques were observed to play a significant role in improving the QoL outcome of NPC survivors. However, the impact size from conventional 2DRT to 3DCRT or IMRT varied on different QoL scales. The therapeutic benefit of IMRT over 2DRT, especially on the swallowing-related QoL scales, is not clear and should be further explored.

One of the main aims of clinical or translational research in cancer is the search for biological factors that could foresee treatment outcomes, in biologic activity and toxic effects. The increasing amount of information regarding the role of genetics in human diseases has led to putative new biomarkers and the development of new fields, as pharmacogenomics (PGx). Pharmacogenomics is a rapidly developing scientific area, especially in oncology. In the most ideal situation, pharmacogenomics will allow oncologists to individualize therapy based on patients' individual germline genetic test results. This can help to improve efficacy, reduce toxicity and predict non-responders in a way that alternative therapy can be chosen or individual dose adjustments can be made. It has been observed that the interpatient variability in response to medications is associated with a spectrum of outcomes, ranging from failure to demonstrate an expected therapeutic effect, to an adverse reaction resulting in significant patient morbidity and mortality, decreasing quality of life, as well as increasing healthcare costs.

The goal of the emerging disciplines of pharmacogenomics is to personalize therapy based on an individual's genotype. To date, the success of PGx has spread across all fields of medicine, although little is known about the genetic profile and its correlation with treatment response and overall survival in nasopharyngeal cancer patients. Genetic information has been used in the identification of disease risk, choice of treatment agents and guiding drug dosing. This is particularly important for chemotherapeutic agents, which in general affect both tumor and non-tumor cells and thus have a narrow therapeutic index, with the potential for life-threatening toxicity. Future work should explore the role of genetic variations in nasopharyngeal cancer patients, in a pharmacogenomics approach.

5. References

Al-Sarraf, M, M LeBlanc, PG Giri, KK Fu, J Cooper, T Vuong, AA Forastiere, G Adams, WA Sakr, DE Schuller and JF Ensley (1998). Chemoradiotherapy versus radiotherapy in patients with advanced nasopharyngeal cancer: phase III randomized Intergroup study 0099. *J Clin Oncol* 16(4): 1310-1317.

Beasly, N, Ed. (2008). Anatomy of the pharynx and oesophagus. Scott-Brown's Otolaryngology Head and Neck Surgery London.

Begum, S and WH Westra (2008). Basaloid squamous cell carcinoma of the head and neck is a mixed variant that can be further resolved by HPV status. *Am J Surg Pathol* 32(7): 1044-1050.

Bhatia, KS, AD King, BK Paunipagar, J Abrigo, AC Vlantis, SF Leung and AT Ahuja (2009). MRI findings in patients with severe trismus following radiotherapy for nasopharyngeal carcinoma. *Eur Radiol* 19(11): 2586-2593.

Bomken, S, K Fiser, O Heidenreich and J Vormoor (2010). Understanding the cancer stem cell. *Br J Cancer* 103(4): 439-445.

Brady, LW, H-P Heilman, M Molls and C Nieder, Eds. (2010). Nasopharyngeal Cancer Multidisciplinary Management. Medical Radiology diagnostic Imaging and Radiation Oncology, Springer.

Bray, F, M Haugen, TA Moger, S Tretli, OO Aalen and T Grotmol (2008). Age-incidence curves of nasopharyngeal carcinoma worldwide: bimodality in low-risk populations and aetiologic implications. *Cancer Epidemiol Biomarkers Prev* 17(9): 2356-2365.

Braz-Silva, PH, S Vitale, C Butori, N Guevara, J Santini, M Magalhaes, P Hofman and A Doglio (2011). Specific infiltration of langerin-positive dendritic cells in EBV-infected tonsil, Hodgkin lymphoma and nasopharyngeal carcinoma. *Int J Cancer* 128(10): 2501-2508.

Breda, E, R Catarino, I Azevedo, T Fernandes, C Barreira da Costa and R Medeiros (2007). [Characterization of the clinical evolution of nasopharyngeal carcinoma in Portuguese population]. *Acta Otorrinolaringol Esp* 58(5): 191-197.

Breda, E, R Catarino, A Coelho, H Sousa and R Medeiros (2008). [Nasopharyngeal carcinoma study: introduction and multidisciplinary perspective]. *Acta Med Port* 21(3): 273-284.

Breda, E, RJ Catarino, I Azevedo, M Lobao, E Monteiro and R Medeiros (2010). Epstein-Barr virus detection in nasopharyngeal carcinoma: implications in a low-risk area. *Braz J Otorhinolaryngol* 76(3): 310-315.

Bull, JW (1969). Tentorium cerebelli. *Proc R Soc Med* 62(12): 1301-1310.

Burkitt, D (1958). A sarcoma involving the jaws in African children. *The British journal of surgery* 46(197): 218-223.

Burkitt, D (1962). A children's cancer dependent on climatic factors. *Nature* 194: 232-234.

Busson, P, C Keryer, T Ooka and M Corbex (2004). EBV-associated nasopharyngeal carcinomas: from epidemiology to virus-targeting strategies. *Trends in microbiology* 12(8): 356-360.

Catarino, R, D Pereira, E Breda, A Coelho, A Matos, C Lopes and R Medeiros (2008). Oncogenic virus-associated neoplasia: a role for cyclin D1 genotypes influencing the age of onset of disease? *Biochem Biophys Res Commun* 370(1): 118-122.

Catarino, R, D Pereira, E Breda, A Coelho, A Matos, C Lopes and R Medeiros (2008). Oncogenic virus-associated neoplasia: a role for cyclin D1 genotypes influencing the age of onset of disease? *Biochemical and biophysical research communications* 370(1): 118-122.

Catarino, RJ, E Breda, V Coelho, D Pinto, H Sousa, C Lopes and R Medeiros (2006). Association of the A870G cyclin D1 gene polymorphism with genetic susceptibility to nasopharyngeal carcinoma. *Head Neck* 28(7): 603-608.

Chan, AS, KF To, KW Lo, M Ding, X Li, P Johnson and DP Huang (2002). Frequent chromosome 9p losses in histologically normal nasopharyngeal epithelia from southern Chinese. *International journal of cancer. Journal international du cancer* 102(3): 300-303.

Chan, AS, KF To, KW Lo, KF Mak, W Pak, B Chiu, GM Tse, M Ding, X Li, JC Lee and DP Huang (2000). High frequency of chromosome 3p deletion in histologically normal nasopharyngeal epithelia from southern Chinese. *Cancer research* 60(19): 5365-5370.

Chan, AT, YM Lo, B Zee, LY Chan, BB Ma, SF Leung, F Mo, M Lai, S Ho, DP Huang and PJ Johnson (2002). Plasma Epstein-Barr virus DNA and residual disease after radiotherapy for undifferentiated nasopharyngeal carcinoma. *Journal of the National Cancer Institute* 94(21): 1614-1619.

Chan, AT, PM Teo and PJ Johnson (2002). Nasopharyngeal carcinoma. *Annals of oncology : official journal of the European Society for Medical Oncology / ESMO* 13(7): 1007-1015.

Chan, SH, NE Day, N Kunaratnam, KB Chia and MJ Simons (1983). HLA and nasopharyngeal carcinoma in Chinese--a further study. *Int J Cancer* 32(2): 171-176.

Chang, ET and HO Adami (2006). The enigmatic epidemiology of nasopharyngeal carcinoma. *Cancer Epidemiol Biomarkers Prev* 15(10): 1765-1777.

Chernock, RD, SK El-Mofty, WL Thorstad, CA Parvin and JS Lewis, Jr. (2009). HPV-related nonkeratinizing squamous cell carcinoma of the oropharynx: utility of microscopic features in predicting patient outcome. *Head Neck Pathol* 3(3): 186-194.

Chernock, RD, JS Lewis, Jr., Q Zhang and SK El-Mofty (2010). Human papillomavirus-positive basaloid squamous cell carcinomas of the upper aerodigestive tract: a distinct clinicopathologic and molecular subtype of basaloid squamous cell carcinoma. *Hum Pathol* 41(7): 1016-1023.

Cho, EY, A Hildesheim, CJ Chen, MM Hsu, IH Chen, BF Mittl, PH Levine, MY Liu, JY Chen, LA Brinton, YJ Cheng and CS Yang (2003). Nasopharyngeal carcinoma and genetic polymorphisms of DNA repair enzymes XRCC1 and hOGG1. *Cancer epidemiology, biomarkers & prevention : a publication of the American Association for Cancer Research, cosponsored by the American Society of Preventive Oncology* 12(10): 1100-1104.

Clarke, MF, JE Dick, PB Dirks, CJ Eaves, CH Jamieson, DL Jones, J Visvader, IL Weissman and GM Wahl (2006). Cancer stem cells--perspectives on current status and future directions: AACR Workshop on cancer stem cells. *Cancer Res* 66(19): 9339-9344.

Cvitkovic, E, M Bachouchi and JP Armand (1991). Nasopharyngeal carcinoma. Biology, natural history, and therapeutic implications. *Hematol Oncol Clin North Am* 5(4): 821-838.

d'Espiney Amaro, C, P Montalvao, P Henriques, M Magalhaes and J Olias (2009). Nasopharyngeal carcinoma: our experience. *Eur Arch Otorhinolaryngol* 266(6): 833-838.

Daniel G. Deschler, TD, Ed. (2008). Pocket Guide To TNM STAGING OF HEAD AND NECK CANCER AND NECK DISSECTION CLASSIFICATION. , Alexandria, American Academy of Otolaryngology–Head and Neck Surgery Foundation, Inc.

Douik, H, A Ben Chaaben, N Attia Romdhane, HB Romdhane, T Mamoghli, C Fortier, W Boukouaci, L Harzallah, A Ghanem, S Gritli, M Makni, D Charron, R Krishnamoorthy, F Guemira and R Tamouza (2009). Association of MICA-129 polymorphism with nasopharyngeal cancer risk in a Tunisian population. *Hum Immunol* 70(1): 45-48.

Epstein, MA, BG Achong and YM Barr (1964). Virus Particles in Cultured Lymphoblasts from Burkitt's Lymphoma. *Lancet* 1(7335): 702-703.

Ereno, C, A Gaafar, M Garmendia, C Etxezarraga, FJ Bilbao and JI Lopez (2008). Basaloid squamous cell carcinoma of the head and neck: a clinicopathological and follow-up study of 40 cases and review of the literature. *Head Neck Pathol* 2(2): 83-91.

Fang, FM, WL Tsai, TF Lee, KC Liao, HC Chen and HC Hsu (2010). Multivariate analysis of quality of life outcome for nasopharyngeal carcinoma patients after treatment. *Radiother Oncol* 97(2): 263-269.

Farrell, PJ (1995). Epstein-Barr virus immortalizing genes. *Trends in microbiology* 3(3): 105-109.

Fukuyama, S, T Nagatake, D-Y Kim, K Takamura, EJ Park, T Kaisho, N Tanaka, Y Kurono and H Kiyono (2006). Cutting Edge: Uniqueness of Lymphoid Chemokine Requirement for the Initiation and Maturation of Nasopharynx-Associated Lymphoid Tissue Organogenesis. *J Immunol* (177): 4276-4280.

Ghisletti, S, C Meda, A Maggi and E Vegeto (2005). 17beta-estradiol inhibits inflammatory gene expression by controlling NF-kappaB intracellular localization. *Mol Cell Biol* 25(8): 2957-2968.

Groome, PA, KM Schulze, WJ Mackillop, B Grice, C Goh, BJ Cummings, SF Hall, FF Liu, D Payne, DM Rothwell, JN Waldron, PR Warde and B O'Sullivan (2001). A comparison of published head and neck stage groupings in carcinomas of the tonsillar region. *Cancer* 92(6): 1484-1494.

Haddad, R, Ed. (2011). Multidisciplinary Management of Head and Neck Cancer, Demos Medical Publishing, LLC.

Henle, G and W Henle (1966). Immunofluorescence in cells derived from Burkitt's lymphoma. *Journal of bacteriology* 91(3): 1248-1256.

Henle, G and W Henle (1976). Epstein-Barr virus-specific IgA serum antibodies as an outstanding feature of nasopharyngeal carcinoma. *International journal of cancer. Journal international du cancer* 17(1): 1-7.

Henle, G, W Henle and V Diehl (1968). Relation of Burkitt's tumor-associated herpes-ytpe virus to infectious mononucleosis. *Proceedings of the National Academy of Sciences of the United States of America* 59(1): 94-101.

Henle, W and G Henle (1976). The sero-epidemiology of Epstein-Barr virus. *Advances in pathobiology*(5): 5-17.

Henle, W, G Henle, M Scriba, CR Joyner, FS Harrison, Jr., R Von Essen, J Paloheimo and E Klemola (1970). Antibody responses to the Epstein-Barr virus and cytomegaloviruses after open-heart and other surgery. *The New England journal of medicine* 282(19): 1068-1074.

Hildesheim, A, LM Anderson, CJ Chen, YJ Cheng, LA Brinton, AK Daly, CD Reed, IH Chen, NE Caporaso, MM Hsu, JY Chen, JR Idle, RN Hoover, CS Yang and SK Chhabra (1997). CYP2E1 genetic polymorphisms and risk of nasopharyngeal carcinoma in Taiwan. *Journal of the National Cancer Institute* 89(16): 1207-1212.

Hildesheim, A and PH Levine (1993). Etiology of nasopharyngeal carcinoma: a review. *Epidemiologic reviews* 15(2): 466-485.

Hui, AB, KW Lo, PM Teo, KF To and DP Huang (2002). Genome wide detection of oncogene amplifications in nasopharyngeal carcinoma by array based comparative genomic hybridization. *International journal of oncology* 20(3): 467-473.

IARC, Ed. (2005). Pathology and Genetics of Head and Neck Tumours. Who Health Organization Classification of Tumours, Lyon.

Jackson, C (1901). Primary carcinoma of the nasopharynx: a table of cases. *JAMA*(37): 371-377.

Jeffery, N (2005). Cranial base angulation and growth of the human fetal pharynx. *Anat Rec A Discov Mol Cell Evol Biol* 284(1): 491-499.

Jiong, L, F Berrino and JW Coebergh (1998). Variation in survival for adults with Nasopharyngeal cancer in Europe, 1978-1989. *Eur J Cancer* 34(14): 2162-2166.

Kalaitzidis, D and TD Gilmore (2005). Transcription factor cross-talk: the estrogen receptor and NF-kappaB. *Trends Endocrinol Metab* 16(2): 46-52.

Kong, QL, LJ Hu, JY Cao, YJ Huang, LH Xu, Y Liang, D Xiong, S Guan, BH Guo, HQ Mai, QY Chen, X Zhang, MZ Li, JY Shao, CN Qian, YF Xia, LB Song, YX Zeng and MS Zeng (2010). Epstein-Barr virus-encoded LMP2A induces an epithelial-mesenchymal transition and increases the number of side population stem-like cancer cells in nasopharyngeal carcinoma. *PLoS Pathog* 6(6): e1000940.

Lee, AW, WM Sze, JS Au, SF Leung, TW Leung, DT Chua, BC Zee, SC Law, PM Teo, SY Tung, DL Kwong and WH Lau (2005). Treatment results for nasopharyngeal carcinoma in the modern era: the Hong Kong experience. *Int J Radiat Oncol Biol Phys* 61(4): 1107-1116.

Lee, N, J Harris, AS Garden, W Straube, B Glisson, P Xia, W Bosch, WH Morrison, J Quivey, W Thorstad, C Jones and KK Ang (2009). Intensity-Modulated Radiation Therapy With or Without Chemotherapy for Nasopharyngeal Carcinoma: Radiation Therapy Oncology Group Phase II Trial 0225. *Journal of Clinical Oncology* 27.

Leung, TW, SY Tung, WK Sze, FC Wong, KK Yuen, CM Lui, SH Lo, TY Ng and SK O (2005). Treatment results of 1070 patients with nasopharyngeal carcinoma: an analysis of survival and failure patterns. *Head Neck* 27(7): 555-565.

Lin, JC, KY Chen, WY Wang, JS Jan, WM Liang, CS Tsai and YH Wei (2001). Detection of Epstein-Barr virus DNA in the peripheral-blood cells of patients with nasopharyngeal carcinoma: relationship to distant metastasis and survival. *Journal of clinical oncology : official journal of the American Society of Clinical Oncology* 19(10): 2607-2615.

List, MA and J Stracks (2000). Evaluation of quality of life in patients definitively treated for squamous carcinoma of the head and neck. *Curr Opin Oncol* 12(3): 215-220.

Liu, MZ, LL Tang, JF Zong, Y Huang, Y Sun, YP Mao, LZ Liu, AH Lin and J Ma (2008). Evaluation of sixth edition of AJCC staging system for nasopharyngeal carcinoma and proposed improvement. *Int J Radiat Oncol Biol Phys* 70(4): 1115-1123.

Lo, KW and DP Huang (2002). Genetic and epigenetic changes in nasopharyngeal carcinoma. *Seminars in cancer biology* 12(6): 451-462.

Lo, KW, KF To and DP Huang (2004). Focus on nasopharyngeal carcinoma. *Cancer Cell* 5(5): 423-428.

Lo, YM, AT Chan, LY Chan, SF Leung, CW Lam, DP Huang and PJ Johnson (2000). Molecular prognostication of nasopharyngeal carcinoma by quantitative analysis of circulating Epstein-Barr virus DNA. *Cancer research* 60(24): 6878-6881.

Lo, YM, SF Leung, LY Chan, AT Chan, KW Lo, PJ Johnson and DP Huang (2000). Kinetics of plasma Epstein-Barr virus DNA during radiation therapy for nasopharyngeal carcinoma. *Cancer research* 60(9): 2351-2355.

Lu, SJ, NE Day, L Degos, V Lepage, PC Wang, SH Chan, M Simons, B McKnight, D Easton, Y Zeng and et al. (1990). Linkage of a nasopharyngeal carcinoma susceptibility locus to the HLA region. *Nature* 346(6283): 470-471.

Marks, JE, JL Phillips and HR Menck (1998). The National Cancer Data Base report on the relationship of race and national origin to the histology of nasopharyngeal carcinoma. *Cancer* 83(3): 582-588.

Molinero, LL, MB Fuertes, MV Girart, L Fainboim, GA Rabinovich, MA Costas and NW Zwirner (2004). NF-kappa B regulates expression of the MHC class I-related chain A gene in activated T lymphocytes. *J Immunol* 173(9): 5583-5590.

Nazar-Stewart, V, TL Vaughan, RD Burt, C Chen, M Berwick and GM Swanson (1999). Glutathione S-transferase M1 and susceptibility to nasopharyngeal carcinoma. *Cancer epidemiology, biomarkers & prevention : a publication of the American Association for Cancer Research, cosponsored by the American Society of Preventive Oncology* 8(6): 547-551.

Niedobitek, G, ML Hansmann, H Herbst, LS Young, D Dienemann, CA Hartmann, T Finn, S Pitteroff, A Welt, I Anagnostopoulos and et al. (1991). Epstein-Barr virus and carcinomas: undifferentiated carcinomas but not squamous cell carcinomas of the nasopharynx are regularly associated with the virus. *J Pathol* 165(1): 17-24.

Niedobitek, G, ML Hansmann, H Herbst, LS Young, D Dienemann, CA Hartmann, T Finn, S Pitteroff, A Welt, I Anagnostopoulos and et al. (1991). Epstein-Barr virus and carcinomas: undifferentiated carcinomas but not squamous cell carcinomas of the nasopharynx are regularly associated with the virus. *The Journal of pathology* 165(1): 17-24.

Parkin DM, BF, Ferlay J, Pisani P (2002). Global cancer statistics. *CA Cancer J Clin. 2005 :* Mar-Apr;55(2): 74-108.
Pathmanathan, R, U Prasad, R Sadler, K Flynn and N Raab-Traub (1995). Clonal proliferations of cells infected with Epstein-Barr virus in preinvasive lesions related to nasopharyngeal carcinoma. *The New England journal of medicine* 333(11): 693-698.
Raab-Traub, N and K Flynn (1986). The structure of the termini of the Epstein-Barr virus as a marker of clonal cellular proliferation. *Cell* 47(6): 883-889.
Rainger, R (1997). Everett C. Olson and the development of vertebrate paleoecology and taphonomy. *Archives of Natural History* 24(3): 373 - 396.
Ripple, MO, WF Henry, SR Schwarze, G Wilding and R Weindruch (1999). Effect of antioxidants on androgen-induced AP-1 and NF-kappaB DNA-binding activity in prostate carcinoma cells. *J Natl Cancer Inst* 91(14): 1227-1232.
Saddlet, TW, Ed. (2009). Langman's Medical Embriology. Philadelphia, Lippincott Wiliams &Wilkins.
Saddlet T, Ed. (1995). Langman's Medical Embryology.
Shao, JY, YH Li, HY Gao, QL Wu, NJ Cui, L Zhang, G Cheng, LF Hu, I Ernberg and YX Zeng (2004). Comparison of plasma Epstein-Barr virus (EBV) DNA levels and serum EBV immunoglobulin A/virus capsid antigen antibody titers in patients with nasopharyngeal carcinoma. *Cancer* 100(6): 1162-1170.
Shikina, T, T Hiroi, K Iwatani, MH Jang, S Fukuyama, M Tamura, H Ishikawa, T Kubo and H Kiyono (2004). IgA Class Switch Occurs in the Organized Nasopharynx- and Gut-Associated Lymphoid Tissue, but Not in the Diffuse Lamina Propria of Airways and Gut. *The Journal of Immunology* 172: 6259–6264.
Sixbey, JW, JG Nedrud, N Raab-Traub, RA Hanes and JS Pagano (1984). Epstein-Barr virus replication in oropharyngeal epithelial cells. *The New England journal of medicine* 310(19): 1225-1230.
Snow Jr, JB and J Ballenger, Eds. (2003). Ballenger's Otorhinolaryngology Head and Neck Surgery. Ontario, BC Decker Inc.
Song, LB, J Li, WT Liao, Y Feng, CP Yu, LJ Hu, QL Kong, LH Xu, X Zhang, WL Liu, MZ Li, L Zhang, TB Kang, LW Fu, WL Huang, YF Xia, SW Tsao, M Li, V Band, H Band, QH Shi, YX Zeng and MS Zeng (2009). The polycomb group protein Bmi-1 represses the tumor suppressor PTEN and induces epithelial-mesenchymal transition in human nasopharyngeal epithelial cells. *J Clin Invest* 119(12): 3626-3636.
Sousa, H, E Breda, AM Santos, R Catarino, D Pinto and R Medeiros (2011). Genetic risk markers for nasopharyngeal carcinoma in Portugal: tumor necrosis factor alpha -308G >A polymorphism. *DNA and cell biology* 30(2): 99-103.
Sousa, H, M Pando, E Breda, R Catarino and R Medeiros (2011). Role of the MDM2 SNP309 polymorphism in the initiation and early age of onset of nasopharyngeal carcinoma. *Molecular carcinogenesis* 50(2): 73-79.
Sousa, H, AM Santos, R Catarino, D Pinto, A Vasconcelos, C Lopes, E Breda and R Medeiros (2006). Linkage of TP53 codon 72 pro/pro genotype as predictive factor for nasopharyngeal carcinoma development. *European journal of cancer prevention : the official journal of the European Cancer Prevention Organisation* 15(4): 362-366.
Standring, S, Ed. (2008). Gray's Anatomy, Curchill Livingstone Elsevier.

Thompson, MP and R Kurzrock (2004). Epstein-Barr virus and cancer. *Clinical cancer research: an official journal of the American Association for Cancer Research* 10(3): 803-821.

Tian, W, DA Boggs, WZ Ding, DF Chen and PA Fraser (2001). MICA genetic polymorphism and linkage disequilibrium with HLA-B in 29 African-American families. *Immunogenetics* 53(9): 724-728.

Tian, W, XM Zeng, LX Li, HK Jin, QZ Luo, F Wang, SS Guo and Y Cao (2006). Gender-specific associations between MICA-STR and nasopharyngeal carcinoma in a southern Chinese Han population. *Immunogenetics* 58(2-3): 113-121.

Tiwawech, D, P Srivatanakul, A Karalak and T Ishida (2006). Cytochrome P450 2A6 polymorphism in nasopharyngeal carcinoma. *Cancer letters* 241(1): 135-141.

Van Hasselt, CA and AG Gibb, Eds. (1999). Nasopharyngeal Carcinoma Hong Kong, Greenwich Medical Media Ltd.

Vasef, MA, A Ferlito and LM Weiss (1997). Nasopharyngeal carcinoma, with emphasis on its relationship to Epstein-Barr virus. *Ann Otol Rhinol Laryngol* 106(4): 348-356.

Wain, SL, R Kier, RT Vollmer and EH Bossen (1986). Basaloid-squamous carcinoma of the tongue, hypopharynx, and larynx: report of 10 cases. *Hum Pathol* 17(11): 1158-1166.

Wei, WI and JS Sham (2005). Nasopharyngeal carcinoma. *Lancet* 365(9476): 2041-2054.

Wenig, BM (1999). Nasopharyngeal carcinoma. *Ann Diagn Pathol* 3(6): 374-385.

Wu, SB, SJ Hwang, AS Chang, T Hsieh, MM Hsu, RP Hsieh and CJ Chen (1989). Human leukocyte antigen (HLA) frequency among patients with nasopharyngeal carcinoma in Taiwan. *Anticancer Res* 9(6): 1649-1653.

Young, LS and AB Rickinson (2004). Epstein-Barr virus: 40 years on. *Nature reviews. Cancer* 4(10): 757-768.

Zhang, F and J Zhang (1999). Clinical hereditary characteristics in nasopharyngeal carcinoma through Ye-Liang's family cluster. *Chin Med J (Engl)* 112(2): 185-187.

Zhang, S, Y Wu, Y Zeng, L Zech and G Klein (1982). Cytogenetic studies on an epithelioid cell line derived from nasopharyngeal carcinoma. *Hereditas* 97(1): 23-28.

Zhu, XN, R Chen, FH Kong and W Liu (1990). Human leukocyte antigens -A, -B, -C, and -DR and nasopharyngeal carcinoma in northern China. *Ann Otol Rhinol Laryngol* 99(4 Pt 1): 286-287.

zur Hausen, H, H Schulte-Holthausen, G Klein, W Henle, G Henle, P Clifford and L Santesson (1970). EBV DNA in biopsies of Burkitt tumours and anaplastic carcinomas of the nasopharynx. *Nature* 228(5276): 1056-1058.